W9-BHW-892

ANATOMY
for Speech and Hearing

Fourth Edition

ANATOMY
for Speech and Hearing

Fourth Edition

John M. Palmer, Ph.D.

Professor Emeritus
Department of Speech and Hearing Sciences
University of Washington
Seattle, Washington

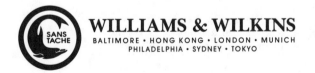

WILLIAMS & WILKINS
BALTIMORE · HONG KONG · LONDON · MUNICH
PHILADELPHIA · SYDNEY · TOKYO

Editor: John P. Butler
Managing Editor: Linda Napora
Copy Editor: Ann Donaldson
Designer: Wilma E. Rosenberger
Illustration Planner: Ray Lowman
Production Coordinator: Anne Stewart Seitz
Cover Designer: Wilma E. Rosenberger

Copyright © 1993
Williams & Wilkins
428 East Preston Street
Baltimore, Maryland 21202, USA

All rights reserved. This book is protected by copyright. No part of this book may be reproduced in any form or by any means, including photocopying, or utilized by any information storage and retrieval system without written permission from the copyright owner.

Printed in the United States of America

Library of Congress Cataloging in Publication Data

Palmer, John M. (John Milton), 1922–
    Anatomy for speech and hearing / John M. Palmer.—4th ed.
      p.   cm.
    Includes bibliographical references and index.
    ISBN 0-683-06737-0
    1. Head—Anatomy. 2. Neck—Anatomy. 3. Neuroanatomy. 4. Speech.
5. Hearing. I. Title.
    [DNLM: 1. Ear—anatomy & histology. 2. Hearing. 3. Larynx—
anatomy & histology. 4. Nose—anatomy & histology. 5. Pharynx—
anatomy & histology. 6. Thorax—anatomy & histology. WV 101
P174a]
QM535.P28   1993
611—dc20
DNLM/DLC
for Library of Congress   91-47928
                                             CIP

                                    93 94 95 96 97
                          1 2 3 4 5 6 7 8 9 10

Preface

In this fourth edition under the auspices of a new publisher, I have made a number of changes. All of these, I hope, will meet the approval of the students using the text. Many of the changes derive from sometimes vigorous input from my own students, but input has been sufficiently positive for the text to continue to a new edition. I draw attention to the differences of the present text from preceding editions.

There is new or revised artwork. The previous artist, Phyllis Wood, was an expert, but retired from medical illustration forcing me to select, serendipitously, Kate Sweeney. To Kate I owe much, for the art is an extremely important part of the text. In no way is she responsible for errors inasmuch as she made originals and I requested changes, so errors fall into my province. However, the purpose of the drawings remains the same: requiring students to identify anatomic landmarks, appropriate terms for which are provided in Appendix I, during which operation it appears that some of the exercise remains in the mind of the students. I also use some of the drawings, as is, for course examinations.

I have added, at the suggestion of the Williams & Wilkins editor, John Butler, Clinical Implications at the ends of chapters. Because some portion of each class using this text eventually is a "major" in speech and hearing sciences, the Clinical Implications might whet some appetites for this aspect of the profession.

Study Questions have been retained with some changes. Students can use them to test themselves on implications of materials, to challenge themselves to seek out other references, and to indicate importance of some content areas. Instructors may use Study Questions for quiz sections or discussion issues in class, or as part of examinations. I have used them in conjunction with submitted drawing assignments to cause students to go beyond the narrow anatomic study the text emphasizes.

Terminology has been updated. I use, to a large extent, Anglicized Nomina Anatomica although I retained some terms for which an Anglicized version might be inappropriate (e.g., "big hole" for foramen magnum). In a related vein, the glossary has been increased. The "layman's" pronunciation guide is utilized, for I rarely have a student knowledgeable about phonetics to use that form of guide. I do, though, strongly recommend the terminology guide by Nicolosi, Harryman, and Kreshek, third edition by Williams & Wilkins, 1989.

From earlier editions, I have included the Physiologic Phonetics material found in Appendix II. It is admittedly very detailed, often based upon educated guessing, but has been recommended by previous users of the text.

I have continued to change emphases in content. Occasional structures (e.g., dilator tubae muscle) received increased attention as the result of my own dissections in that area. Other changes in emphasis stem from clinical experience as much as anatomic study; here, I refer to such examples as the cricopharyngeal muscle, otherwise known as the esophageal sphincter, which receives considerable attention from dysphagia specialists.

I have made no changes in the sequence of the contents. Beginning the text, and the course as I teach it, with the bones of the skull provides me with an opportunity to explain a number of anatomic concepts that are basic to understanding of later areas. For example, the hierarchy of structure from cell, through tissue, to organ, and so on, can commence rather easily with bone cells and connective tissues. Then, other anatomic concepts can be laid down. Here I point to such terms as "process" or "spine" to which later will be attached muscles or ligaments. I am also able to introduce anatomic spaces as part of the study of anatomy, especially later when I focus on the vocal tract. So, the paranasal sinuses, the nasal passages, and the oral cavity are introduced early, as are entrances (e.g., naris, choana, isthmus) to and from those spaces.

I am well aware that many such anatomy courses begin with respiration and its supporting anatomy. I have no argument with instructors who do so, and know full well that they can and will commence the course with appropriate chapter reference at that time.

Because of the apparent increase in recent years in clinical emphasis in disorders of the nervous system resulting in communication disorders, I have amplified some aspects of that chapter. Some increase in content area (e.g., midbrain control regions for swallowing) is noted. However, this chapter is but a cursory exploration of the area for many students in the basic anatomy course who will go on to an advanced and specialized neuroanatomy course, as well as later neuropathology courses.

I repeat the debt I owe to present and former students, especially those performing dissection tasks for demonstration laboratory experience for beginning students. I recognize Nancy Whitmore, Billie Garber, Kurt Herzog, and several other dedicated young scholars in this respect. The manuscript was prepared by Arlene Chaussee of my department, whose word processing skills are unsurpassed and whose patience is wonderful to behold. My department has been most patient with me during this work and I thank Chairman Wes Wilson for setting the tone and encouragement for much that makes this a fine department. I am proud to be an emeritus member.

John M. Palmer

List of Illustrations

List of Tables

Contents

Chapter 1
Preliminaries

THE TEXT

This text is written for the student. It assumes no prior knowledge of anatomy or physiology, but it does acknowledge the need for outside help. In studying anatomy, the usual procedure is to have a class with an instructor and perhaps the luxury of a laboratory. The help you will need should come, first, from the instructor. The laboratory should provide clarification. A library should provide other texts. Any body of scientific knowledge is explained in different ways by different authors; seek out another explanation of troublesome areas.

This text provides one source of additional help: the drawings. These are a major part of the text. Numbered lines point to important landmarks of the region illustrated for general orientation, a few landmark names are provided.

One way of using the drawings would be to list the numbers for each drawing and try to name the landmark pointed to. Another approach would be to seek out the alphabetized list of landmarks for each drawing (see Appendix I) and to name the numbered lines on each drawing by pulling from the list the appropriate term and placing that term directly on the drawing. The thorough student will go beyond the given list of terms and add other landmarks. You may wish to repeat terms on different drawings, using different views to test your understanding of the anatomy. The addition of color to portions or divisions often helps in reviewing anatomic drawings.

The student anatomist must quickly become aware that not only are structures (such as bones and muscles) important to know and understand, but the spaces often formed or affected by these structures are equally important. This is especially true in the vocal tract where those spaces in which air flow and pressure and sound events are produced create the acoustic events of speech. Even the entryways, the doorways, into spaces are named and become important.

Studying from a text alone is extremely difficult; outside help can facilitate learning. Other textbooks, lectures, laboratory assistants, and knowledgeable professionals are sources that the questioning student might seek out. Students who have already studied the material can be helpful. A few helpful references are offered at the ends of the chapters, as well as study questions that have been designed to emphasize important points made in the chapter. Answering those can be a helpful study activity.

The organization of this text differs from that of some others. It begins with the bones of the skull, not the respiratory system for speech. There are a number of reasons for this beginning. It introduces important bones and landmarks that later will be used for muscle and other attachments. It affords first use of numerous terms (e.g., process and superior) basic to an understanding of anatomy. It introduces the notion of paired and unpaired structures. This format also develops the concept of structures forming spaces, and spaces are what the vocal tract is all about.

1

As one of the oldest of the sciences, the study of anatomy has become an important part of many disciplines. It has been a scholarly pursuit in many parts of the world and, as such, has been served by many languages. As knowledge increased, so did the terms used to represent structures and spaces. At one point some anatomic landmarks had as many as 50 different names throughout the scholarly world. For an anatomist of one language group to speak or write to another, must have been difficult!

THE LANGUAGE OF ANATOMY

The first comprehensive systematic organization of anatomic nomenclature was adopted by the German Anatomical Society when it met in Basel, Switzerland, in 1895. The Latin name for this terminology system is *Basel Nomina Anatomica,* or *BNA.* Some national groups, however, failed to accept this system. In 1933 scientists in Great Britain developed the Birmingham Revision (BR), in part because they approached terminology from the standpoint of human anatomy, while the Germans and others approached it from the standpoint of comparative anatomy (i.e., by looking at other animals of the vertebrate group and attempting to develop a terminology that would cover all vertebrates).

In 1937, anatomists met in Jena, Austria, and a revision of the BNA was adopted, the *Jena Nomina Anatomica,* or JNA (in languages without the letter J it is known as the INA). Later committees and groups continued to examine anatomic terminology. In 1955 in Paris the international association of anatomists heard their nomenclature committee present another revision, which was accepted. It was then known as either the *Nomina Anatomica* (NA) or the *Paris Nomina Anatomica* (PNA). The designation NA has become standard, because it encompasses subsequent revisions. The official language is Latin, but most language groups translate the Latin terms into their own languages.

This text uses the accepted Anglicized version of the NA. There are changes in terminology from the earlier editions. Older terminology has been replaced by newer, more generally acceptable terms. Significant changes include the terms for four of the muscles around the mouth, the term for the Eustachian tube, and the terms for the external and internal auditory canals. Some spellings have also been changed.

Perhaps one of the major problems in learning anatomic terminology is the use of eponyms, where anatomy landmarks are named after persons associated with research in that area. This is a way of honoring important workers and, as such, is understandable, although not entirely in keeping with the objective approach scientists take to other aspects of their work. Thus, the names of many anatomic landmarks must simply be memorized.

For example, in speech and hearing sciences, we have Eustachian tube, organ of Corti, ventricle of Morgagni, Deiters' cell, and Reissner's and Shrapnell's membranes. These are but a few of the many eponyms in all of anatomy. Although many or even most anatomic terms derive from the Latin, there are a number of Greek origin. In fact, some structures are identified in reference to both languages. For example, the Anglicized "tongue" may use the Latin "lingua" or the Greek "glossa" in referring to its parts or actions.

Other terms, even some with which students already feel familiar in other contexts, can cause problems. For example, consider the word process. In anatomy this word denotes a structure, usually a projection from a bone or cartilage. Other common terms that appear to be used in special ways should be looked up. The present text has a glossary that provides brief explanations of how terms are used herein. For more thorough explanations, a medical or scientific dictionary is the best resource. A recent edition of Dorland's, Blakiston's, Melloni's, Stedman's, or of other medical dictionaries will help with spelling, pronunciation, and meaning; often, line drawings and tables and charts of muscles and nerves are also provided in such references. A good dictionary can be of considerable assistance as one reads textbooks and professional journals. The language of anatomy is not an easy language, but it serves its science well in its logic and its systematic formation.

Directions and Locations

One aspect of studying anatomy is learning to find and locate landmarks. It is important to place the landmark in the correct region, as well as to locate it in relation to other landmarks. The terms used to locate landmarks are in part based upon comparative anatomy and can be used to locate similar structures on dogs or pigs or humans. However, a basic difference is that the human landmarks are located with the human body standing erect. This stance creates some differences in the words used in describing similar structures or spaces in different animals.

The reference posture of the human body is known as the *anatomic* or *cadaveric position.* The body is upright on its two feet, the eyes and the head are oriented horizontally, and the palms of the hands face forward. Obviously, there would be some differences in the words used to describe landmarks in relation to each other if one were describing the anatomy of a dog rather than a human. For example, in the dog the neck might be said to be posterior to the nose, while in the human the neck might be said to be inferior to the nose. The term *caudal* can apply to either creature in locating a landmark toward the tail.

There are many such terms that are very specifically used in locating landmarks. As new terms of location are encountered, the glossary or a dictionary should be used to ensure accurate understanding. A few of the more common terms of location in reference to the human body are listed.

Term	General Meaning
Anterior	Toward the front
Posterior	Toward the rear
Ventral	Toward the belly
Dorsal	Toward the back
Inferior	Below
Superior	Above
Caudal	Toward the tail
Cephalad	Toward the head
Lateral	Away from the midline
Medial	Toward the midline

Body Planes

It is often helpful to present the body as if it had been sectioned—that is, divided, or cut (Fig. 1.1). Three basic planes are often used to depict body parts. The *sagittal plane* parallels the midline of the body from front to back. It divides the body into a right and a left portion. If the section is made at the midline itself, it is sometimes termed a *midsagittal plane.* If the cut is made to one side of the midline, the term *parasagittal plane* is used.

The *coronal plane* (or *frontal plane*) is at a right angle to the sagittal plane. It is a section made from side to side, dividing the body into a front and a back portion. Because there is no midline from the front to the back of the human body, there is no plane identified as "midcoronal."

The *transverse plane* (or *horizontal plane*), again at a right angle to the others, divides the body into an upper and a lower portion. Again, there is no midline for this section. Sometimes the term *cross-section* is used for this cut, such as when describing a picture of a blood vessel or another tube in the body. In this case it is not essential that the body orientation be considered, for a tube could travel a winding route.

The labels on illustrations should provide the viewer with sufficient information to identify not only the object, but also the aspect of the object being studied. The plane or orientation is used to direct the observer. Illustrations not depicting a cutaway section may present a view of an object's outer surface from one direction or other. In such a case, the term *frontal view,* or *superior surface,* for example, could help orient the observer toward the drawing. An illustration can present only part of what the object really is, because it can offer only two dimensions and those on only one side of the object.

Pairings

Generally, bilateral symmetry is assumed when presenting information about anatomic structures. In reality, the body is only approximately symmetrical. The right arm is very similar to the left arm; the same is true of the eyes, the ears, muscles moving bones, and nerves traveling through the body. When describing anatomic parts we commonly assume the parts are "paired," one on the left side and one on the right side. A single description of one side is presented. When it is not, the term "unpaired" will be used in the uncommon instance. The student might guess that unpaired structures are frequently found near the body midline.

THE TISSUES OF THE BODY

The study of anatomy and physiology can start with the study of individual cells—that is, with cytology. Individual human cells do nearly everything that bodily systems do as a whole. A cell ingests nutrients and excretes waste products. Cells reproduce themselves. There are exceptions, and there are differences among cells, as might be expected, but these generalizations can be useful in describing structures and activities important in understanding the body as a whole and the vocal tract in particular.

Cells must connect with other cells; otherwise they could not acquire oxygen, for example. Cells differ in their structure and in what they do. Similar cells can group together to provide unique functions. Such a grouping of similar cells is called a *tissue.* A number of different tissue types occur within the vocal tract. This text will present only those tissue types more commonly associated with structures forming the vocal tract, the ear, and the related neurologic structures.

Connective Tissue

Osseous tissue (or *bone tissue*) is a kind of *connective tissue.* Bone tissue is composed of living cells that are bound together in a tough and rigid network of mineral salts. Osseous tissue connects, supports, and protects parts of the body. Bone tissue is related to *cartilage tissue.* Cartilage is living cellular material that has a solid matrix more flexible than that of bone. Cartilage is sometimes seen as the precursor of bone; some bones or parts of bones in the adult were cartilaginous prenatally or even in early childhood and adolescence. In its fully developed forms, there are three types of cartilage: *hyalin, elastic,* and *fibrous.*

Other connective tissue types of interest to speech and hearing students are *ligaments* (connecting bone to bone or cartilage to cartilage) and *tendons* (connecting muscle to bone or cartilage). Connective tissue is named by varying techniques. *General location* of the bone is represented by the unpaired frontal bone of the skull. The *shape* of the structure is shown by the arytenoid (scoop-like) cartilage. The name may come from *connections* that are made; e.g., we find the stylohyoid ligament interconnecting the styloid process of the temporal bone with the hyoid bone. Some medical dictionaries give the English form of the word, whether of Latin or Greek derivation.

Some bones and cartilages have a region called its *body.* From this may extend *portions* or *processes.* The body of a bone may be of any shape or size, for there

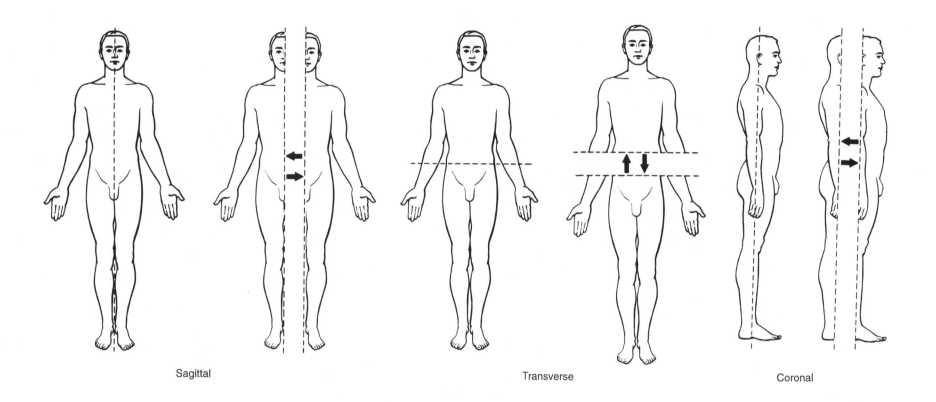

Sagittal   Transverse   Coronal

Figure 1.1 Body Planes

is nothing regular about this aspect. It is, of course, continuous with its processes, with little indication where one ends and the other begins. These processes are named and identified because of important characteristics. For example, the condyloid processes of the mandible bone make possible chewing and even talking, while the alveolar process of the maxilla bone houses the upper teeth. Tendons and ligaments and muscles are attached to the bodies or processes of bones and cartilages.

Where two bones or cartilages meet, a *joint* (or *arthrosis,* NA) is formed. The two are said to *articulate* with each other. There are different types of bony joints: fibrous, cartilaginous, and synovial.

Fibrous joints generally have layers of periosteum and fibrous tissue uniting the bones. Such joints, in which little if any movement is permitted *(synarthrosis)*, are found, for example, in the articulation among the various cranial bones, where such joints are *sutures.*

Cartilaginous joints are not common and are usually midline; they consist of a plate of hyaline cartilage (with some fibrous content) firmly connecting the bones. Such joints include the symphysis at the pubic bones and the vertebral joints.

Synovial joints, also called *diarthrodial joints (diarthrosis),* permit relatively free movement. Characteristic of the anatomy of such joints are smooth, articular cartilage covering the joint surfaces and an articular capsule connecting the two bones, forming an articular, or joint, cavity lined by synovial membrane, which secretes lubricating synovial fluid that fills the cavity. Most synovial joints are protected from separation by (accessory) ligaments that impart some elasticity to the joint. Synovial joints are provided with sensation (kinesthesis); thus, the individual has continuous awareness of joint position, and reflex function is made possible. The ligaments of joints also have sensory nerve endings, among which are those indicating pain.

An outstanding example of a synovial joint is the *temporomandibular (TM) joint.* It allows the condyloid process of the mandible bone to move on the mandibular fossa of the temporal bone. This important joint has the usual characteristic of diarthroses, plus an articular disc on the articulating surfaces and two accessory ligaments. To move the mandible, as in chewing or speaking, the two temporomandibular joints must be bilateral in structure and nearly identical in function. The movements of the mandible through this two-sided arthrosis are depression (or downward movement) and a forward gliding movement, as well as a somewhat rotational movement (grinding) made possible by alternate actions of muscles on opposite sides.

Clinical Note

The movements of the mandible bone, whether in biting, chewing, swallowing, or speaking, are of considerable impor-tance. Disorders of the TM joint can be serious, and at times dental specialists find problems of this joint difficult to alleviate. Speech clinicians find that limited mandibular excursion around the TM joint decreases the volume of the oral cavity and may affect the production of speech sounds.

Muscle Tissue

The movement of bones and cartilages is effected by *muscle tissue,* a massing of similar cells that are unique in that they are contractile (i.e., they shorten when stimulated). These cells are thread-like fibers that combine into bundles. In one kind of muscle *(striated muscle,* or *skeletal muscle)* they are arranged in parallel bundles so that there is a beginning (origin) and an end (insertion) to the muscle. In another kind of muscle *(smooth muscle,* or *nonstriated muscle)* they form networks that surround tubes, such as arteries and the intestinal tract; they narrow the tube when they contract.

Muscles are attached to bones, to cartilages, to skin, or to other muscles. The muscle bundles have membranous connective-tissue coverings that gather at the ends of the muscle. This connective tissue then becomes a part of another tissue to which it attaches. Such connective tissue is called a *tendon* and is found in several forms, depending upon the kind of muscle and its location and function.

Muscles of the type associated with the vocal tract are striated, or skeletal, and can be voluntarily commanded to contract. Hence, they are sometimes called *voluntary muscles*. Muscles are commonly described by naming the muscle and identifying its origin, its insertion, often its direction (or course), its action, and its nerve supply. Muscles are usually paired. The names of the muscles derive from differing references as noted above; for example, their shapes (trapezius muscle), their functions (tensor palatine muscle), their interconnections (stylohyoid muscle), their combination forms (digastric or two-bellied or biceps or two-headed), and so on.

The *origin* of a muscle is the relatively fixed, or nonmoving, attachment. A muscle coming from the skull to the tongue would be said to have its origin on the skull, for that end would not be moving much. The structure providing the origin of the muscle may give its name to the muscle. The end of the muscle at the origin is known as the *head* of the muscle. It is entirely possible for a muscle to have multiple origins and thus to have several heads.

The *insertion* of a muscle is the structure to which it attaches and that moves when the muscle contracts. A muscle may divide and insert into several landmarks. The insertion of a muscle can be a bone, a cartilage, another muscle, or soft tissue, including skin.

The *course* a muscle takes, along with its form, is sometimes given in its description. One might say that a muscle passes downward as a thick bundle, for example.

The *action* of a muscle is the effect it has when it contracts. In the case of muscles that are named by their actions, the effect may be fairly apparent. But muscles can have different actions depending upon

changes in origins and insertions and on whether other muscles cause the moving end to become fixed or the nonmoving end to move.

The *nerve supply* to a muscle is the source of the stimulus (the nerve impulse) that causes the muscle to contract.

Anatomy texts frequently oversimplify the actions of muscles by assigning activities to a single muscle at a time. This can lead the student to assume that a single muscle alone accomplishes a certain task. Although the present text often will seem to support that notion, muscles function in groups and in different manners within groups, and groups of muscles function together. The action assigned to a single muscle might be said to be its *primary function*.

A second or third muscle may be described as having a function similar to the function of another muscle already presented. The second or third muscle probably has a slightly different manner of functioning, however. When the student finds that several muscles have similar actions assigned, there is every likelihood that careful study will disclose slight differences that allow for subtle movement differences.

Another way of looking at the same phenomenon is to note that an action can be the product of more than one muscle. Muscles can team up in moving a structure, but when studying the elements of the activity or the elements of the anatomy, one takes them one at a time. Each muscle is described individually.

There is another aspect to the activities of muscles and muscle groups. This involves the notion of *agonist muscles* and *antagonist muscles*. The muscles that perform an action (agonist) usually are opposed by other muscles that perform a nearly opposite, or antagonistic, action. Of course, such oppositions should be controlled so they do not interfere with, but actually help each other in, the jobs they have to do.

Usually, the antagonistic musculature gradually relaxes to allow an agonist to do its work. This keeps an action in check. The antagonistic muscle guides, or steers, the movement and checks against rapidly accelerating movements of structures. In this explanation, the antagonist is presented as another muscle or a muscle group. However, opposing forces can be something other than muscles; gravity, cavity contents, and elastic forces are common antagonists. Thus, it is an oversimplification to think of muscle-to-muscle relationships as agonist-antagonist pairings, and this is hardly the basis of real functioning.

Synchrony in movement develops as the person learns patterns that are coordinated, smooth, and well timed. As children develop, they learn to control various body parts so they can walk, feed themselves, play with toys, and above all, speak.

Nerve Tissue

Nervous tissue is composed of cells called *neurons.* They have a surrounding or supporting tissue *(neuroglia)* that is a type of connective tissue making up a large portion of the entire nervous system. Nerve cells are unique. Once formed, they generally last the life of the individual. Their primary characteristic is that they are irritable, which means they quickly respond to stimuli.

Some nerve cells form the *central nervous system,* great collections of nerve centers and of nerve fibers interconnecting these centers in the brain and spinal cord. They are housed within the bones of the cranium (the brain) and within a canal in the chain of vertebrae (the spinal cord). They form a continuous central unit with peripheral connections to and from body tissues. Those nerves connected to the brain are *cranial* nerves. Those nerves connected to the spinal cord, from within the vertebrae are called *spinal* nerves.

The nerves stimulating muscles are *motor* (or efferent) nerves, while those nerves carrying sensation—for example, vision or pain—are sensory (or afferent) nerves. The nerves coming to muscles are outside the brain and spinal cord passing through other body tissues (bone, fat, glands) and are called *peripheral nerves.*

The names of nerves differ in other ways, also. Cranial nerves are both named and numbered in Roman numerals. For example, the cranial nerve stimulating the muscles around the mouth opening is called the facial nerve; it is numbered V. Other cranial nerves are named by their locations (e.g., hypoglossal, XII) or by their functions (e.g., olfactory, I), or by their shapes (e.g., trigeminal, V), and other ways.

Spinal nerves are usually identified by the adjacent vertebrae by which they exit (or enter) the spinal cord. Thus, we have Thoracic 3 (or T3), or Lumbar 5 (or L5), and so on. Each major nerve may have subdivisions, each having its own name. So, we find Inferior Laryngeal Nerve to the vocal folds and the Phrenic Nerve to the Diaphragm Muscle, for example.

Important tissues of the vocal tract include, then, bone, cartilage, muscle, and nervous tissue. Also, lining the passageways and the chambers of the airway is a tissue called *mucous membrane,* which produces a fluid called *mucus.* This important fluid lubricates tissues that otherwise would dry. Mucus also moistens the passing air and assists in warming the air. Mucous membrane is an important type of *epithelial tissue,* or *epithelium.* The cells of epithelial tissue can arrange themselves in a variety of ways to form layers such as skin, while the lining of the vocal tract (respiratory epithelium, or mucous membrane) is another. The membrane of the respiratory tract varies from end to end.

DEVELOPMENTAL ANATOMY

Time and growth are required for cells and tissues to organize into the orderly patterns that characterize the mature organism. The tissues, the arrangements they take, and the organs and organ systems formed develop from the moment of fertilization. The study of the development of individual organisms is called embryology, or developmental anatomy.

Embryology is largely the study of the first 2 or 3 months of development after the union of the nucleus of the sperm and the nucleus of the ovum—that is, after fertilization. This period, the embryonic period, involves the development of at least the rudiments of all the principal organs of the adult body. The developing human in this period is called an *embryo*. After this period, it is called a *fetus*.

The fertilized cell, the zygote, starts to divide rapidly and forms a mass of cells, the blastocyst. This structure forms three primary germ-cell layers called the *ectoderm, endoderm,* and *mesoderm.* From these layers will develop all of the tissues and organs of the body; anatomic structures are frequently identified as being of ectodermal or endodermal or mesodermal origin. This characterizes tissues with important similarities.

From the ectoderm develops the skin and the nervous system. The mesoderm produces the lining of the abdominal cavity, muscle tissue, and bone and other connective tissues. The lining of the digestive tract and other important organs develop from the endoderm.

By the end of the 1st month of embryonic life, the embryo is about 5 mm (approximately 3/16 inch) in length. The vertebral column and vertebral canal (for the spinal cord) have formed, as has the heart. The arms and legs are tiny buds. There are no signs of eyes, ears, or nose.

During the 2nd embryonic month, the embryo grows to as much as 3 cm (1/4 inch) in length. Arms and legs, as well as fingers and toes, have formed by this time. Eyes are formed and are in approximately the right spacing, although the interposed nose remains little more than a slightly elevated area. Internal organs and blood vessels are well on their developmental paths. The upper lip is formed by the fusion of facial parts surrounding the mouth and nose. The palate remains unfused, but it closes in the next few weeks, by the end of the 3rd month. From the beginning of the 3rd month, when the embryo becomes a fetus, eyelids form, nails appear on toes and fingers, and of course the fetus continues to grow in size. The closing of the palate separates the nasal and oral cavities.

The formation of the openings of the body, especially those associated with the vocal tract, occurs early in embryonic life. The development of these head-end entrances to the gut is closely associated with the differentiation around the pharyngeal arches, which are arc-like swellings in what may be identified as the neck region. These arches, also called branchial (related to gills) arches or bars, have associated grooves and pouches. There are six pharyngeal arches, numbered from above; numbers five and six are little developed.

The first pharyngeal arch is the mandibular arch, having a cartilage (Meckel's) that forms the mandible bone and other structures, including the malleus and incus bones of the middle ear. The second pharyngeal arch, the hyoid arch, contributes to the hyoid bone and other structures, including the anterior portion of the tongue, the stapes bone, and perhaps some of the laryngeal cartilages. The third arch, with no distinctive name, also contributes to the hyoid bone and the posterior portion of the tongue. The fourth arch forms part of the larynx (thyroid cartilage), while the fifth arch may give rise to the cricoid and arytenoid cartilages of the larynx.

The pharyngeal grooves and pouches give rise to the external ear, the auditory tube and middle ear, the tonsil depressions, and other cavities. These spaces persist into later life and generally develop from the first two grooves or pouches. The spaces developed by lower pouches and grooves often disappear with development. It should be seen, though, that early in embryonic life there is a close association between what will ultimately develop as hearing mechanisms and the apparatus that produces speech.

The last 6 months of fetal life consist of further development of organs and organ systems whose foundations are already well prepared. Small features of the body, some of extreme importance, develop—for example, eyelids with eyelashes, billions of nerve cells, and reproductive organs. At birth, the individual still has not completed all aspects of development. Some bony portions are not complete until the 2nd or even the 3rd decade of life. For example, at birth the bones of the cranium have not ossified but are partially cartilage, especially at the corners of the parietal bone. These soft spots, called *fontanelles,* serve to allow growth of the brain within the cranium for the first few months of extrauterine life.

By age 7 years, a number of the cranial bones have grown to full size. After that, until puberty, growth is slower. It accelerates rapidly at puberty, especially in the facial region. There is a plate of cartilage between the sphenoid and occipital bones at puberty, but this ossifies at around age 25 years. Some cranial sutures, where the bones of the cranium articulate, do not fuse until around age 40 years.

All of these bony changes may be associated with spatial changes in the vocal tract. The sizes, shapes, and relationships of the cavities of the vocal tract may change during various stages of growth and development, although there is not much data available that would allow us to state the rate or extent of such change at various ages. Such changes in structure of both bony and other tissues and of the spaces within the vocal tract are mirrored by changes in physiology and in function. A few studies of such changes have been done, but many more remain to be performed.

THE VOCAL TRACT

The *vocal tract* (Fig. 1.2) consists of the sound generator, the resonance chambers, and the articulators. The sound (voice) generator consists of the vocal folds within the larynx, which is located at the top of the airway into and out of the lungs. Air passes through the larynx quietly when one simply breathes. Air flowing from the lungs may create the vocal tone, or phonation, when the vocal folds are moved into the path of the flowing air. The vocal tone can be described as a buzzing sound that is delivered into vocal tract regions above.

The chambers above the vocal folds—that is, the cavities within each individual's head and neck—modify, or resonate, the original noise. This determines the quality of the voice. This is resonance and this is the product of the chambers. The pharynx, above the larynx, is a major chamber. The mouth, through which the sound then passes, is also a major resonating cavity. The nose may be used to add resonance in certain speech sounds.

The mouth also moves its parts to form speech sounds. The soft palate moves into position. The tongue elevates, protrudes, or lowers. The flowing air is interfered with or stopped or allowed to pass freely. The teeth, the lips, and the tongue articulate the modified or resonated sound and direct the flowing air stream when necessary to produce the many different noises called speech sounds.

The vocal tract, then, consists of those changeable spaces that phonate, resonate, and articulate to make speech sounds. It is the purpose of this study to understand the nature of the instrument. With further study, one can delve deeply into the nature of every aspect of the vocal tract and its partner, the auditory system.

Spaces and Valves

The spaces, or chambers, of the vocal tract can be considered in sequence. Starting inferiorly, there are the two (or more) spaces within the larynx; these communicate with the pharynges above; the pharynges communicate with the mouth and with the nose; the mouth and the nose communicate with the outside environment. Between each of these neighboring spaces there is a doorway: the aditus ad laryngis, the faucial isthmus, the velopharyngeal port, or isthmus, and so on.

In combination with the unique character of the walls of the spaces, their angulations, and so on, valves or constrictors change the chambers in a moving, dynamic manner. The volumes of the chambers change, as does their availability to flowing air and to resonating sound. Such changes make possible the production of many kinds of sounds.

The valves may completely close off one space from another space. For example, the lips can close off the mouth, as in the production of [p] and [m] sounds.

The tongue can lift itself and contact any of a number of other oral structures to make a constriction, or valve, as in the [d] and [k] sounds. The soft palate and the epiglottis operate within their environs with adjacent structures to close off spaces. Thus, spaces are coupled, or joined in relationships, and in this way different sounds are produced.

A chamber changes internally because of valvings or constrictions. The tongue is very flexible; it can assume a number of different postures and provides an outstanding example of how the oral cavity can be changed internally to produce different sounds. These valvings and constrictions in the oral cavity are sometimes termed *articulation,* the production of specific speech sounds.

ASSOCIATED SYSTEMS

The *auditory system* has important anatomic and physiologic connections with the voice-producing system. The auditory system senses acoustic events (i.e., sounds) in the environment. The speech we learn to produce is modeled after that which we hear.

The child learns to manipulate his/her vocal tract, to close off chambers, to create valves and constrictions, and so to produce the vowels and consonants that s/he hears in the environment. These are the sounds of the language that the other human beings around are using. The child and the adult use their auditory systems to monitor their speech productions and maintain a quality-control system.

None of the sounds that become part of the speech code can be made without some means of energizing the vocal tract. This energy comes from air flowing

under pressure through the tract and both acting upon the tract and being acted upon. This air is usually associated with the respiratory system.

The *respiratory system* brings environmental air, with its oxygen content, into the body and expels air back out of the body. During inhalation, the air pressure within the lungs is less than the outside air pressure, so outside air flows into the lungs. The surface tissues of the internal chambers remove oxygen from the air and transfer the oxygen to a transport system (red blood cells). The oxygen then travels to where it is processed, becoming part of the metabolic program of the body.

The same transport system removes waste products from various parts of the body and returns these to the lungs, where the waste products (mainly carbon dioxide) pass out of the red blood cells into the environmental air found within the lung spaces. This exchange of oxygen and carbon dioxide is the essential function of the lung tissues. The walls of the lung spaces are then squeezed, and the air with the waste products is forced out into the atmosphere by the increased pressure.

The pressurized air flows outward utilizing the vocal tract as its passageway. This exhaled (expired) air is essential in the production of sounds of speech. Thus, the respiratory system is important both in supporting life and in energizing the sound-producing machinery during speech.

Another associated system already described is the *nervous system;* it is extremely sensitive, flexible, and complex. The nervous system has the ability to sense the body and the environment in which the body exists. When necessary, it transmits impulses that cause body parts to function. The nervous system makes it possible for the body to see, hear, smell, feel weight, taste, identify temperatures, and so on. All of these provide the body with means of relating to the environment. The nervous system protects the body by identifying undesirable elements. It aids the body by locating food.

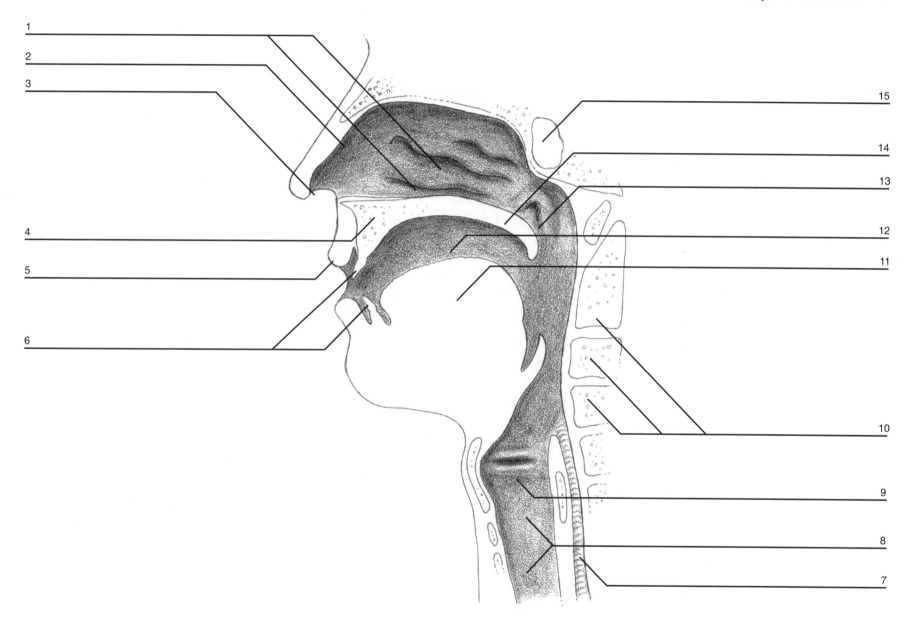

Figure 1.2   Vocal Tract

It assists in perpetuating the species by identifying mates and predators.

Not only does the nervous system sense the external environment, but it combines that awareness with an awareness of the multitudinous states and activities of the internal body. It is aware when there is a need for nutrition. It knows when oxygen is in demand or when there is an overabundance of waste products. It knows when the body is standing, sitting, prone, or when it is walking, running, or climbing a tree. It knows when a muscle contracts or a joint is used.

These external and internal sensing devices allow the nervous system to collect information. It can file the information, and it can make information meaningful by collating or grouping different kinds of information. It can recall information already gathered, and if it determines that the information deserves to be acted upon, it can program appropriate action.

Movement of body parts is coordinated as well as initiated by the nervous system. A movement is best done when a contrary movement or position is eliminated. For example, it is difficult to lift the right foot to take a step when the left foot is lifted and taking a step; it is difficult for a person to speak a phrase or sentence efficiently when inhaling. Thus, awareness and coordination of activities to produce an efficient mechanism is the function of the nervous system.

Other bodily systems and organs that play a role in maintaining the health of the organism can also be thought of as associated systems. There is no doubt about the importance of the glandular system, the vascular system, the reproductive system, the locomotor system, and others. However, because of their relatively remote connection with the acts of speaking and hearing, they will not be considered here.

Our study, then, is mainly concerned with the vocal tract and commences with the structural elements—the materials that form the walls of the chambers, the muscles that move the valves and produce the constrictions, and the nerves that cause the movements to happen.

SUMMARY

This is an elementary college text on the anatomy of the speech and hearing systems. It does not assume any background by the student in anatomy or physiology. The drawings are an important aid in understanding the text, and it is assumed that the student will seek out other texts and reference works in trying to come to grips with the material herein.

The language of anatomy has a long and varied history. The student must master the NA nomenclature used in this text. The terms used in talking about directions and locations and in establishing body planes are highly important. In describing the body, bilateral symmetry is generally assumed. The various ways in which body parts are named can shed light on their structure and function. Cells of similar types form tissues. Tissue types forming the speech and hearing systems include connective, muscle, and nervous. Of some interest is embryology and postnatal growth and changes.

The vocal tract is an interconnected series of chambers in the head and neck that produce and modify sound to form articulate speech. The anatomy of these spaces consists largely of the anatomy of the walls forming them, of the valves that are found between them, and of the structures that produce constrictions within them. The associated auditory, respiratory, and nervous systems also play important parts in the production of vowels and consonants.

Clinical Implications

The speech and hearing scientist, whether interested in the normal aspects of oral communication or the disorders, is well founded in the anatomic bases of oral communication. It becomes highly important to the speech/language pathologist, especially those who serve in medical environments (such as hospitals and nursing homes), and to those concerned about the communication skills of infants with problems associated with disorders of body systems.

Examples of some of the interest areas, anatomic and physiologic areas that fail to provide adequate means of oral communication, are the following. Bony defects include those where the embryo has failed to complete an important speech structure; here, an outstanding event is cleft palate, but another can be advanced bony fusion of the cranial bones (craniostenosis), among other conditions. Other bony defects are *iatrogenic* in that they result from surgical intervention, such as surgery to remove a portion of a bone for cancer. Of course, traumatic bone defects occur from vocation, motorcycle and automobile, war, and other events that severely damage bony structures.

Muscle-based communication disorders may be related to congenital (present at birth) defects with muscles failing to form properly to abnormality of the stimulating nerve impulses. In older individuals, there are several degenerating conditions of the muscular system (e.g., myasthenia gravis) and, of course, damage or loss of muscular tissue from accident or surgery.

An increasingly important area in speech and language pathology is associated with disorders of the nervous system associated with oral communication. The most common is probably degeneration of the nervous elements of the auditory system, but of nearly equal proportion are those disorders associated with degenerative neurologic conditions (e.g., Alzheimer's disease) that cause deterioration of memory and cognitive functions. Other neurologic-based communication problems are those stemming from accident, such as blows that damage the nervous system, or from strokes and tumors and the like. Brain damage can create speech and language disorders; hearing problems; injury or destruction of the nerves serving special areas related to oral communication can be similarly damaging.

The modern speech/language pathologist, like the physical therapist and the physician and the nurse, must know that s/he is dealing with a normal or an abnormal anatophysiologic organism when dealing with the person who demonstrates a communication disorder. To know what is abnormal, it is essential to know what is normal. The purpose of your study here is to acquire a fundamental knowledge of normal!

Study Questions

1. *When we discuss anatomic pairing (there's a similar structure on both sides of the body), just how similar are the two? Examine a friend's face, either by photograph or directly, and closely note the right and left eyes and how much alike they may be. Or, look at the corners of the mouth. You may find there is considerable difference between right and left anatomic parts. Would you guess that this is also demonstrated internally, such as the right and left sides of the brain?*

2. *Consider the names of anatomic structures internationally. Is it important for there to be some agreement among language groups (e.g., French, German, and English) that a common term for, say, mouth, is oris? Why could not each language group have its own term and ignore what others call the structure?*

3. *You are interested in how an artery travels through the body. What kind of section (cuts through the body) would you make to follow the twists and turns of the blood vessel in its travels? Would a sagittal section suffice?*

4. *What about the midline? A structure or a space that is located at the midline of the body is usually unpaired. If you were the engineer, would you make the throat or the stomach paired and move each of the two to the sides?*

5. *Again, if you are considering the midline as a geometric concept, how many midlines are there in the human body? Can you have a midline from front to back, in a coronal section? Can there be a midline in a horizontal (transverse) section?*

SUGGESTED REFERENCES

Human Anatomy Texts

There are numbers of such texts. What is identified below is only a start. It is suggested that a medical library be examined to note the proliferation of such reference. Each year, new ones and revised old ones appear. Anatomy does need updating!

Agur A: Grant's atlas of anatomy. 9th ed. Baltimore: Williams & Wilkins, 1991.

This is a popular atlas, predominantly illustrations with little text. An atlas is always helpful, especially in identifying anatomic landmarks.

Anson BJ, ed: Human anatomy: A complete systematic treatise. 12th ed. New York: McGraw Hill, 1966.

Morris' text, also known as "Morris' Human Anatomy, is organized by systems. You can quickly cover the digestive or respiratory systems this way.

Clemente C, ed: Anatomy of the human body. 30th American ed. Philadelphia: Lea & Febiger, 1985.

This book is commonly known as "Gray's Anatomy." Note the first chapter, Introduction, as it covers much of the same material as this text does. How is the figure drawn that represents the various planes of the body? Note the organization of the information from chapter to chapter.

Perkins WH, Kent RD: Functional anatomy of speech, language, and hearing. A primer. San Diego: College Hill, 1986.

Romanes GJE, ed: Cunningham's textbook of anatomy. 12th ed. New York: Oxford University Press, 1981.

Again, note the first chapter with introductory information about the nature of anatomic study. In the preceding section, Preface, there is a paragraph about International Anatomical Nomenclature; you'll note what British anatomists identify as BR (Birmigham Revision) of the Nomina Anatomica referred to in the text and elsewhere. Note also the organization of chapters.

Tortora GJ: Principles of human anatomy. 6th ed. New York: Harper and Row, 1990.

This is probably the most commonly used anatomy text in the United States. It is widely accepted as an introductory text, and examination of Chapter 1 (and preceding materials) will clearly indicate why. Broad principles of anatomy are introduced as well as basic matters including pronunciation of terms, spatial orientation, and other important considerations. The illustrations are excellent.

Zemlin WR: Speech and hearing science. Anatomy and physiology. 2nd ed. Englewood Cliffs, NJ: Prentice-Hall, 1981.

Chapter 2
The Skull

GENERAL INTRODUCTION

The speaking and hearing acts are largely centered in the head, with the neck and the thorax as indispensable partners. The head has its skeletal or bony support in what is commonly called the *skull* (Figs. 2.1 and 2.2). The bones of the skull not only contribute to spaces, but also provide for the attachment of muscles and ligaments.

The spaces include the air-filled cavities that actually participate in the speech act, such as the oral cavity, the nose, and the pharynx. These spaces are outlined and supported not only by bones but also by such "soft" tissues as muscles and membranes. Other chambers of the skull region are potential spaces in that they are volumes that contain anatomic materials. An outstanding example is the cranial vault of the skull, which houses the brain.

The muscles of the head have specific bony landmarks for attachment, which one should know because their physiologic functions are largely determined by the locations of these attachments. There are numerous muscles and muscle groups associated with the skull. Some of these play little part in the speaking act, but there are many of direct importance.

Beginning your study with the skull is an exercise in the language of anatomy. The terminology used to identify skull bones is also used in naming other structures. For example, the styloglossus muscle is attached to the skull at the styloid process at one end and to the tongue (glossa) at the other. Several of the bones of the cranium have names that are also applied to the lobes of the brain within (e.g., the frontal bone and the frontal lobe).

In studying the skull from the speech perspective, one must also become familiar with the teeth, of course. In a later chapter, the structure of the auditory system will be presented. In what follows, selected aspects of the skull (those that pertain primarily to human communication) are discussed. It is necessary at the outset to understand that the bones of the skull are studied in two divisions: the cranium and the facial skeleton.

THE CRANIUM

The *cranium* encloses the brain within its cranial vault. This relationship is obvious in the case of some cranial bones (e.g., the frontal bone and the parietal bones). In other cases (the ethmoid bone, especially), the relationship to the brain may be less obvious. There are eight bones forming the cranium: one frontal, one ethmoid, one sphenoid, two temporal, two parietal, and one occipital.

The Frontal Bone

The *frontal bone* (Figs. 2.1 and 2.2) provides the smooth, convex surface of the forehead. Inferiorly, it extends from the superior margin of the orbit of the eye; laterally, it extends through the *temporal fossa (temple)*; and superiorly, it extends to the *vertex (crown)*. The frontal bone is significant, first, because it houses the *frontal sinus,* which is of some importance to the functioning of the nasal area and ultimately to the health of the individual; second, because it serves as the attachment for muscles related to speech activities; and third, because it houses the frontal lobes of the brain.

The frontal sinus is a part of the *sinus system* of the skull. This system is a series of spaces within the skull bones; its function has been the subject of considerable debate. Among the suggested purposes of the sinuses are lightening the skull, providing for better balance of the skull, resonating for the voice, and expanding the area served by the nose in warming, moistening, and filtering incoming air.

Clinical Note

There are several sinuses in the vicinity of the nose—the paranasal sinuses. They are found within bone, are air-filled, and are lined with mucous membrane, which produces fluid mucus that drains into the nasal passages.

Little is known about the contribution of the sinuses to normal speech; perhaps they mainly contribute to the resonance of the voice, providing a chamber that either vibrates sympathetically or functions as a cul-de-sac. More important, however, are the pathologic aspects of the sinuses. Inflamed, infected, and structurally defective sinuses are major contributors to various speech and hearing disorders. It is common to find sinus trouble in the histories of individuals who suffer from loss of hearing, as well as among those with some type of speech disorder, especially voice problems.

The frontal sinus itself is composed of paired spaces located at each side of the midline and extending to various heights in the frontal bone. The total effect is pyramidal; one wall of this pyramid separates the right from the left frontal sinus. The frontal sinus communicates with the nasal passage through the *frontonasal duct* and opens into either the *frontal recess* or the *middle meatus* of the nose. The frontal sinuses are two of several that are located in close proximity to the nasal passages. Other *paranasal sinuses* are found in the ethmoid bone, in the sphenoid bone, and in two maxilla bones of the facial skeleton group.

The Ethmoid Bone

The *ethmoid bone* (Figs. 2.2 and 2.3) is found immediately inferior and posterior to the frontal bone. It is a single midline bone, light in weight, spongy in composition, and cuboidal in shape. This bone forms important surfaces of the cranial floor, the framework of the nose, and the two eye orbits. The bone is composed of four parts: a *horizontal,* or *cribriform, plate* (forming part of the cranial floor), a *perpendicular plate* (contributing to the structure of the nasal septum), and the two *lateral labyrinths* (containing the ethmoid air cells).

Protruding medially from the lateral labyrinths, and thus into the air spaces of the nasal passageways, are three (sometimes four) curved, shelf-like *nasal conchae (turbinates):* the *superior,* the *middle* and the *inferior.* When a fourth concha is found on this bone, it is termed the *supreme concha.* These conchae are covered by mucous membrane, as is the entire respiratory tract. The major purposes of this membrane are to warm, moisten, and filter inhaled air. The filtering is effected by hairs, the moistening by the mucus produced, and the warming by the capillary beds of blood near the surface. The mucous membrane also contains nerve endings that serve in olfaction (smell). Adjacent conchae and the walls of the nasal passageways form spaces, which are the meatuses or air channels. The spaces of the nose serve both to conduct air into and out of the respiratory tract and to resonate the voice.

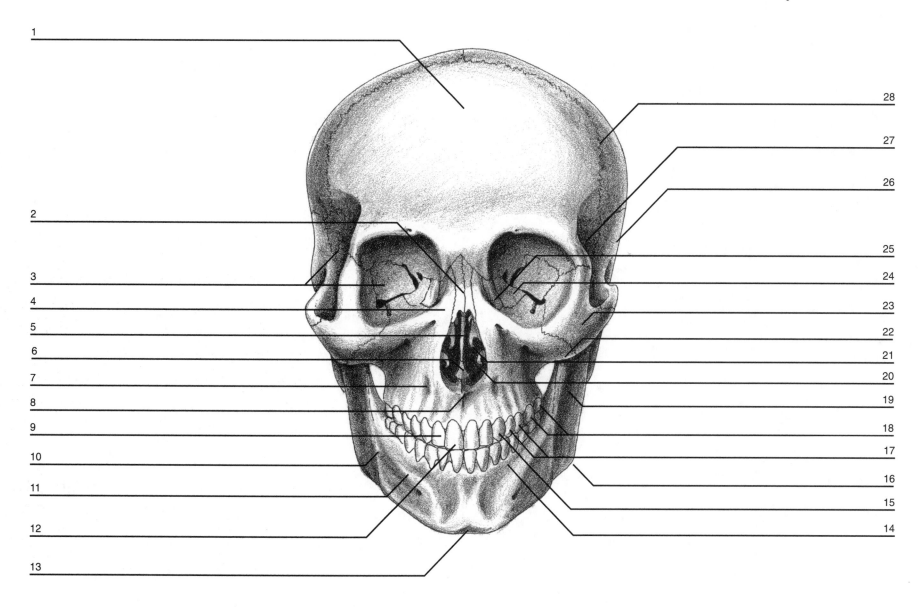

Figure 2.1   Skull: Frontal View

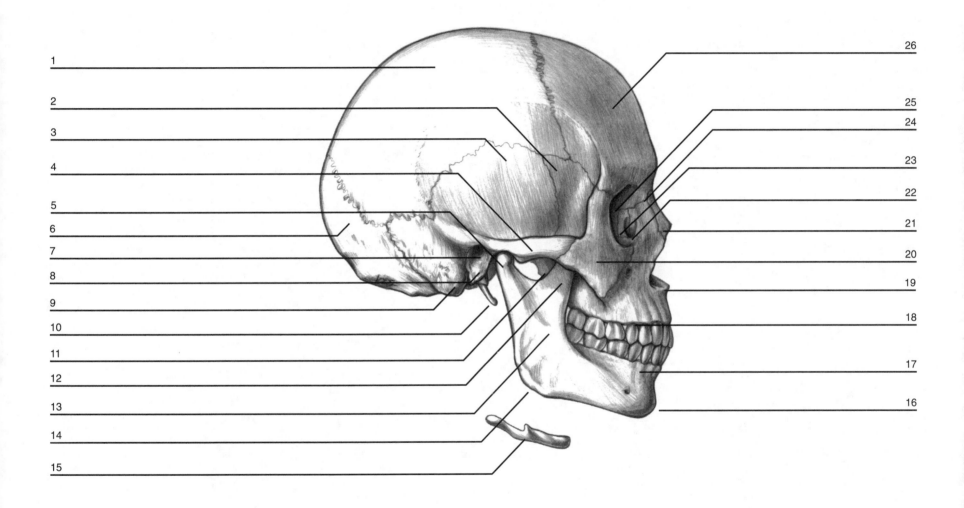

1

2

3

4

5

6

7

8

9

10

11

12

13

14

15

26

25

24

23

22

21

20

19

18

17

16

Figure 2.2   Skull: Lateral View

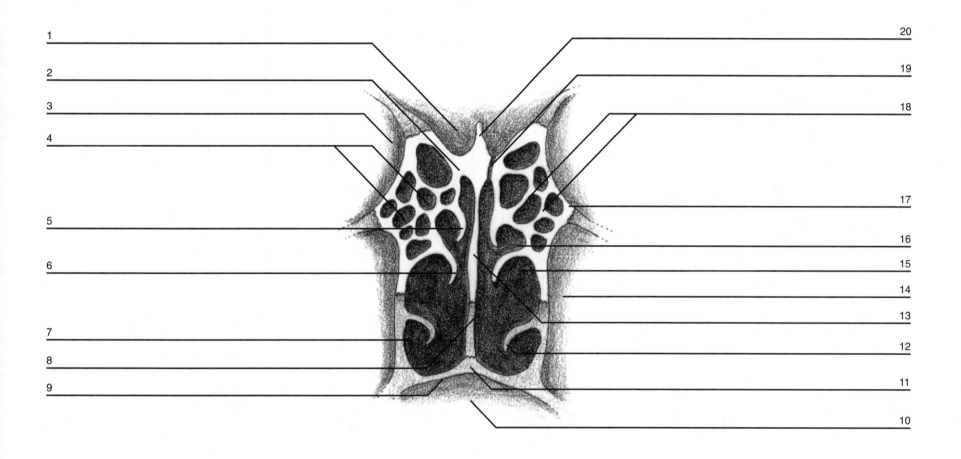

Figure 2.3   Ethmoid Bone: Coronal View

The horizontal plate is cribriform, meaning perforated, to provide passage through the bone for the sensory nerve fibers for olfaction. Immediately upon leaving the plate, the nerve fibers penetrate the olfactory bulb resting in its paired depressions on the superior surface of the plate. The anterior tip of the horizontal plate provides for a midline elevation, the crista galli, to which is attached a part of the dura mater covering the brain.

The *ethmoid air cells* are sinus-like spaces lined with mucous membrane. They occupy the space between the orbits and are extremely variable (as to size and number) cavities. They may number as few as 3 or as many as 18; the larger the number, however, the smaller are the individual cells. Occasionally, a cell will invade a bordering bone; thus, such a space as the anterior ethmoid cell could well be named the posterior frontal sinus because of its location in the frontal bone.

Clinical Note

The contribution of the nasal passages to speech is small, but disturbances have obvious results in speech. When the mucous membrane swells, as in a bad cold, or when the nasal septum is badly deviated, the resonating chamber normally provided is diminished or lost. The result is a voice that is denasal or hyponasal.

The Sphenoid Bone

The *sphenoid bone* (Figs. 2.1, 2.2, and 2.4) is immediately posterior to the ethmoid and frontal bones. This complex and irregular bone forms part of the base of the skull, just anterior to the temporal bones and to the basilar part of the occipital bone. The sphenoid bone is a relatively large midline structure, with projections from its body oriented to give the entire bone a strong resemblance to a bat with its wings outstretched, each side having a greater wing and a lesser wing. There are two pterygoid processes projecting inferiorly that are of considerable importance to structures and tissues affecting speech and hearing.

The body of the sphenoid is hollowed into two separate spaces, the *sphenoid sinuses*. These paranasal sinuses have their openings into the nasal passages. The body of the sphenoid bone has a smooth superior surface, deeply indented (*sella turcica*) for housing the pituitary body. The body articulates anteriorly with the cribriform plate of the ethmoid bone and posteriorly with the basilar part of the occipital bone. The lateral surfaces of the body are united with the great wings. The anterior surface, forming a part of the wall of the nasal cavity, is divided at its midline by the *sphenoidal crest*, a small vertically oriented ridge of bone that articulates with the perpendicular plate of the ethmoid and forms a part of the nasal septum. Inferiorly, the body of the sphenoid presents a rough surface for the soft tissues of the pharynx, as well as providing for articulation with the vomer bone.

The *great wing* of the sphenoid is attached to part of the lateral surface of the body and extends laterally, then superiorly. The wing makes up part of the floor and outer wall of the cranium, supporting parts of the convolutions of the temporal lobe of the brain. In addition, the great wing serves as a portion of the eye orbit and as the attachment for the cartilaginous auditory tube.

The *lesser*, or *small*, *wing* of the sphenoid bone is composed of two thin, triangular plates of bone arising from the upper and anterior parts of the body and projecting laterally or horizontally. This structure serves to support part of the frontal lobe of the brain and forms a part of the roof of the orbit.

Descending inferiorly from the juncture of the body and great wing on either side are the *pterygoid processes* with their two plates, the *lateral pterygoid plate* and the *medial pterygoid plate*. Anteriorly at their upper ends these plates are fused, creating two posterior-facing V-shaped spaces. These are a larger, lower *pterygoid fossa* and a smaller, upper *scaphoid fossa.* From these fossae and their pterygoid plate walls arise two muscles, the internal (medial) pterygoid and the tensor (veli) palatine.

The lateral pterygoid plate is a broad, thin sheet forming part of the infratemporal fossa on its lateral surface and part of the scaphoid fossa on its medial surface; its lateral surface also gives origin to the external pterygoid muscle, while its medial surface gives rise to the internal pterygoid muscle.

The medial pterygoid plate is a longer and narrower sheet of bone than the lateral plate; it curves at its extremity into a hook-like process, the *pterygoid hamulus,* around which the tensor (veli) palatine muscle tendon passes and from which the dilator tubae muscle originates. The lateral surface of this plate forms part of the boundary of the posterior nares of the nasal passage. The posterior border of this plate provides attachment for pharyngeal structures, especially the superior constrictor muscle.

Clinical Note

The sphenoid bone is not commonly seen as a source of problems. Certainly, sinusitis involving the sphenoid sinus can cause difficulties in the upper airway. Too, the *hamular process* has been of historic interest as it relates to the tensor (veli) palatine muscle in patients with cleft palate; it provides origin for the dilator tubae muscle so important for opening the auditory tube. It has been noted that the angulation formed between the body of the sphenoid bone and the basilar portion of the occipital bone creates spatial differences in the nasopharynx that might test the efficiency of the valving system in that region. Lastly, the space for the pituitary body (sella turcica) is often a landmark visible in radiographs and becomes most important in measurements determining bony relationships in the skull.

The Temporal Bones

On either side of the cranium are the two *temporal bones* (Figs. 2.1, 2.2, and 2.5) contributing to the lateral walls and the base. The temporal bone contributes significantly to speech and hearing processes, affording attachment to muscles of mastication of the neck, tongue, and pharynx; it also houses the major portion of the peripheral hearing mechanisms, as well as the equilibrium (vestibular) end organs.

Although authorities variously divide this bone into from three to five parts (pars), or portions, here it will be presented as having four portions with some extremely important subdivisions and processes. The first is the squamous portion with its zygomatic process, temporal fossa, and mandibular fossa. The second is the mastoid portion, with its mastoid process and mastoid air cells. The third is the tympanic portion, with its scroll-like plate forming a large part of the external acoustic canal. The fourth portion is the petrous portion, containing important canals housing the auditory system's end organ, as well as those end organs serving the sensory function for equilibrium, or balance (the vestibular system). The inferior aspect of the petrous portion has not only attachments for several important muscles but also the distinctive, spike-like styloid process.

The *squamous portion* of the temporal bone is the relatively large, fan-shaped, thin part that also forms part of the temporal fossa. This smooth and convex area provides origin for the *temporal muscle,* a muscle of mastication. Projecting anteriorly from the lower part of the squamous portion is the long and arched *zygomatic process;* the inferior border of this process provides origin for the *masseter muscle,* another masticatory muscle. The end of the zygomatic process is rough and serrated for articulation with the zygomatic (cheek) bone, an important member of the facial skeleton. The undersurface of the zygomatic process and the adjacent area of the

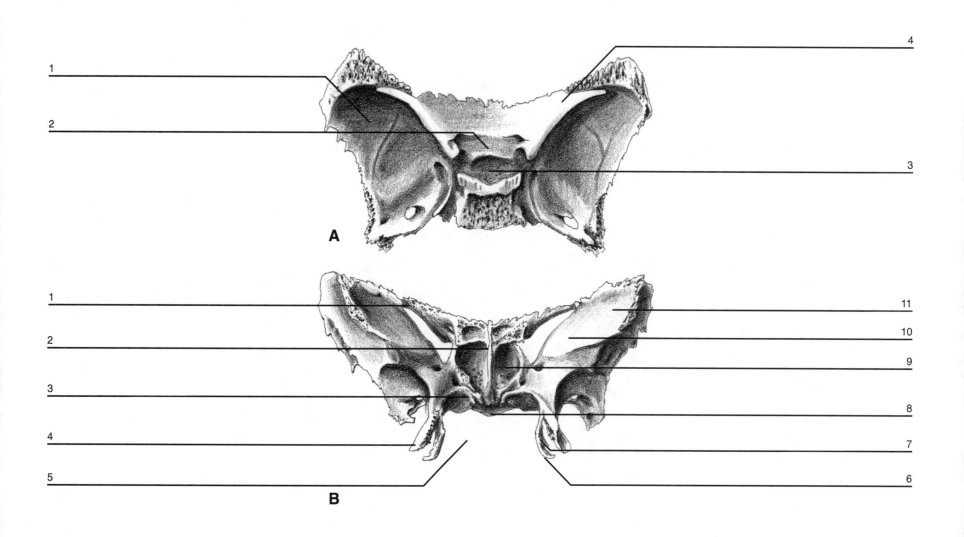

Figure 2.4A   Sphenoid Bone: Superior Surfaces

Figure 2.4B   Sphenoid Bone: Anterior Surfaces

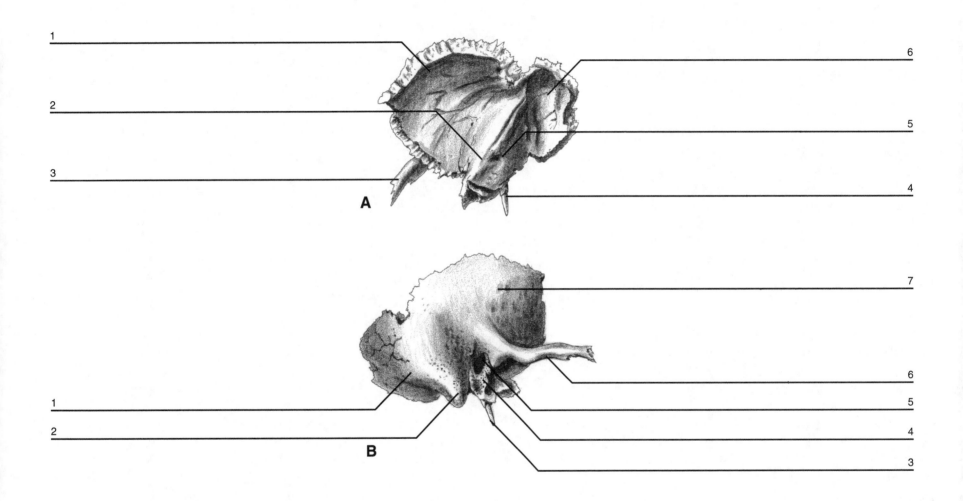

1

2

3

A

6

5

4

7

6

5

4

3

1

2

B

Figure 2.5A   Temporal Bone: Superior View

Figure 2.5B   Temporal Bone: Lateral View

squamous portion provide for the *mandibular fossa,* the site of the important articulation (joint) with the mandible bone. A little of the squamous portion acts as the ceiling of the external acoustic meatus.

Inferior to the squamous portion is the large and bulky *mastoid portion* of the temporal bone; this is the most posterior part of the bone. A large conical projection beneath this portion is the *mastoid process,* giving attachment to several muscles, the *digastric* of the suprahyoid group and *sternocleidomastoid* of the cervical region. The mastoid process is composed of many internal air cells of irregular size, shape, and number. At the uppermost region is a larger, irregular cavity, the *tympanic antrum,* communicating with the mastoid air cells in one direction and with the middle ear cavity in the other. All of these cavities are lined with mucous membrane.

The *petrous portion* of the temporal bone is a pyramid-shaped structure found at the floor of the cranium and projecting medially between the occipital and the sphenoid bones. The sides of the pyramid are oriented somewhat anteriorly and posteriorly; the anterior surface presents marks for the convolutions of the brain, a prominence (the *arcuate eminence*) under which is found the superior semicircular canal of the vestibular system, and a very thin portion of bone, the *tegmen tympani,* beneath which is the tympanum, or middle ear, of the hearing system. The posterior surface of the petrous portion presents orifices of importance, including the opening to the internal acoustic meatus (canal). Within the petrous portion are the canals of the inner ear, the cochlea and semicircular canals.

Another surface, part of the anterior one, presents a wall of the middle ear. This medial wall continues posteriorly to form part of the tympanic antrum and anteriorly to form part of the auditory tube that ultimately opens to the pharynx. The under or inferior surface of the petrous portion is highly irregular, not smooth as are the other walls. This aspect provides for passage of blood vessels and nerves, as well as providing

attachment for muscles of the pharynx and neck. Also from this undersurface projects the highly variable *styloid process,* from which derive three important muscles associated with the speaking act and a suspensory ligament to the larynx. The internal acoustic meatus, on the posterior surface, carries the facial (Cranial VII) and the auditory (Cranial VIII) nerves and other nerves and blood vessels.

At the angle of the joining of the petrous and squamous portions of the temporal bone are two canals that pass into the *tympanum* (middle ear cavity). The upper one carries the tensor tympani muscle, which is housed within this canal and is attached through its tendon to the *malleus bone.* The lower canal is larger; it is the bony portion of the auditory tube (formerly called the Eustachian tube).

The *tympanic portion* of the temporal bone is a thin and somewhat curled structure that forms all of the anterior and inferior and part of the posterior walls of the bony portion of the external acoustic meatus. The remainder of the canal wall, the superior and part of the posterior walls, is composed of the *temporal squama.* More medially, the canal is grooved through part of its circumference; this groove is the tympanic sulcus, which receives the tympanic membrane.

The *external acoustic meatus* is composed of both cartilaginous and bony sections. The former will be discussed later in association with other cartilaginous structures of the external ear. The bony portion of the canal is the internal two-thirds of the entire canal, oriented forward and somewhat downward, and most narrow at its medial or internal end.

The Parietal Bones

The paired parietal bones (Figs. 2.1 and 2.2) contribute to the roof and the sides of the cranium. Each is a curved plate of bone having essentially two surfaces and four angles. It is at these angles that the newborn infant demonstrates the membranous fontanelles, or soft spots, as ossification continues postnatally. A large portion, variably sized depending upon the sex and size of the person, of the outer surface of the parietal bone contributes to the temporal fossa; observable ridges indicate the arc-like attachment of the temporal muscle across this surface.

The Occipital Bone

The single *occipital bone* (Fig. 2.2) has been described as leaf-shaped and trapezoid-like; it forms the back of the cranium and an important part of the base of the entire skull. The portion curling upward at the back of the cranium is the *squamous portion.* This curves anteriorly to form at the undersurface of the skull a rather large opening *(foramen magnum).* This foramen provides for communication between the cranium above and the vertebral canal below, in effect allowing for continuity of the two parts of the central nervous system, the brain and the spinal cord. On the anterolateral rim of this foramen will be found the two *condyles,* serving as the support pedestals for the skull as it articulates with the uppermost vertebra *(atlas).* Anterior to the foramen magnum is the midline basilar portion that, as it fuses with the body of the sphenoid bone, forms a portion of the roof and posterior wall of the nasopharynx as the sphenoccipital angle. The occipital and sphenoid bones fuse at about age 28 years; at that time, the fused structure is named the *clivus.* Numerous muscles of the neck for head posture and movement are attached to various landmarks of the occipital bone.

THE FACIAL SKELETON

The *facial skeleton* is formed by 14 bones of the skull that surround the nose and mouth and thus a major portion of the vocal tract. These 14 bones do not include those of the middle ear (ossicles) or, usually, the hyoid bone. The latter will be included in the present discussion because of its importance to the upper vocal tract and the mobile structures therein. The bones of the facial skeleton are the zygomatic, nasal, lacrimal, vomer, inferior nasal concha, palatine, maxilla, and mandible. All are paired except the vomer and mandible.

The *zygomatic bone,* or *cheek bone* Figs. 2.1 and 2.2), is quadrangular and forms the prominence of the cheek and the floor of the eye orbit. The *nasal bones* (Figs. 2.1 and 2.2) are two small, oblong bones placed together at the bridge of the nose. The *lacrimal bone* (Figs. 2.1. and 2.2) forms part of the anteromedial wall of the eye orbit. It is the smallest and most fragile of the facial bones and contributes to the lacrimal groove and the nasolacrimal duct.

The *vomer bone* (Figs. 2.1 and 2.3; see Fig. 2.10) is an unpaired bone that forms the lower and posterior part of the nasal septum. It is a midline structure, thin, roughly quadrilateral, and frequently bent or deflected to one side at its anterior end. The long, sloping anterior border articulates in its lower portion with the triangular *septal cartilage* and in its superior portion with the perpendicular plate of the ethmoid bone. Its superior border, which is the thickest part of the bone, divides into two alae, with an intervening groove that receives the *sphenoid rostrum.* Its posterior border is free and forms the operating wall between the posterior nares. The inferior border is received into the groove formed by the two halves of the maxilla and the palatine bones; this groove is part of the (superior) *nasal crest.*

The *inferior nasal concha (inferior turbinate) bone* (Fig. 2.3) is a scroll-like bone horizontally oriented along the lateral wall of the nasal cavity and separating the inferior from the middle meatus. It is more pointed at its posterior end than at its anterior. This bone is attached by its superior border to the conchal crest of the maxilla bone.

The *palatine bone* (Fig. 2.6; see Figs. 2.8 and 2.10) is an L-shaped bone situated at the posterior end of the nasal cavity between the maxilla bone, which is

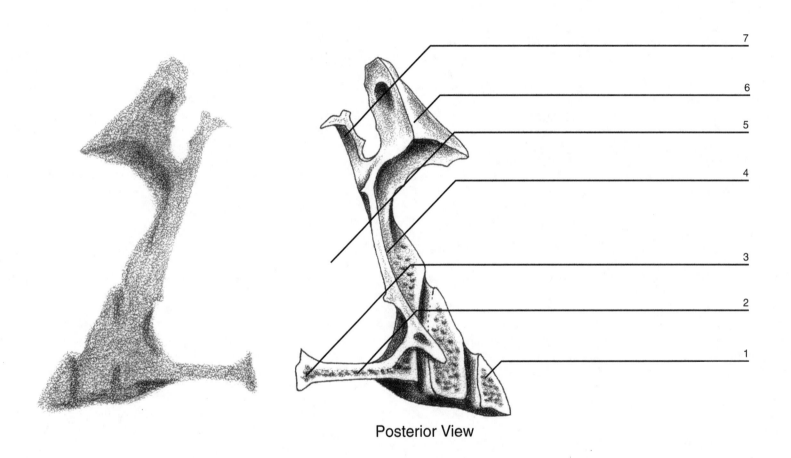

Posterior View

Figure 2.6   Palatine Bone

forward, and the medial pterygoid plate of the sphenoid bone, which is behind. It has two parts, the vertical (or perpendicular) and the horizontal. There are also three processes, the pyramidal, orbital, and sphenoidal. The perpendicular part of the palatine bone forms a major part of the posterior nasal cavity.

The horizontal part of the palatine bone forms the posterior part of the floor of the nasal cavity, thus it is the posterior one-third of the bony palate. Its superior, or nasal, surface is smooth and concave. Its inferior, or oral, surface is likewise concave but roughened. The anterior border of the horizontal part is roughened and articulates at the transverse suture with the palatine process of the maxilla bone. Its medial border is roughened for articulation with its opposite side palatine bone and is thickened on its nasal surface to provide a continuation of the nasal crest (to receive the vomer bone). The lateral margin of the horizontal part of the palatine bone is united with the lower margin of the perpendicular part. The posterior border of this part is concave and free; it forms the attachment for the soft palate, and presents the midline posterior nasal spine. The three processes of the palatine bone provide for articular surfaces with other facial and cranial bones.

The *maxilla bone* (Figs. 2.1, 2.3, and 2.7; see Fig. 2.10) (informally known as the *upper jaw*) forms an important part of the upper vocal tract. One portion of it makes a major contribution to bounding the mouth, while other portions of the maxilla provide landmarks to which are attached muscles and soft tissues important to the speaking act.

The two maxillae provide boundaries of four cavities: part of the roof of the mouth, the floor and lateral wall of the nose, a portion of the eye orbit, and the *maxillary sinus (antrum of Highmore)*. Each maxilla has a body and four processes. The pyramidal body has its base pointed toward the nasal cavity and contains the air-filled sinus lined with mucous membrane.

Of some significance to speech are the four max-

illary processes: frontal, alveolar, zygomatic, and palatine. The *frontal process* forms part of the lateral boundary of the nose. The *alveolar process,* thick and spongy, is shaped like a crescent and contains eight alveoli (cavities) in which the upper teeth in the adult are lodged. (A young child has but five alveoli.) The *zygomatic process* is small, rough, and triangular, articulating with the zygomatic bone.

The fourth maxillary process, the *palatine,* forms the greater portion of the floor of the nose and the roof of the mouth in its horizontal and medial projection from the sides of the crescent. This forms about two-thirds of the hard palate, or bony palate (Fig. 2.8; see Fig. 2.10). The horizontal part of the palatine bone completes the hard palate. The medial border of the palatine process is roughened, or serrated, for articulation with its opposite; this suture line commences anteriorly at the *incisive foramen.* Extending laterally and anteriorly from this point to the region between the lateral incisor and the canine tooth is the suture line fusing the palatine process of the maxilla with the embryonic *premaxilla (incisive) bone,* the fusion being completed postnatally.

The posterior border of the palatine process articulates with the horizontal portion of the palatine bone; this line of articulation is the *transverse suture.* The previously mentioned midline suture continues through the palatine bone and terminates in the posterior nasal spine; this is the *longitudinal,* or *palatine, suture.* Superiorly on the nasal surface along this suture, a raised portion presents the *nasal crest,* receiving the vomer bone; the crest extends anteriorly to form the *anterior nasal spine.*

Clinical Note

Some of the people seen by speech and hearing clinicians are those with palatal defects. These defects stem from developmental failure of fusion of the lines (sutures) of articulation. More commonly, clefts are found along the midline suture, with one process failing to grow and fuse with the opposite side; also occurring are clefts along the maxillary-premaxillary suture line, unilaterally or bilaterally separating the premaxilla and its soft tissues from the rest of the structures. Concomitant defects, such as dental or nasal deformities, frequently accompany the basic palatal failure. Further related problems result from faulty skeletal support of various muscle groups, so that problems may be found in deglutition, respiration, and even audition.

The *mandible bone* (Figs. 2.1, 2.2, and 2.9), which fuses into a single bone about the time of birth, is the largest and strongest of the bones of the face. Its major biological function is to support the lower teeth. The mandible is made up of a body shaped somewhat like a horseshoe; from each end a ramus ascends at nearly a right angle to articulate with the temporal bone at the mandibular fossa. The two halves of the mandible fuse at the ventral midline at the *symphysis menti,* which protrudes at the point of the chin to form the *mental protuberance.* The arch-like bend of the mandible bone is the *genu.* There are two lines on the mandible: the *oblique line,* which is a slight ridge running externally from low anteriorly to high posteriorly, and the *mylohyoid line (ridge),* running on the internal surface upward and backward toward the ramus. The lower, or mandibular, teeth are found on the alveolar process (ridge) of the mandible, each side having eight cavities in the adult and five in the child.

The *ramus* (perpendicular portion) extends upward, ending in two prominent processes: the coronoid and the condyloid. The *coronoid process* is the more anterior of the two and provides attachment for the temporal and masseter muscles. The *condyloid process* rises to meet the articular disc of the temporomandibular joint of the mandibular fossa of the temporal bone. The external (lateral) pterygoid muscle attaches to the neck of this process. Inferiorly, the ramus terminates in the *angle* of the mandible, an important landmark.

The *hyoid bone* (Figs. 2.2; see Figs. 3.1, 4.3, and 5.3 to 5.6), located in the anterior part of the neck between the larynx and mandible, is sometimes called the *lingual bone* because it is the major supporting structure for the tongue. This bone is U-shaped; the bottom of the U is directed horizontally anteriorly, and the two pairs of processes are directed laterally and dorsally. Not only is the hyoid bone intimately related to the tongue, but it also provides numerous attachments for muscles and membranes of the laryngeal region. It is suspended in its position by two thin ligaments from the tips of the *styloid processes* of the *temporal bones.* The hyoid bone has a body, and the two pairs of processes are the greater and the lesser cornua. It is not a skull bone and articulates with no other bone.

The *body* of the hyoid bone is roughly quadrilateral and is oriented across the midline of the neck ventrally. The larger of the two processes of the hyoid bone is the *greater cornu,* which is directed laterally and posteriorly, tapering from front to back and ending in a tubercle. Until middle life, the connection between the greater cornu and the body of the hyoid bone is cartilaginous; ossification occurs thereafter.

The *lesser cornua* are smaller, conical bodies that project upward and backward from their points of attachment at the junction of the body and the greater cornu. This attachment is usually fibrous in nature, and some authorities feel there is a true diarthrodial joint with the body and/or the greater cornu. The apex of the lesser cornu serves as the point of attachment for the *stylohyoid ligament.*

CARTILAGES

The cartilages of the cranium and facial skeleton are few and have only modest relationship with the act of speaking, except for the nasal cartilages. The carti-

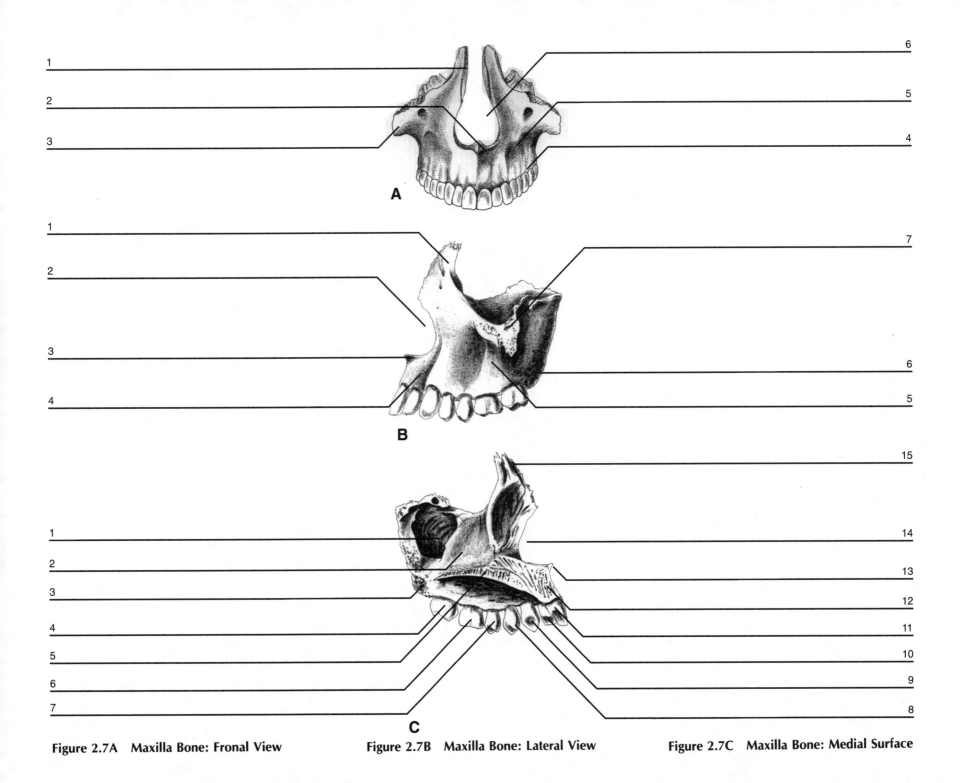

Figure 2.7A   Maxilla Bone: Fronal View   **Figure 2.7B   Maxilla Bone: Lateral View**   **Figure 2.7C   Maxilla Bone: Medial Surface**

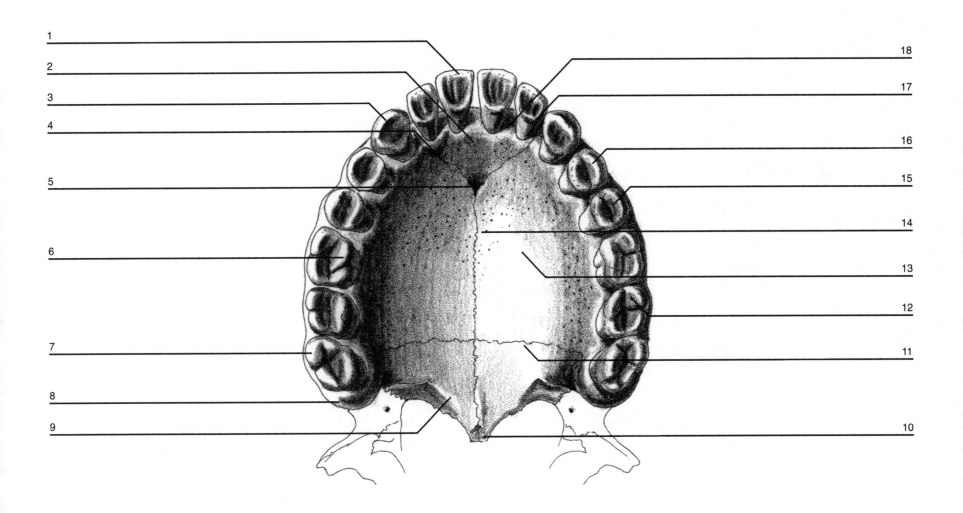

Figure 2.8   Bony Palate and Maxillary Teeth

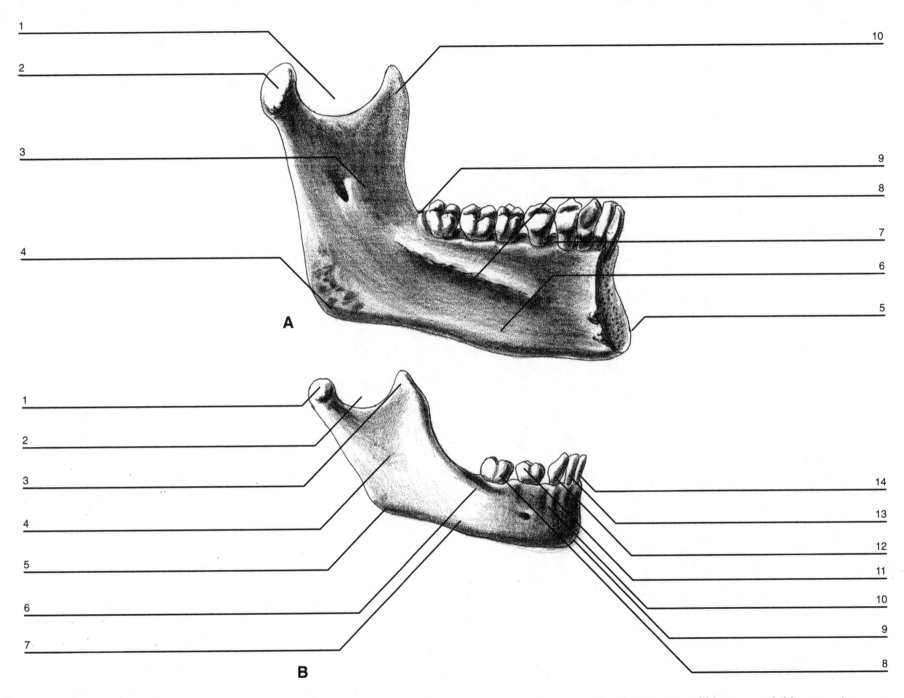

Figure 2.9A Mandible Bone (Adult): Internal Aspect

Figure 2.9B Mandible Bone (Child): Lateral Aspect

laginous portions of the ear and auditory tube, although part of the facial skeleton, are discussed in Chapter 7.

The supporting structure of the nose is composed of both bone and cartilage; the bony structures have already been described. There are five larger cartilages of the nose and several smaller ones. These vary considerably from individual to individual and determine an aspect of facial profile. There are two lateral nasal cartilages, two greater alar cartilages, and the single nasal septal cartilage. There are also the lesser alar, the vomeronasal, and the sesamoid cartilages.

The *greater alar cartilages* form the medial and lateral walls of the anterior nares on each side. A part of these walls is also formed by the lesser alar cartilages. The flaring of the nares, thus the nature of the nasal entrance, is the product of the form of the ala (wings).

Immediately superior and somewhat dorsal to the alar cartilages is the *lateral nasal cartilage,* which forms the side wall of the nose. This cartilage is interposed between the greater alar cartilage inferiorly and the nasal bone superiorly. It meets the nasal septal cartilage at the "bridge" of the nose.

The *nasal septal cartilage* (Fig. 2.10) is an unpaired midline structure that continues the separation of the two nasal passages in an anteroposterior direction. It is generally quadrilateral. The septal cartilage runs from the nasal bone forward between the two lateral nasal cartilages and thereafter between the two greater alar cartilages. The posterior portion of the septal cartilage is attached to the vomer and to the nasal crest of the maxilla bones. A portion of its anterior dimension forms the cartilaginous skeleton of the columella, the skin-covered separation between right and left nares.

The *lesser alar cartilages* are three or four in number. The *vomeronasal* is a part of the septal cartilage. The *sesamoid cartilages* vary in occurrence, number, and size, but generally are found as small, thin plates interposed between the lateral nasal cartilages and the greater alar cartilages.

DENTITION

The two jaws in which the teeth are found are the maxilla and the mandible bones. In each of these, the *alveolar processes* house the dentition. The *alveolus* is the socket, or hole, in which the tooth normally resides. The alveolar processes are crescent-shaped, with the closed end of the crescent oriented anteriorly and the open end posteriorly toward the pharynx. Normally, the teeth are arranged around the crescent. They differ from anterior to posterior in number and type, but bilateral and upper-lower symmetry pertains.

Because the teeth are arranged in the same order on both sides from midline back to the most posterior tooth, each side is termed a *quadrant.* When viewing the teeth and identifying surfaces, the outermost surface is the *facial surface,* while the surface directed inward toward the tongue is the *lingual surface.* Sometimes the surfaces of the anterior teeth (incisors), being oriented toward the lip, are termed the *labial surfaces,* while the more posterior (in dental parlance, *distal*) teeth surfaces, facially oriented, are the *buccal (cheek) surfaces.*

The first teeth of the two sets the human being develops are generally temporary and are replaced by the second, more permanent set. These first dental structures, the *deciduous teeth,* are 20 in number (Fig. 2.9B; Table 2.1). In each deciduous segment, then, there are 10 teeth, while each quadrant has 5 teeth. The arrangement of the 5 is mirrored from one quadrant to the other.

There are only three types of deciduous teeth, repeated in patterns in the upper and lower jaws. The most anterior teeth, the cutting and slicing teeth, are appropriately named the *incisors;* there are two of these in each quadrant, making a total of eight for the individual. There is a tearing and ripping tooth in each quadrant, *the canine tooth;* the individual has four canines. Finally, there are two grinding teeth, the *molars,* in each quadrant, giving a total of eight molars (each being identified from front to back as the first or second molar tooth).

The so-called *permanent teeth* number 32 (Figs. 2.1, 2.2, 2.7, 2.8, 2.9A; Table 2.2) because of the addition in each quadrant of one molar tooth and two *premolar teeth* distal to the canine tooth. The permanent teeth gradually replace the deciduous teeth. By the time of adolescence there should be a reasonably full complement of teeth, but individual variations and heredity play major roles.

The Eruption of Teeth

Both sets of teeth erupt through the alveolar processes and their covering mucous membrane (gingiva). The deciduous teeth are exfoliated (shed) as the child grows and develops. The bony housing (alveolar ridge) expands to provide for two new kinds of teeth in each quadrant, for a fairly common *third molar,* and for permanent teeth that are larger in size and that have other anatomic differences among themselves.

The child erupting the deciduous teeth could have by the first birthday the mandibular central incisor (first tooth to erupt), its maxillary counterpart (second tooth), and the maxillary lateral incisor (third tooth). Shortly thereafter, by about 1½ years of age, the child should erupt the lower lateral incisor (fourth tooth), the first molar (fifth tooth), and perhaps the canine, or cuspid, tooth (sixth tooth). By the second birthday or a few months later, the second molar (seventh tooth) should complete the dental complement.

The deciduous teeth should serve the child for 4 to 10 years. At varying times, depending upon the individual, the new and larger permanent teeth make their appearance, sometimes as early as the 6th year and usually by a few months past that birthday. Erupting early, between the ages of 6 and 8 years, will be the upper and lower central incisors, the upper and lower first molars (6–year teeth), and the lower lateral incisors, while the upper lateral incisors develop around 8

years of age, if not later. Around 10 years of age, the child should erupt the mandibular canines and both the upper and lower first premolars. About a year later the upper canines erupt, along with the upper and lower second premolars. A year or so after that, between the ages of 11 and 13, the second molar erupts in both dental arches. The third molar teeth will not erupt until well after puberty, between 17 and 25 years. All of these ages for the eruption of both deciduous and permanent teeth are averages; variation among sexes, races, and individuals can be expected.

Dental Occlusion

One definition of *dental occlusion* is "the contact between the teeth of both jaws when closed or during those excursive movements of the mandible which are essential to the function of mastication." Dental specialists identify different types of occlusion, both normal and abnormal *(malocclusion),* and the highly specialized field of orthodontics places heavy emphasis upon this aspect of dentition.

In normal occlusion, first, the two segments are not exact duplicates, either in size or shape; second, the curves the two segments take are not symmetrical; and third, the role of the maxilla bone, which is somewhat larger than the mandible bone, is not identical to that of the mandible bone.

In occlusion, the maxillary incisors labially overlap the mandibular incisors, which effects the cutting or slicing function. The upper canines similarly tend to overlap the lower ones, although somewhat posteriorly. There may be a slight overlap of the maxillary premolars over the mandibular, while the upper molars become more buccally situated. Generally, with some exceptions, each tooth meets two teeth in the other arch while the buccal cusps only of the lower premolars and molars contact the surfaces, not the cusps, of the occluding opposite teeth. It is of some importance to consider tooth position and arch relationship in light of

1

2

3

4

5

6

7

18

17

16

15

14

13

12

11

10

9

8

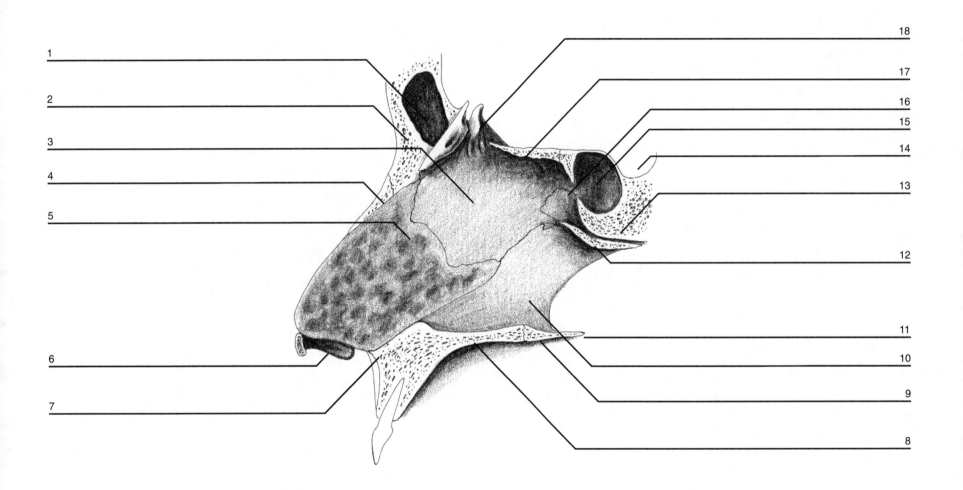

Figure 2.10   Nasal Septum

Table 2.1. Deciduous Teeth[a]

	Molars	Canines	Incisors	Midline ↓	Incisors	Canines	Molars
Maxilla	2	1	2		2	1	2
Mandible	2	1	2		2	1	2

[a] Total, 20.

the maxilla and the mandible bones and their alveolar processes.

Clinical Note

The teeth are vocal-tract articulators. Malocclusion, missing teeth, malplaced teeth, and other dental problems can occasionally relate to speech problems. The young child shedding his or her deciduous teeth, the teenager undergoing orthodontic treatment, and the older adult losing teeth (and gaining dentures) can all experience related speech disorders.

SUMMARY

The skull consists of two divisions, the cranium and the facial skeleton. Both contribute significantly to the vocal tract, in different ways. The cranium contributes to a portion of the upper vocal tract, particularly the nasal passages and the nasopharynx, and provides important anatomic landmarks for muscle and other tissue attachments. The other role of the cranium is to house the brain portion of the central nervous system.

The facial skeleton, besides its obvious role in forming the facial features, also forms part of the vocal tract, including the mouth and aspects of the nasal passages. It provides for changes in the vocal tract (i.e., the mouth opens and closes), with the important temporomandibular joint allowing for depression and elevation of the mandible bone. The facial skeleton also

contributes numerous important landmarks that will serve as muscle and other attachments, as well as having sensory surfaces for various monitoring purposes.

The maxilla and mandible bones also house the dentition. Biting, chewing, and grinding are aspects of mastication. The teeth, whether deciduous or permanent, assist in the formation of speech sounds.

Clinical Implications

As noted at the outset, the text begins with this chapter on the skull and bones. This is to assist the student in introduction to terminology, in preparing the student for anatomic conditions such as processes and sutures, to identify important bone structures sometimes associated with abnormalities, and lastly to locate bony landmarks for muscle attachments, among other reasons.

The cranial bones attract immediate interest because of their association with the brain within. Brain lobes derive their names from the bones encasing them; thus, the *frontal* lobe, the *parietal* lobe, the *occipital* lobe, and the *temporal* lobe. The adjectives for each of these lobes must be remembered because of the important brain functions generally subsumed: frontal is associated with (among other functions) initiation of nerve impulses leading to speech muscle activity; parietal causes one to consider body sensations such as pain, pressure, and touch; occipital should call to mind vision; and, of considerable importance to speech and hearing students, temporal conjures up the sensation of audition.

Table 2.2 Permanent Teeth[a]

	Molars	Pre-molars	Canines	Incisors	Midline	Incisors	Canines	Pre-molars	Molars
Maxilla	3	2	1	2		2	1	2	3
Mandible	3	2	1	2		2	1	2	3

[a]Total, 32.

The facial skeleton has more functions than those associated with facial appearance! One can consider it as forming two major entranceways for food and air: the mouth and nose. It also contributes no small portion of the housing for the eye orbits. Considering the airway, the pathway through the nose causes the air to be warmed, moistened, and filtered before it passes into the lower unprotected respiratory system. On the other hand, food is acquired, sliced, broken, pulverized by the teeth. Mastication is an important initial step in the ingestion of nutrients. The oral cavity, formed by the facial bones in part, also serves as the region for the first steps in deglutition (swallowing). And, of course, these bones forming both the nasal and oral chambers provide ample mechanisms for the production of speech.

There is deliberate limitation of discussion of the temporal bone as it relates to hearing. It is such a major and important aspect of human communication that a separate chapter (Chapter 7) is reserved for delving deeply into it. It is of interest, however, that there are several processes and landmarks of the temporal bone of importance to speech production. We will attach muscles to the styloid process, the mastoid process, the zygomatic process, the temporal fossa, and so on. The sphenoid bone, too, will demand attention because of its pterygoid processes. We will find that landmarks of the maxilla and mandible bones serve as origins for the muscles of facial expression. We will also see the maxilla bone makes a major contribution to the palate, the roof of the mouth, which is critical to good speech.

Study Questions

1. *Identify, by locating the bones participating, at least two synarthroses in the skull.*

2. *What bone might be called the <u>auditory bone</u> because of its extremely important role in hearing?*

3. *Identify the bones that form the bony palate, noting the specific portions and what fractions of the bony palate they form. Note their specific processes.*

4. *Consider the movements of the mandible around the temporal bone and how opening and closing the mouth relates to that movement. Move your own mandible in its various manners and visualize the activity of the temporomandibular joint while doing so.*

5. *What type of joint is the temporomandibular joint? List its characteristics.*

6. *If a child is shedding some teeth and erupting others (mixed dentition) about what age should s/he be? Explain.*

7. *What is the difference between the anterior and posterior nares? Between the anterior and posterior nasal spines?*

8. *How do sinuses drain into the nose? Identify the sinuses.*

9. *Locate the spheno-occipital angle (where the two bones unite) in relationship to the nasopharynx portion of the vocal tract.*

10. *Which anatomic spaces in the head have been identified to this point? Are they all part of the vocal tract?*

Chapter 3
Oral Cavity

GENERAL INTRODUCTION

The vocal tract, that series of interconnected and varying cavities associated with the speaking act, begins with the oral cavity. Its vital functions are several, but the main one is the ingestion of food. It can also act as a passageway for air to the respiratory tract.

In humans and other mammals, the mouth is used by infants in sucking. More mature humans use the mouth to masticate ingested food in preparation for digestion. The mouth is capable of thrusting the pulverized, masticated bolus of food into the pharynx to start the next phase of swallowing. In speaking, the oral cavity acts as a continuously variable volume for modifying the tone produced at the larynx in vowel production and as an obstructable chamber through which exhaled air is directed to create some consonants. Both acoustic events have linguistic significance. These two types of speech-sounds, vowels and consonants, plus combinations of them, form most of the speech-sounds of languages. Other chambers, specifically the nose and pharynx, also may serve as sites of origin for speech-sounds.

Clincal Note

The vital functions of the mouth are studied by speech clinicians trying to understand the physiology of the speech system. An early philosophy, considered too limited today, viewed the speaking act as a function overlaid on the vital functions. From that point of view developed schools of therapy and of remediation based upon those vital functions. Approaches oriented toward chewing, sucking, and swallowing have long been used to alleviate certain speech problems by some specialists.

GENERAL DESCRIPTION OF THE ORAL CAVITY

The mouth has two spaces. The outermost space is generally a potential space, meaning that it is not always filled with air but may actually be collapsed or otherwise not easily available to air. This outermost space is the *vestibule,* or the *buccal (cheek) cavity.* The other, with larger volume, is the *oral cavity proper.*

The vestibule's lateral, or external, boundary is the *cheek.* This muscular sheet lined with mucous membrane is the outer and movable covering of the vestibule. Anteriorly, the vestibule is bounded by the *lips* and the mouth opening *(rima oris).* The *upper* and *lower lips* have thick muscle bundles within and are covered by mucous membrane internally and by integument (skin) externally, with a thin, blood-filled, and sensitive intermediary type of tissue bounding the rima itself, the vermilion border. Medially, or internally, the vestibule is bounded by the alveolar ridge and its covering gums *(gingiva)* and the exposed buccal surfaces of the teeth. Sometimes, an upper region of the vestibule is identified as the *fornix.* The fornix might be interrupted medially and laterally with thin flaps of mucous membrane interconnecting the lip and alveolar mucosa, the *labial frenula.* The vestibule may also be called the *(alveolabial) sulcus.*

The *oral cavity proper* is usually not a large air-filled chamber when the teeth are in occlusion, for the tongue nearly fills the cavity. The boundaries of the oral cavity proper start anteriorly with the mouth opening, between the upper and lower teeth, and with the teeth themselves. Their gingiva-covered alveolar processes (ridges) hold the teeth to form important anatomic landmarks, especially for speech purposes. In the upper, or maxillary, region the mucosa often has several irregular transverse folds, the *rugae,* or *plicae.* In the gingiva between the two central incisors will be found the *incisive papilla,* immediately anterior to the now-covered *incisive foramen* of the maxilla bone.

The *alveolar ridge* slopes up to the roof of the mouth, the *palate.* Its anterior two-thirds is the bony partition, described earlier, while its posterior portion is the *soft palate,* or *velum,* terminating in the finger-like *uvula* at the midline.

The oral cavity at the posterior midline joins with the pharynx behind via the *isthmus of fauces* (or just the *fauces*). This communicating doorway, then, is bounded above by the velum and uvula and laterally by two *faucial pillars* and the *palatine tonsils.* Of course, masticated food and sometimes air during breathing pass through this faucial isthmus into the pharynx and beyond.

The oral cavity proper is largely filled with the *tongue.* This large muscular structure covered with mucous membrane is attached inferiorly (the *root*) and is relatively free anteriorly, at its *apex.* The lateral margins, like the apex, are relatively free and highly mobile. The tongue is attached via muscles and other tissues to the palate, the epiglottis, the hyoid bone, the styloid process, and the mandible, among other structures. It is an extremely important structure for mastication, deglutition, and speech articulation, and

it provides a structure for gustatory (taste) and other sensations.

The movements of the mobile mouth structures that are important in speaking have certain parallels in the movements necessary in various life-supporting behaviors. The tongue can change its position in the mouth and alter its contour or shape to keep pieces of food between the occlusal surfaces of the teeth to be crushed and pulverized. The tongue also collects the pulverized food *bolus* and presses itself against the bony and soft palates sequentially dorsally to pressure the bolus posteriorly across the dorsum until the food is thrust into the pharynx from where the contractile pharyngeal muscles propel *(peristalsis)* the bolus onward.

The lips close against the possible exit of food during mastication and deglutition. The cheeks are made to press against the facial surfaces of the teeth so as to prevent food from falling into the vestibule. The sloping and pendulant soft palate moves actively during the oral swallowing phase. As the bolus of food travels dorsally over the upper tongue surface, the soft palate swings up and back, meeting the moving lateral and posterior pharyngeal walls effectively to close off the nasopharynx and nose. Thus, food and drink are kept from these chambers during eating.

During the speaking act, the tongue and velum execute extremely refined maneuvering. The tongue directs, or "nozzles," the stream of air; it also elevates or lowers to form a resonance chamber for vowel sound production. The soft palate and pharyngeal walls close off the nose and nasopharynx (most speech-sounds are nonnasal) and thus allow fine control to be maintained over the oral cavity at times and create air turbulence that may be part of speech-sound production. The mandible moves up and down to provide support for the tongue and to allow for oral opening and closing during speech-sound production.

These general functions of the structures of the mouth are made possible by contracting muscles. The muscles of the oral cavity and the vestibule are grouped for study purposes, but of course act in varying degrees of concert within and among groups to produce their effects. As individual muscles are studied and their functions described to depict a primary activity, it must be remembered that support and cooperation among all of the muscles of a region are needed to produce the desired result, the speech act.

LANDMARKS OF THE ORAL CAVITY

Before plunging into the detailed anatomic makeup of the oral cavity, one should have some concept of the chamber as if one were looking into it. Doing so should provide a basis for going on to study the bones and muscles found within. Although diagrams and pictures can be helpful, the interested student would be wise to find a willing subject, child or adult, or perhaps both, who might demonstrate the surface structures and spaces described in the following paragraphs.

We start at the facial surface and identify the mouth opening *(rima oris)* between the upper and lower lips. This opens into the *oral vestibule,* noted earlier. Most of the time this is a "potential" space, with the two lips resting against the teeth and alveolar ridge. Its pink mucous membrane lining is very similar to that elsewhere in the oral cavity, including that which covers the alveolar ridge. Note the other areas mentioned earlier, especially the fornix and the labial frenula. Then, depressing the mandible provides a wider opening into the oral cavity and with appropriate lighting, the landmarks therein can be seen.

Mucous membrane lines the oral cavity (see Fig. 1.2) as it does a good deal of the digestive and respiratory tracts. The *palatal rugae (plicae)* are folds of tissue running laterally across the anterior palate just posterior to the incisor teeth. They tend to smooth out with increasing age. On the gingiva (the mucous membrane covering the alveolar ridge) of the upper arch, lingually, will be found the *incisive papilla,* a small prominence of mucous membrane immediately behind the space be-

tween the two upper central incisor teeth. Posterior to that, perhaps as much as a centimeter, may be found evidence of the *incisive foramen* in the form of a slight depression in the mucosa of the palate. The *palatine raphe,* indicating midline adjoining of the two sides of the palate, sometimes can be seen extending posteriorly from the region of the incisive foramen.

The end of the bony palate is sometimes seen in faint outline beneath the mucous membrane. Behind that, in the *soft palate,* an occasional functional dimple occurs during *velopharyngeal closure;* this near-midline indentation, slightly behind the posterior border of the hard palate, is an indication of the insertion of the levator (veli) palatine muscle. The palatine raphe sometimes continues faintly through the soft palate. At its terminus, the finger-like *uvula* is suspended into the *faucial isthmus;* the uvula is an extremely variable structure, being sometimes long and thin like a pencil, sometimes very short and stout, and even sometimes unobservable.

The faucial isthmus is a space, an entryway, between the oral cavity and the pharynx. It has several landmarks: the uvula and posterior velar border superiorly, the two pillars and tonsillar landmarks laterally, and the dorsum of the tongue inferiorly.

The *anterior pillar of the fauces* is a vertically oriented ridge covered with mucous membrane; it runs in a slightly arc-like route from the posterior border of the velum and disappears posteriorly beneath the lateral borders of the tongue below. This pillar, of course, is the external evidence of the palatoglossus (glossopalatine) muscle and should show some medial movement during contraction. In the adult, on the backside of this pillar is a depression, the *tonsillar fossa;* in childhood, this fissa houses the *palatine tonsil,* a part of the ring of lymphoid tissue *(Waldeyer's ring)* surrounding the oral and nasal entryways into the body. On the back side of this fossa will be seen the *posterior pillar of the fauces,* which derives from the posterior border of the soft palate and then curves outward and downward and disappears behind the pharyngeal portion of the tongue in the lateral pharyngeal walls. This pillar houses the palatopharyngeal (pharyngopalatine) muscle and can be seen to move medially during contraction.

The *tongue* is the major structure within the oral cavity. It has a somewhat narrow apex oriented toward the mouth opening. Its superior surface, the *dorsum,* is covered with mucous membrane; this membrane is highly specialized, serving as a container for the several kinds of *papillae* that cover its surface. Papillae house *gustatory end organs,* serving the various sensations of taste. The dorsum often demonstrates an anteroposterior depression called the *sulcus,* possibly an external sign of an internal *lingual septum;* the latter is a midline structure of fibrous tissue that sometimes serves as a muscle attachment, especially for intrinsic muscles. The tongue widens posteriorly developing into the lateral borders, or margins, sometimes quite mobile and free. The undersurface of the apex, still covered with mucous membrane, may show the *lingual frenum* (or *frenulum*) as a thin film of membrane vertically oriented at midline and connecting the apex to the floor of the mouth.

Posteriorly, the dorsum of the tongue abruptly changes its plane, descending nearly vertically to form a wall, the *pharyngeal portion* of the tongue. As the dorsum becomes pharyngeal portion, there appear a half-dozen or more *vallate papillae,* fairly prominent circular structures arranged in a V across the back of the tongue. Beneath the point of the V, dorsally, may be seen the depression for the *foramen cecum,* an indicator of a vestigial duct. In this pharyngeal portion of the tongue may also be seen the *lingual tonsils,* a scattering of lymphoid pads across the back of the tongue that are further partners in Waldeyer's ring of lymphoid tissue. At the midline of the pharyngeal portion, a fold of mucous membrane is elevated to join the middle of the rising *epiglottis.* On either side of this *glossoepiglottic membrane* will be found the moderate depression, the *valleculae* (also known as the *pill pockets*) that serve to collect liquids before they pass down the pharynx via the pyriform sinuses. There is also a lateral glossoepiglottic membrane that is sometimes lost in the array of pillars and tonsils laterally.

MUSCLES OF FACIAL EXPRESSION

There are 10 muscles of a larger number in the oronasal region that together form the muscles of facial expression (Fig. 3.1). Use of the term *facial expression* stems from the common anatomic practice of ascribing specific emotional appearances to the action of these muscles. However, such an approach is not useful in discussing speech. This group of muscles is associated with the mouth. As such, they play a role in such biological functions as maintaining closure (fixing the oral aperture), retaining the food bolus, as well as speech. They differ from most other muscles in that they may have their origins on bones, but their insertions are often in soft tissues, such as skin or other muscles.

The paired muscles of facial expression are the levator labii superior, levator anguli oris, zygomatic, risorius, depressor anguli oris, depressor labii inferior, mental, orbicularis oris, buccinator, and platysma. All receive their innervation from the *facial nerve (Cranial VII).* Table 3.1 provides pertinent facts about this group of muscles.

Clinical Note

In certain pathologies in which the speech clinician plays a rehabilitative role, the muscles (all or part, bilateral or unilateral) are direct effectors of a speech disorder. For example, certain neurologic disorders (palsies, Parkinson's disease, and others) are characterized by facial paralysis. The muscles cannot make the fine movements required for the articulation of many speech-sounds. As a result, speech is often slurred, imprecise, or even unintelligible. When the lips cannot be moved, the speech disorder is obvious and disturbing.

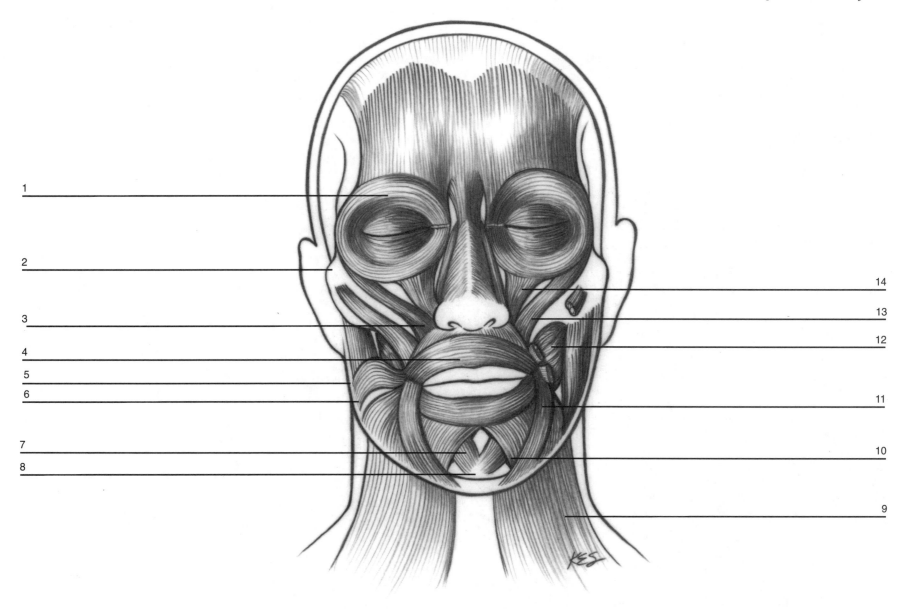

Figure 3.1 Muscles of Facial Expression

Table 3.1. Muscles of Facial Expression

Muscle	Origin	Insertion	Action	Nerve
Levator labii superior	Frontal process of maxilla bone; lower margin of orbit; zygomatic bone	Upper lip at midline	Elevates portion of upper lip	Cranial VII
Levator anguli oris	Canine fossa of maxilla bone	Angle of mouth, upper lip	Elevates portion of upper lip	Cranial VII
Zygomatic	Zygomatic bone	Angle of mouth, upper lip	Draws corner of mouth up and back	Cranial VII
Risorius	Fascia over masseter muscle	Skin at angle of mouth	Retracts corner of mouth	Cranial VII
Depressor anguli oris	Oblique line of mandible bone	Angle of mouth, lower lip	Depresses corner of mouth	Cranial VII
Depressor labii inferior	Oblique line of mandible bone	Lower lip between angle and midline	Depresses lower lip	Cranial VII
Mental	Mandible alongside symphysis	Integument of chin	Protrudes lower lip, wrinkles chin	Cranial VII
Orbicularis oris	(A sphincteric muscle, deriving from others of the area, with no definite origins or insertions.)		Closes mouth, puckers lips	Cranial VII
Buccinator	Alveolar processes of maxilla and mandible bones, pterygomandibular raphe	Angle of mouth, mingling with fibers of muscles forming upper and lower lips	Flattens cheek	Cranial VII
Platysma	Thoracic fascia over pectoralis major, deltoid, and trapezius muscles	Mental protuberance of mandible, skin of cheek, corner of mouth	Depresses mandible and corner of mouth, wrinkles skin of neck and chin	Cranial VII

The *levator labii superior muscle* (also known as the *quadratus labii superior muscle*) is the most median of the superior lip muscles in its origin. It has three heads, which some anatomists label as entirely separate muscles. The origin of these heads is, in general, from the side of the bony nose, which is made up of the frontal process of the maxilla bone, the lower margin of the orbit, and the zygomatic bone. The three muscle bundles run inferiorly to insert into the upper lip close to its midline and along its upper boundary. The levator labii superior participates in elevation of the lateral half of the upper lip.

The *levator anguli oris muscle* (also called the *canine muscle*) has its origin in the canine fossa just below the infraorbital foramen of the maxilla. Its fibers descend into the angle of the mouth in a nearly vertical direction, so that when it contracts it elevates the lateral portion of the upper lip.

The *zygomatic (major) muscle* begins at the zygomatic bone, lateral to the origin of the levator anguli oris, with its fibers descending rather obliquely into the upper lip at the angle, or corner, of the mouth. It draws the corner of the mouth up and backwards. There is often a lesser slip of muscle, *zygomatic minor,* adjacent to the major.

The *risorius muscle* originates in the fascia (connective tissue) overlying the masseter muscle, still lateral to the muscles previously described. It runs nearly horizontally superficially to the platysma, into the skin at the angle of the mouth. Its action is to retract the angle of the mouth.

The *depressor anguli oris muscle* (also known as the *triangular muscle*) has its origin in the oblique line of the mandible, but somewhat lateral to the origin of the depressor labii inferior muscle. Its fibers radiate into the lower lip at the angle of the mouth, so that upon contraction it depresses the angle.

The *depressor labii inferior muscle* (sometimes called the *quadratus labii inferior muscle*) originates from the oblique line of the mandible, anteriorly. Its fibers pass medially and upward into the lower lip. Its action is to draw the lateral portion of the lower lip directly down.

The *mental muscle* is close to the midline of the mouth of the lower lip. Its origin is near the midline of the mandible, with its fibers coursing into the integument, or skin, of the chin. It acts to protrude the lower lip when the integument is fixed or to wrinkle the skin of the chin.

The *orbicularis oris muscle* is a complex muscle of the mouth area. It is essentially a layer of muscle fibers derived from the other muscles that are inserted into the lips; technically, it is said to have no origin or insertion. These muscle fibers continue on from their originating muscle, bypass the insertion location at which other fibers stop, and pass along the border of the lip. In this way a circular muscle is formed encompassing the periphery of the mouth. As a sphincter-like muscle, upon contraction it acts somewhat as a drawstring, closing the mouth and upon extreme contraction, pursing or puckering the lips. It is possible to view this muscle as paired—that is, as a *superior* and an *inferior orbicularis oris muscle* (not as left and right).

The *buccinator muscle* is the principle muscle of the cheek, the lateral wall of the vestibule. Its origin is in the outer surfaces of the posterior alveolar processes of the maxilla and mandible, as well as in the pterygomandibular raphe. The fibers pass forward in a con-

verging fashion to insert or blend with the deeper stratum (layer) of the muscle fibers of the corresponding lip. Its action, then, is to compress the cheek, forcing air from the mouth. By performing this compression, it also acts as an accessory muscle of mastication, keeping the food from slipping out from between the teeth, while the tongue operates from within holding the food between the chewing surfaces of the teeth.

The *platysma muscle* is a variable muscle of facial expression. It is composed of thin scatterings of muscle bundles found along the sides of the neck from the upper thorax to the sides of the chin and mandible. It is a superficial muscle, originating in the coverings of the muscles of the thorax (the pectoralis major, deltoid, and trapezius muscles), with its fibers running obliquely upward and medially over the side of the neck and inserting into the protuberance of the mandible, the skin of the lower cheek, and the corner of the mouth (with the depressor labii inferior). The action of these muscle bundles is to wrinkle the skin of the neck and chin, to depress the corner of the mouth, and to assist in depressing the mandible in opening the mouth.

Clinical Note

Defects and differences in the muscles of facial expression occur in certain paralytic conditions, as well as in some congenital musculoskeletal deformities. A unilateral paralysis of the facial muscles leads to an easily observable facial asymmetry, often accompanied by a speech disorder as a form of dysarthria. Bilateral in effect is Parkinson's disease, which often attacks more than just the facial structures. The facial configuration of the upper lip region is often disturbed in congenital cleft lip, extending variously from the anterior nares to and through the vermilion border of the upper lip.

MUSCLES OF MASTICATION

The muscles of mastication (Fig. 3.2), also known as the *craniomandibular muscles,* are four in number and are paired. In general, they originate on the bones of the cranium and insert into the mandible. Their actions effect masticatory (chewing) movements, essentially vertical and horizontal (grinding) movements of the mandible against its opposite bone, the maxilla. The four pairs of muscles are the temporal, masseter, internal (medial) pterygoid, and external (lateral) pterygoid (Table 3.2). Each is supplied by the trigeminal nerve (Cranial V).

The *temporal muscle* has as its origin the whole of the temporal fossa of the temporal bone and its covering fascia. The muscle fibers radiate and converge downward, forming a tendon that passes internal (deep) to the zygomatic arch. This tendon inserts on the anterior borders of the coronoid process and the ramus of the mandible bone externally. The action of this muscle is to elevate and retract the mandible, which closes the mouth and brings together the lower and upper teeth.

The *masseter muscle* is a two-part muscle, having a superficial and a deep portion. These originate from the zygomatic arch. The fibers pass downward and insert into the lateral surface of the ramus and of the angle of the mandible. The action of the masseter muscle is to raise the mandible (close to the mouth) against the maxilla bone in mastication.

The *internal (medial) pterygoid muscle* has its origin at the lateral pterygoid plate, with slips from the palatine bone and the tuberosity of the maxilla bone. Its fibers pass downward, laterally, and backward and insert in the ramus and angle of the medial surface of the mandible bone internally. This muscle elevates the mandible (closes the mouth) in chewing and speaking, as well as protruding the mandible during these and other activities.

The *external (lateral) pterygoid muscle* arises by two heads. One comes from the infratemporal fossa of the great wing of the sphenoid bone and the other from the lateral surface of the lateral pterygoid plate of the sphenoid bone. They run horizontally and insert into the neck of the condyle of the mandible bone and the articular disc. The action of this muscle is to depress the mandible (opening the mouth), to protrude the mandible, and when operating unilaterally, to assist in lateral movement (grinding) of the mandible.

As a group, the muscles of mastication function to slice, bite, grind, and chew food. Closing the mouth is accomplished by the temporal, masseter, and internal pterygoid muscles working together. Biting is performed mainly by the masseter and internal pterygoid muscles, whereas chewing requires all three. Opening the mouth is accomplished by gravity (and contribution of the platysma muscle) and by the contraction of the external pterygoid muscle, through its forward pull on the condyle moving the mandible about an axis located at the angle. Other muscles, especially the suprahyoid group, also contribute to depression of the mandible bone and thus to the opening of the mouth.

Clinical Note

Weakness, paralysis or injury of these muscles initially will produce a disorder of mastication, of course, but one could expect accompanying speech disturbances. In some cases, a dysarthria may result, evidenced by more or less severe articulatory and resonance disturbances. Fairly good mouth closure (via jaw, lips, and tongue maneuvers) must be available to produce many speech-sounds (e.g., the plosives and some of the fricatives), and the size and shape of the oral cavity is one of the prime determinants of vowel resonance. A unilateral paralysis of the muscles of mastication might cause protrusional deviation of the mandible rather than a smooth up-and-down movement of the mandible paralleling the midline.

Table 3.2 Muscles of Mastication

Muscle	Origin	Insertion	Action	Nerve
Temporal	Temporal fossa and its covering fascia	Anterior borders of mandibular ramus and coronoid process	Raises and retracts mandible	Cranial V (mandibular division)
Masseter	Zygomatic arch	Lateral surface of angle and ramus	Raises mandible against maxilla	Cranial V (mandibular division)
Internal (medial) pterygoid	Lateral pterygoid plate, palatine bone, maxillary tuberosity	Ramus and angle of medial surface of mandible	Raises and protrudes mandible	Cranial V (mandibular division)
External (lateral) pterygoid	Upper head arises from infratemporal fossa and great wing of sphenoid bone; lower head arises from lateral aspect of lateral pterygoid plate of sphenoid bone	Mandibular condyle and articular disc	Depresses mandible, draws mandible forward and sideways	Cranial V (mandibular division)

MUSCLES OF THE SOFT PALATE

The *soft palate,* or *velum,* is a soft-tissue extension of the hard (bony) palate. It is a musculomembranous shelf that is mobile in several planes, thus providing for changes in the volume and shape of two cavities (the nose and mouth), as well as being a major contributor to the action separating the nasal from the oral pharynx. This action is called *velopharyngeal* or *palatopharyngeal closure* and is very important in swallowing and in speaking.

The soft palate is mainly composed of various muscles (Fig. 3.3) entering the palate from structures in the immediately surrounding vicinity. Because of the various origins—some superior, some inferior, and some posterior—it is possible for the velum to be moved in a cephalad, caudad, dorsad direction, or a combination of these. Five muscles make up the major part of the soft palate, with a sixth muscle importantly contributing when present from its pharyngeal muscle beginnings. The five muscles that are primarily soft palate muscles are the levator (veli) palatine, tensor (veli) palatine, uvula, glossopalatine, and pharyngopalatine (Table 3.3).

The *levator (veli) palatine muscle* derives its name from its action upon the velum. It has its origin from the petrous part of the temporal bone. A second attachment is sometimes said to come from the pharyngeal end of the auditory tube cartilage. The muscle fibers then pass downward and medially and insert into the midline of the velum, the *palatal raphe* (or *aponeurosis*). Some of the fibers do cross the midline to blend with the fibers of the opposite muscle. The levator palatine muscle contracts to raise the velum toward the posterior wall, to narrow the pharyngeal isthmus in velopharyngeal closure, and possibly to widen (dilate) the orifice of the auditory tube to ventilate the middle ear. The nerve supply to this muscle comes from the pharyngeal plexus, a network of nerve branches of several cranial nerves, but here primarily the *vagus nerve (Cranial X).*

The *tensor (veli) palatine muscle,* also named for its apparent effect on the soft palate, has been described as having a twofold origin: at the medial pterygoid plate and the lateral walls of the auditory tube. It is possible, however, that a more accurate description would yield origins at the medial pterygoid plate and the scaphoid fossa. The fibers from the superior origins pass forward and downward, continue as a tendon around the ha-

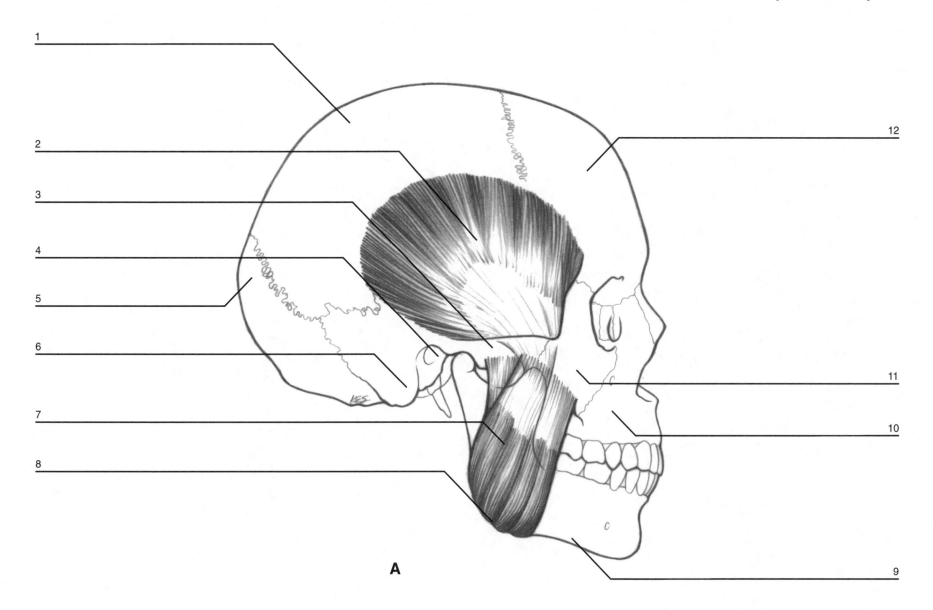

Figure 3.2A Muscles of Mastication: Masseter and Temporal Muscles

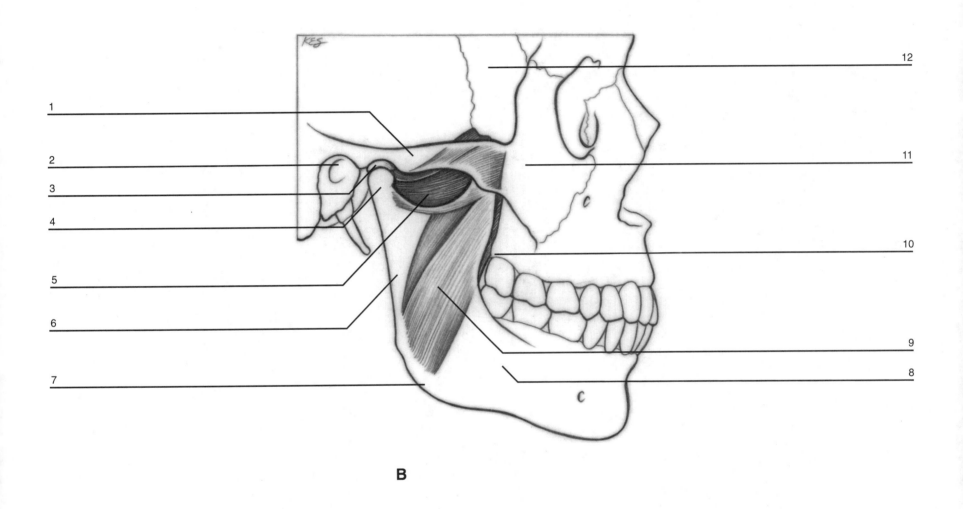

Figure 3.2B   Muscles of Mastication: Internal and External Pterygoid Muscles

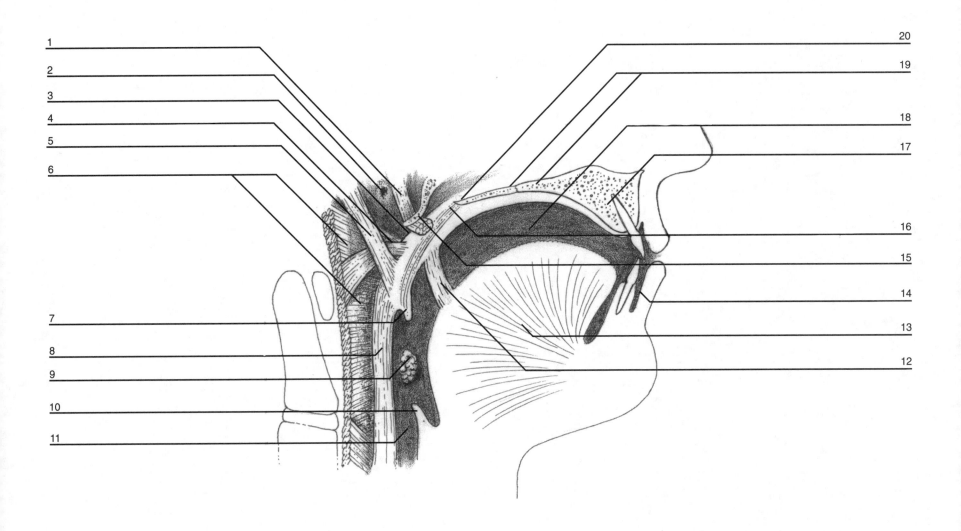

1

2

3

4

5

6

7

8

9

10

11

20

19

18

17

16

15

14

13

12

Figure 3.3 Muscles of the Soft Palate

Table 3.3. Muscles of the Soft Palate

Muscle	Origin	Insertion	Action	Nerve
Levator (veli) palatine	Apex of petrous portion of temporal bone, auditory tube	Palatal raphe	Raises soft palate to meet posterior pharyngeal wall	Cranial X (pharyngeal plexus)
Tensor (veli) palatine	Scaphoid fossa, medial pterygoid plate, posterior border of hard palate	Palatal raphe, auditory tube	Tenses soft palate, opens auditory tube during swallowing	Cranial V (mandibular division)
Uvula	Posterior nasal spine, palatal raphe	Mucous membrane of uvula	Raises and shortens uvula	Cranial X (pharyngeal plexus)
Glossopalatine (palatoglossus)	Merges with transversus and superficial muscles of side and undersurface of tongue	Palatal raphe	Raises posterior portion of tongue, constricts isthmus of fauces, depresses side of palate	Cranial X (pharyngeal plexus)
Pharyngopalatine (palatopharyngeal)	Posterior thyroid cartilage; pharyngeal walls	Palatal raphe	Depresses soft palate, aids in elevating larynx and pharynx, constricts faucial isthmus	Cranial X (pharyngeal plexus)

mulus, and then enter the velum to terminate at its raphe, much as the levator muscle does. The action of the tensor palatine muscle is said to make the velum taut (in swallowing). The nerve supply comes from the mandibular division of the trigeminal nerve (Cranial V).

A muscle in this region that has been somewhat ignored is the *dilator tubae muscle* (Fig. 3.4). It is not strictly a palatal muscle, but serves to dilate the auditory tube. Its origin is at the hamular process (hamulus), and it passes as a thin layer of muscle up to and along the edge (anterior crus) of the cartilaginous auditory tube. Its function is to draw anteriorly the cartilage, thus dilating (opening) the tube to ventilation and

drainage of the middle ear. Earlier, this function was attributed to the tensor (veli) palatine muscle, but it is now thought to be exclusively in this little known muscle. Its nerve supply is the same as that for tensor palatine, i.e., Cranial V.

The *uvula ("little grape") muscle* consists of paired bands of muscle fibers passing dorsally through the soft palate. Their origins are alongside the posterior nasal spine and at the palatal raphe anteriorly. The two muscle bundles pass as narrow strips of muscle fibers along each side of the midline until they terminate in, or insert into, the uvula itself. It is believed that this free-swinging, pendulous structure is vestigial and serves no important function in the human. Usually it swings upward and backward upon contraction. The uvula muscle has its nerve supply from the pharyngeal plexus (from the vagus nerve).

The *glossopalatine (palatoglossus) muscle* passes from the tongue to the palate along the sides of the oral cavity, making a large bundle called the *anterior pillar of the fauces* (also termed *glossopalatine pillar* or *arch*). Its origin is in the superficial layer of muscles of the side and undersurface of the tongue and from the transverse muscle of that structure. The fibers pass from the side of the tongue in the bundle mentioned, beneath the mucous membrane of the mouth, and up toward the velum. They enter the side of the velum and finally insert into the palatal raphe, again with some fibers crossing the midline to blend with fibers of the opposite muscle. Upon contraction, this muscle draws down the sides of the soft palate or draws up and back the sides of the tongue, depending upon which end of the muscle is the more fixed end. Thus, it can be identified as a velum depressor or as a tongue elevator and can be associated with either structure. The nerve supply comes, as in the case of the levator and uvula muscles, from the pharyngeal plexus (Cranial X).

The *pharyngopalatine (palatopharyngeal) muscle* is similar to the glossopalatine muscle in that it has an attachment inferior to the velum and forms a noticeable bundle beneath the mucous membrane lining of the oropharynx. Its origin is considered to be the posterior border of the thyroid cartilage near the base of the superior cornu and a broad expansion of the fibrous layer of the pharynx at its lowest part. The fibers pass up the lower part of the pharynx, along with the stylopharyngeal muscle, until they form the *posterior pillar of the fauces* (also termed *pharyngopalatine pillar* or *arch*). From here the bundle divides into two fasciculi, a lower one and an upper one. The lower band of muscle fibers follows the posterior curve of the soft palate; the upper one enters the palate directly. Both insert into the midline of the soft palate at the palatal raphe. This muscle acts to constrict the pharyngeal isthmus, to depress the soft palate, or to elevate the pharynx and larynx in swallowing. It, too, is supplied by the pharyngeal plexus of the vagus nerve.

The sixth muscle, the *velopharyngeal sphincter muscle,* is a palatal muscle, but because of its intimate relationship to a pharyngeal muscle (the superior pharyngeal constrictor), it is described later with the pharynx.

The muscles of the soft palate do move the soft palate. Also, under certain conditions they move other structures to which they are attached. Thus, the origins and insertions suggested are to some extent arbitrary. In the soft palate, the coordinated manner in which muscles and muscle groups must operate can be observed. The soft palate is complex and varies somewhat among individuals in both structure and function.

Clinical Note

Knowledge of the palatal muscles is basic to therapeutic procedures applied to a number of disorders. In many cases of dysarthria, of resonance problems, and of cleft palate, it is important to evaluate the position and the functioning of these muscles individually and as a group. For example, the postsurgical cleft palate that demonstrates disorders might well do so because of the malplacement of muscles congenitally or because of surgical disturbances. In other cases, muscles may be paralyzed, injured, or disturbed in such ways as to require special attention, both in evaluation and in therapy. Here, defects in muscles of the soft palate are emphasized, but some of the disorders observed in cases of cleft palate stem from causes other than abnormalities of the muscles, such as defects in supporting or other tissues in the vicinity.

MUSCLES OF THE TONGUE

In structure, the tongue is almost entirely muscular (Fig. 3.5). Four muscle pairs make up the majority

1

2

3

4

5

6

7

8

9

13

12

11

10

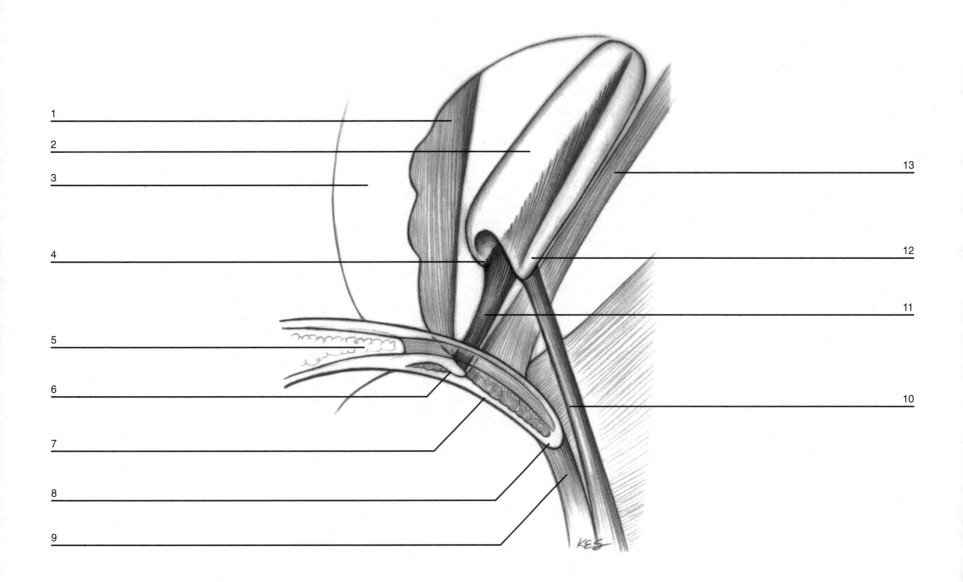

Figure 3.4   Auditory Tube-Related Muscles and Structures

1

2

3

4

5

6

7

8

14

13

12

11

10

9

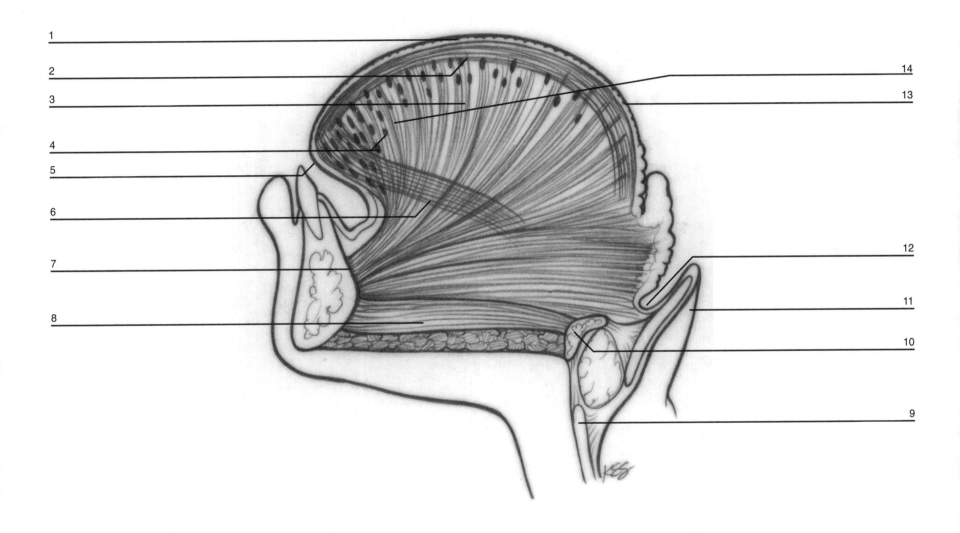

Figure 3.5A   Tongue Muscles: Intrinsic (Lateral View)

1

2

3

4

5

10

9

8

7

6

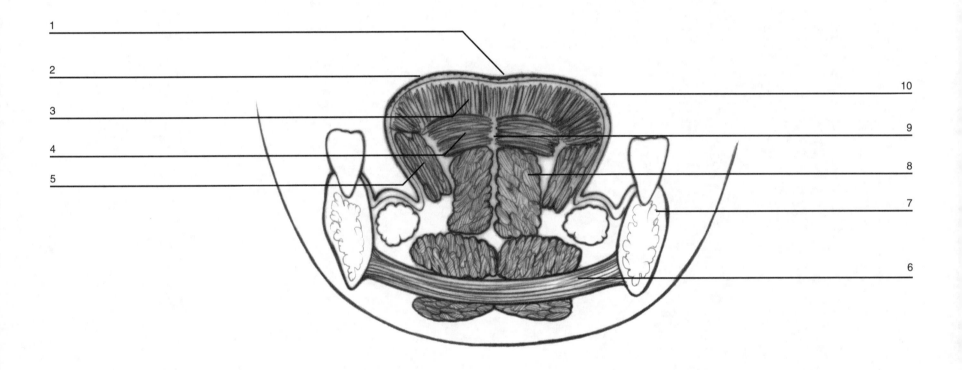

Figure 3.5B   Tongue Muscles: Intrinsic (Coronal View)

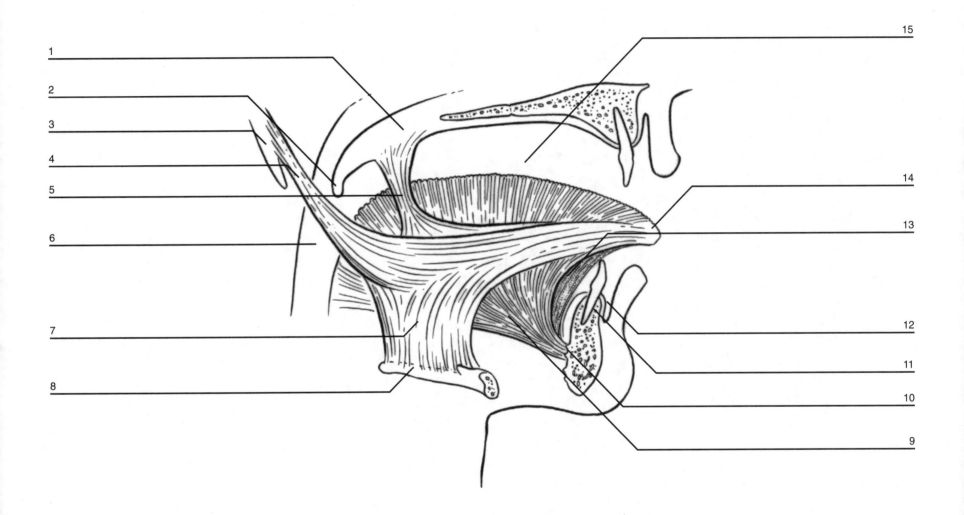

Figure 3.5C   Tongue Muscles: Extrinsic (Sagittal View)

of the intrinsic muscle group. Four other pairs, that come from adjacent skeletal areas, make up the extrinsic group of muscles. An overgeneralization but somewhat of a guide, is the notion that the intrinsic muscles provide for changes in the shape or contour of the tongue, while the extrinsic muscles are largely responsible for changes in its position within the oral cavity (Fig. 3.6). In most activities involving the tongue, the two muscle groups function together cooperatively.

Clinical Note

Defects of either or both groups of tongue muscles may cause speech disorders. The tongue muscles can be limited by paralyses or injuries, and they may malfunction from congenital or hereditary influences. In paralysis, for example, if the innervation to the intrinsic muscles were disturbed (not very likely to happen as an isolated event, however). it would become very difficult for the tongue to assume the contour required to produce certain speech-sounds. As an example, the [s] sound requires a very fine control of the tongue to produce a narrow groove through which the turbulent air stream passes to strike the central incisor teeth. Again, the extrinsic muscles could be related to speech-articulation disorders, due to interruption in the nerve supply; resonance changes in the voice might result because of the tongue's important role in changing the size and shape of the resonating cavities. The two problems could be combined (e.g., a nerve injury could limit muscle activity), so that resonance problems in the form of vowel disorders and problems with consonant sound production might both be present. Such neuromuscular problems might be bilateral, attacking both sides of the tongue, or unilateral. In the latter case, tongue movement would occur, but in such activities as protruding the apex there would be an obvious deviation toward the side of the weakened muscles. This also could interfere with speech production.

Intrinsic Muscles

The paired intrinsic muscles of the tongue are named according to their orientation within the tongue. Thus, there are the vertical, the transverse, the inferior longitudinal, and the superior longitudinal muscles (Table 3.4; Fig. 3.5, *A* and *B*). These are largely separate, sparse accumulations of muscle fibers, with some parts of each being composed of fibers entering the tongue from certain of the extrinsic muscles. This arrangement provides for a firm yet flexible coordination between the shape and the position of the tongue.

The *vertical lingual muscle* is found at the borders of the tongue, near the apex. It runs from the upper surface to the undersurface of the structure, interlacing its fibers with those of the other muscles. The fibers of the *transverse lingual muscle* pass horizontally laterally between the two longitudinal muscles. The origin of this muscle is considered to be the lingual septum, and its insertion is the mucosa of the dorsum and the lateral margins, or borders, of the tongue.

The *inferior longitudinal lingual muscle* is a narrow band of fibers on the undersurface of the tongue between the genioglossus and hyoglossus muscles, running from the hyoid bone and the muscles below the tongue to insert into the lingual apex. The fibers at the apex blend with the styloglossus muscle, and the posterior fibers may pass inferiorly to attach to the hyoid bone. The *superior longitudinal lingual muscle* is a thin layer of superficial fibers running from the pharyngeal portion to the apex of the tongue beneath the mucosa. These muscle fibers arise (originate) near the epiglottis and insert along the sides of the tongue as they pass anteriorly.

The actions of these four muscles, when artificially viewed separately, can be described in a simplistic manner. The vertical muscle flattens and broadens the tongue. The transverse muscle narrows and elongates the tongue and elevates its lateral borders. The inferior longitudinal muscle shortens the tongue, turns down

Table 3.4. Intrinsic Muscles of the Tongue

Muscle	Origin	Insertion	Action	Nerve
Vertical	Borders of tongue near tip edges	Inferior surface of tongue	Widens and flattens tongue tip	Cranial XII
Transverse	Lingual septum	Mucosa at sides of tongue	Elongates, narrows, and thickens tongue; lifts sides	Cranial XII
Inferior longitudinal	Hyoid bone; internal portion of tongue	Apex of tongue	Creates convex dorsum, depresses tip	Cranial XII
Superior longitudinal	Pharyngeal portion near epiglottis	Sides and apex of tongue	Shortens tongue, raises tongue tip and edges, forms concave dorsum	Cranial XII

the tip, and makes a convex dorsum. The superior longitudinal muscle shortens the tongue and turns up the apex and sides to form a concave dorsum.

All four of these intrinsic muscles, as in the case of the extrinsic group, receive their nerve supply from *Cranial XII*, called the *hypoglossal nerve* because it approaches the musculature of the tongue from beneath it.

Extrinsic Muscles

The extrinsic muscles of the tongue are responsible for the movement of the tongue from place to place within the oral cavity. They function together with the intrinsic muscles and with others. The extrinsic tongue muscles are attached to the skull and to the hyoid bone and effect positional changes necessary for biological and speech functions (Table 3.5).

There are three extrinsic tongue muscles. An important fourth muscle acting to change the position of the tongue is the glossopalatine (palatoglossus) muscle, described earlier as a muscle of the soft palate. It should be considered as a muscle of both the tongue and the velum. The three primary extrinsic muscles of the tongue are the styloglossus, the genioglossus, and the hyoglossus muscles.

The *styloglossus muscle* runs from the styloid process of the temporal bone obliquely forward and downward, and somewhat medially, to the lateral border of the tongue. Here it divides into a longitudinal and an oblique portion. The longitudinal portion enters the side of the tongue and runs to the apex along the lateral border, blending with the fibers of the inferior longitudinal muscle, and inserting its fibers into the mucosa of the sides along the length of the structure. The smaller, oblique portion of the styloglossus muscle enters the tongue transversely in a number of small muscle bundles that penetrate the hyoglossus muscle and finally reach the midline of the tongue internally. Here they decussate (cross) and terminate with their fellow tongue-muscle fibers from the opposite side. The styloglossus muscle retracts the tongue and draws its sides upward, thus raising both the posterior portion of the tongue and the hyoid bone below, because of the hyoid bone's other attachments to the tongue.

The *genioglossus muscle* forms a large part of the tongue. Its shape and position resemble a vertically oriented fan (Fig. 3.5, *A* to *C*). Its origin is near the midline of the lingual surface of the mandible bone, at the superior mental spine. This origin is immediately superior to that for the geniohyoid muscle of the suprahyoid muscle group, to be discussed in Chapter 5.

1

2

3

4

5

6

7

8

9

16

15

14

13

12

11

10

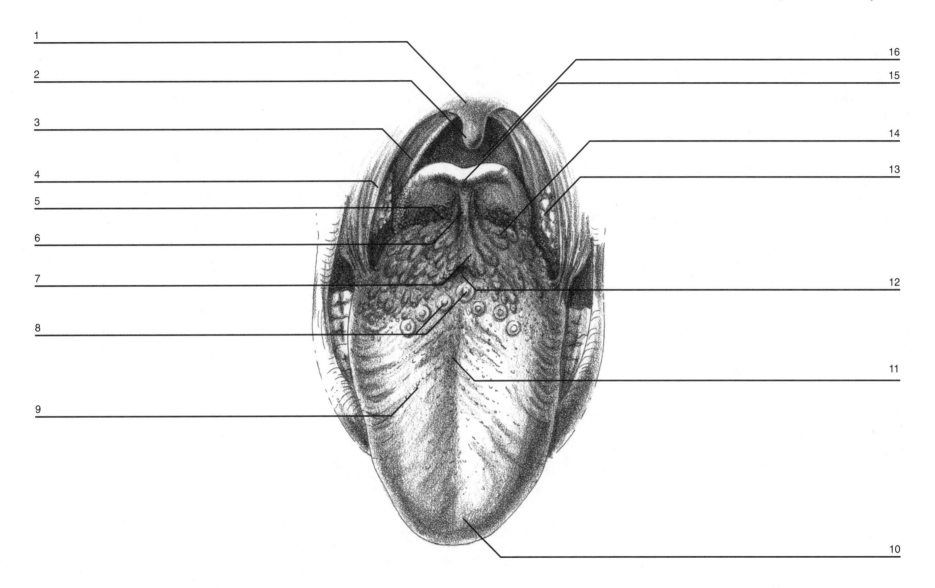

Figure 3.6   Oral Cavity (Anterior View)

Table 3.5. Extrinsic Muscles of the Tongue

Muscle	Origin	Insertion	Action	Nerve
Styloglossus	Styloid process of temporal bone	Lateral border of tongue	Elevates rear of tongue, retracts protruded tongue	Cranial XII
Genioglossus	Superior mental spine on lingual surface of mandible bone	Lingual fascia, dorsum of tongue, body of hyoid bone	Various fibers work to depress, retract, and protrude tongue	Cranial XII
Hyoglossus	Greater cornu of hyoid bone	Posterior half of side of tongue	Depresses and retracts tongue	Cranial XII
Glossopalatine	(See Table 3.3)			

Fibers of the genioglossus muscle fan out from this point along either side of the midline fibrous septum of the tongue. The most anterior fibers curve upward and forward to the apex of the tongue and insert into the lingual fascia. The middle fibers pass up and back and insert along the dorsum. The inferior fibers may curve back and downward to insert into the upper part of the body of the hyoid bone as well as into the posterior pharyngeal portion of the tongue.

The genioglossus muscle has a number of tasks to perform. The most anterior portion, running to the tip of the tongue, withdraws the tip into the mouth and depresses it. This portion, acting with the middle portion, also draws downward the entire superior surface of the tongue into a concave shape, producing a channel from front to back. This channel is used primarily for sucking purposes, but is also used in forming certain speech-sounds. The middle portion, if acting alone, draws forward the posterior portion of the tongue and thus causes the tip to protrude through the teeth, which is also important in speech (in the [TH] sounds). The inferior group of fibers acts upon the less fixed end, the hyoid bone, to elevate it and move it forward, an important activity in deglutition. The genioglossus muscle on one side causes the tongue apex to deviate to the opposite side, as when one moves the tongue tip to the corner of the mouth.

The *hyoglossus muscle* is a thin sheet extending from the upper borders of the greater cornu of the hyoid bone upward into the posterior half of the sides of the tongue. The fibers pass medially and interlace with intrinsic muscle fibers as they insert into the fibrous septum of the tongue. Penetrating the hyoglossus muscle are some of the oblique fibers of the styloglossus muscle. The hyoglossus muscle will act, when the hyoid bone is fixed, to depress the sides of the tongue and contribute to its retraction, as well as to return the tongue to its rest position following its elevation (as in swallowing).

All three of these muscles, plus the intrinsic group, are supplied by the hypoglossal nerve (Cranial XII).

Clinical Note

The use of the term *organ of speech* to refer to the tongue is indicative of popular, though distorted, ideas about the speaking act. Disorders of speech are many times thought to arise from defects of the tongue, a hypothesis not always supported by anatomic or physiologic evidence. For example, the lingual frenum, connecting the inferior surface of the tongue with the floor of the mouth, is often considered to be "too short" and is sometimes clipped, or cut. This shortened lingual frenum *(tongue-tie)* may be, but rarely is, the cause of a speech disorder. More serious speech problems that do arise from tongue deviations are those that stem from neurologic problems that give rise to paralyses or pareses of the tongue musculature. In such instances the clinician sees failures in such acts as tongue protrusion, deviations of the tongue from the midline, tremors, and the like. In some rare instances, either congenitally or arising from the other (e.g., hormonal) conditions, the clinician may see a tongue abnormal in size or shape. *Macroglossia* (enlarged tongue) is one such rare condition. The clinician considers the tongue size and shape in relationship to the space it occupies and to its behavior within that space in determining it to be an abnormality.

SURFACE LANDMARKS

It is of considerable importance to understand the skeletal support—the bones and cartilages that form the outlines of the cavities and spaces that create speech—for the vocal tract. It is equally important to have an accurate idea of the muscles that attach to various elements of the skeletal support, so as to better understand how the volumes and shapes of the various vocal tract cavities change. Lastly, because it is impossible to examine visually these bony and muscular components without special instruments, assessment must be done by studying the surfaces of the spaces and by noting changes in surface landmarks that accompany cavity changes and, ultimately, speech changes.

The surface landmarks of the facial region include some landmarks observable around the nasal cavities and those around the mouth. The interrelationship of nose and mouth becomes clear in closely observing normal faces and faces having important structural differences. Surface landmarks can be external and internal (extraoral and intraoral).

The External Nose

The external nose represents only a small portion of the internal cavities served by this entryway to the respiratory tract. The *bridge* of the nose, formed by the two nasal bones, is interposed between the bones of the skull surrounding the eye orbit and the cartilaginous skeleton of the nose. This midline ridge continues to the *tip* of the nose, usually a somewhat thin and relatively pointed termination. From this landmark flare out bilaterally the two *nasal alae*, arching down from the tip to attach to the skin of the face. These are supported by the alar cartilages, which maintain the patency of the *anterior nares*. In turn, the nares open to the *nasal vestibule* within.

Each naris is protected to some extent by the presence of hairs, especially in postadolescent individuals. The two nares are further separated by the single, midline *columella*. This is the skin-covered termination of the nasal septal cartilage internally. The columella is continuous above with the nasal tip and below with the integument of the upper lip. Internally, the two nasal passages (right and left) are completely separated by the *nasal septum*, which is cartilaginous anteriorly and bony posteriorly.

The Lips

The skin of the *upper lip* generally is like that of the remainder of the facial integument. The central region of this lip is formed embryologically from the prolabium, which fuses with the lateral regions to form the entire lip. In the center of this region, running vertically from the columella to the border of the lip, is the grooved indentation called the *philtrum*. Its lowermost end forms the midportion of the *cupid's bow*, the heart-shaped line at the midline of the upper lip.

At the lip border, the skin of both lips changes

its form into a reddish *vermilion.* This is an adapted continuation of the mucous membrane lining the mouth. The extremely sensitive vermilion is found on both lips, and is highly variable in its extent from individual to individual. It is more abundant at the midportion of the lips, and narrows considerably to the lateral boundaries, the angles of the mouth. From here, the cheeks extend bilaterally to cover the sides of the mouth within, with tissue folds indicating demarcation areas between muscle groups and tissue-type changes.

The Tongue and Oral Cavity

Surface landmarks of the oral cavity itself are generally encased in mucous membrane. The tongue's upper surface *(dorsum)* has a mucosal covering that contains multitudinous *papillae* of differing kinds (e.g., filiform and fungiform), some of which have taste buds associated. Posteriorly, as the tongue changes to a more vertical direction (the *pharyngeal portion*), are the 10 to 12 *circumvallate* papillae, all having taste buds. Just inferior to the point of the V formed by the line of papillae is the midline *foramen cecum,* a vestigial duct. The lingual *sulcus* runs anteriorly along the midline of the tongue dorsum.

The tongue appears to be somewhat ovoid, narrower at its *apex* or tip, which is relatively free for limited movement, as in curling the tongue. The undersurface of the lingual apex displays the midline lingual *frenum* (frenulum). This is a thin membrane from the floor of the mouth up to the midregion of the apex, but may in some few persons run as a rather thick membrane to the apex. It is possible for this membrane to tether the tongue tip, thus a *tongue-tie* (or *ankyloglossia*).

There are three bilateral salivary glands emptying into the oral cavity. The *parotid gland's* entrance is a small opening in the cheek wall just opposite the second molar tooth. The *submandibular gland* drains into the posterior region of the oral cavity, while the *sublingual gland* enters in the anterior portion.

Posterior to the tongue and attached to its pharyngeal portion is the epiglottis. The attachments are by three glossoepiglottic membranes. Between the tongue and epiglottis and contained by these membranes are the two *valleculae* (or pill pockets). Saliva produced in the oral cavity drains into these valleculae; from these, the fluids pass alongside the epiglottis via the *pyriform sinuses* to by-pass the entrance to the larynx into the esophagus below.

Other landmarks of the oral cavity include the alveolar process (ridge) containing the teeth. Covering this ridge is a form of mucous membrane; the gingiva. Mucosa covers the remainder of the oral surfaces in different forms. The palate has a relatively thick covering in its highly variable arching. Posteriorly, the arch continues laterally inferiorly in the *anterior pillar* and the *posterior pillar.* These guard the opening from oral cavity into oral pharynx, the *faucial isthmus.* Between the two pillars, at least in the prepubertal, child is the palatine tonsil.

Clinical Note

The surface landmarks of the body often indicate the nature of what lies inside. For example, scarring of the upper lip may well suggest an internal defect, such as a cleft palate. The muscles of one side of the face might well "sag" and demonstrate little movement in speech activities; inside the oral cavity a similar muscle weakness (or paralysis) might be found that would provide a better understanding of a speech disorder. On occasion, such surface evidence of disorder might well become the primary complaint of a patient, as in the case of one who feels a strong need to have his/her upper lip "made more normal," a largely cosmetic change perhaps, but one which must be acknowledged by rehabilitation specialists.

NEUROMUSCULAR CONSIDERATIONS

The many movements of the oral structures (and other structures of the body) are produced by muscles. Muscles contract when they are stimulated to do so by nerves. The following outline exemplifies the sequence of steps that compose such an action.

Action studied:	Opening the mouth.
Basis:	The individual wishes to open his/her mouth.
Step 1.	The cerebral cortex region in the brain, having been affected by the wish, issues the general command (in the form of nerve impulses) to open the mouth.
Step 2.	Other brain centers investigate whether it is a possible activity (e.g., if the mouth is free to be opened).
Step 3.	Parallel facilitating orders are sent (e.g., mouth-closing muscles, antagonistic to the wished-for opening movement, are ordered either to relax completely or to lessen their influence).
Step 4.	The order to open the mouth is sent to the muscular system via the primary nerve.
Step 5.	The nerve impulse reaches the muscle at the point of contact, the neuromuscular junction (or the motor end plate).
Step 6.	Individual muscle cells throughout the muscle are stimulated, and the muscle as a whole contracts.
Step 7.	The movable end (insertion) of the muscle is pulled toward the fixed end (origin), and the action is done.
The muscle:	External (lateral) pterygoid muscle, inserting into the condyloid process of the mandible bone and originating in the sphenoid bone. The nerve: Cranial V (trigeminal). The action: Depression of the body of the mandible bone. The effect: Opening of the mouth.

There are many variations of this simple representation of muscles doing the will of the brain (i.e., of the individual). For example: (*a*) A single muscle will not always be involved. In the case of mouth opening just presented, other muscles (the suprahyoid group especially) would play a role. (*b*) The participation of antagonistic muscles is important in checking any overextensive movement of the primary muscle, allowing for a controlled movement. (*c*) The brain may fail to put a wish into action because if has information that makes the action undesirable at the moment (e.g., it would resist causing the mouth to open when the mouth is engaged in another activity such as swallowing).

The efferent nervous system, or motor system, makes up the command system throughout the body. The efferent nerve supply to the craniomandibular muscles and to the external pterygoid muscle in the example above is provided by Cranial V, the trigeminal nerve.

In contrast, information concerning the state and condition of the body is provided by the afferent, or sensory, nervous system. In the case of opening the mouth, if the brain had received sensations indicating that the mouth should not be opened because it was full of water needing to be swallowed, awareness of that condition would have precluded mouth opening. The afferent nerve signals from the sensory system in the mouth are carried back to the brain, in this case, by other components of the same Cranial V. So, Cranial V carries both motor and sensory stimuli for parts of the mouth.

Clinical Note

Some people cannot move a structure important to the act of speaking because of paralysis. In paralysis, the nerve that normally carries stimuli to a muscle or a group of muscles is not functioning. Muscles do not receive commands to contract, and the action cannot take place in the normal fashion. Clients who have had brain injuries (e.g., stroke) or who have had nerves damaged in accidents may have such paralytic conditions. Some people do not have certain sensations and so cannot monitor the status or position of speech structures, which could lead to speech differences. For example, many normal persons note temporary speech problems while under the influence of dental anesthesias; a more permanent effect of the same kind might occur with real damage to the nerves or the brain centers serving those sensations. The person cannot monitor, does not know, what condition or position his/her speech structures may be in. Medications, drugs, alcohol, and other ingested materials can produce similar effects in the monitoring or feedback systems.

The Efferent System of the Oral Area

The oral musculature is controlled by several cranial nerves. They are called *cranial* because they exit from the central nervous system, the brain, in the cranium. The cranial nerves are identified by Roman numerals, as well as by names. In all, there are 12 cranial nerves, which differ in their division, structure, and functions. The act of oral communication does not demand the use of all 12; in fact, only 6 are necessary for speaking and 1 more for hearing. They are numbered sequentially as they are located in the brain anteroposteriorly.

As was seen earlier, different cranial nerves go to different groups of muscles. The muscles of facial expression are supplied (innervated) by Cranial VII (the facial nerve). It is both efferent (motor) and afferent (sensory). The muscles of mastication (the craniomandibular muscles) are supplied by Cranial V (the trigeminal nerve); it too contains both efferent and afferent fibers.

The muscles of the soft palate are not as clearly neurologically identified as other muscles of the oral region, for there are some differences of opinion among the various authorities as to which cranial nerve has primary responsibility. It is reasonably clear that the tensor (veli) palatine muscle is stimulated by Cranial V. The other three muscles (the levator palatine, glossopalatine, and pharyngopalatine) receive their nerve supply from a nearby subcenter called the *pharyngeal plexus*. Confusion arises concerning the source of the nerves entering that plexus. In this book, we arbitrarily assign that source to Cranial X (the vagus nerve).

The motor supply to the tongue is provided by Cranial XII (the hypoglossal nerve). This cranial nerve is predominantly efferent, although there is some evidence that it has a sensory component also.

The Afferent System of the Oral Area

The sensations served by the afferent system are several (see Chapter 8 for further discussion). In the oral area, there are both general and special sensory components. The general sensations include several varieties of touch, pressure, and a muscle sense with several subtypes. The general sensory organs are often broadly distributed throughout the body. In contrast, the special senses are located at one or two fairly restricted regions. In the mouth, the tongue fulfills an important special sensory function, taste (the gustatory sense). Other special senses include audition and vision.

The special sense of taste is served by the facial nerve (Cranial VII) in the anterior portion of the tongue, while the posterior areas are served by the glossopharyngeal nerve (Cranial IX).

Two cranial nerves serve most of the general senses of the oral cavity. The trigeminal nerve (Cranial V) seems to serve the anterior two-thirds of the tongue surface, the lips, the teeth and gingiva, the mucous membrane covering the hard and soft palates and that of the vestibule, and the skin of the cheeks around the mouth opening. The glossopharyngeal nerve serves general sensation for the posterior portion of the tongue, as well as for areas beyond (the pharynx).

Some sensations of the mouth that are important in the monitoring and control of speaking activities are the tactile sensations of the surfaces of various structures. These sensations are those of light touch, surface pressure, and deep pressure. Other important sensations related to speaking skill are those that are used to monitor muscles, tendons, and joints. These sensations are those of kinesthesia (sensing the movement of anatomic units) and proprioception (sensing the position or posture of body parts). There is overlap between these two types of sensation.

As might be expected, given the way in which speech-sounds are produced, there is considerably more tactile sensitivity in the anterior parts of the mouth than in the posterior regions.

SUMMARY

The mouth portion of the vocal tract is a chamber, or cavity, that serves the important speech functions of resonating the voice and manipulating the air stream during articulation by changing in both continuous and discrete fashion. The main purpose of the mouth is to participate in the ingestion of food.

The mouth is broadly divided into two spaces, the vestibule and the oral cavity proper. The latter is nearly filled by the tongue, which together with the lips and other structures of the mouth, performs many movements important both in eating and in speech.

These movements are made possible by the actions of certain muscles and muscle groups.

The 10 paired muscles of facial expression are found around the mouth and have their effects on the lips and the areas immediately around the lips.

The four paired muscles of mastication move the mandible in order to effect chewing movements.

The major part of the soft palate is composed of and moved by five muscles, with a sixth sometimes important.

The tongue is almost entirely muscular, being composed of an intrinsic and an extrinsic group of muscles. In general, the intrinsic muscles effect changes in the shape of the tongue, while the extrinsic muscles change the position of the tongue within the oral cavity.

The surface landmarks of the facial region, both extraoral and intraoral, give information about the support for the vocal tract.

Neuromuscular considerations enter into an analysis of how muscles effect movements. The simple action of opening the mouth is seen to be highly complex and variable. The cranial nerves carry the signals that result in movements of the oral musculature, with the nerves serving both efferent and afferent functions.

Clinical Implications

Speech/language pathologists, as well as other professionals in the helping professions, find numerous disorders of human functioning stemming from problems with the mouth. Dentists, pediatricians, and physicians are among those dealing with a great variety of abnormalities. The speech-language pathologist might well find anatomic and physiologic bases for speech problems such as articulation and resonance disorders.

Because of lack of neurologic control of the muscles of the tongue, as in Parkinson's disease, the slurring and the difficulty in initiating speech (among other problems) give persons with this disorder important communication limitations.

Tumor growths in and around the oral region may require surgical removal, which leaves the patient with missing articulators such as the tongue or the palate.

There are some anatomic differences that might be only temporarily or minimally important to communication disorders. For example, when a child passes through the mixed dentition stage (losing deciduous for permanent teeth), a minimal or even no speech problem might be observed. Another temporary type may occur when dental work requiring anesthesia takes place leaving the patient with, perhaps, an indistinct articulation ability.

As part of major conditions that have a broader field of effect, we might find paralysis of the oral musculature resulting from a stroke or from an injury to the nerves serving those muscles, sometimes unilaterally (on one side) or bilaterally (both sides). Degenerative conditions, such as myasthenia gravis or multiple sclerosis, interfere with muscle function, in the oral region as well as elsewhere in the body, with the resulting speech disorder as a part of the overall deterioration.

In clinical assessments, speech/language pathologists generally make at least a cursory if not a detailed (depending upon the speech problem) examination of the structures and functions of the oral region in speech. With increasing numbers of such professionals actively engaged in services in medial settings (i.e., hospitals and clinics), one would expect to find increasing importance placed upon both the normal and the disordered character of the mouth region.

Study Questions

1. Without allowing any part of the mouth or chin to touch anything else, open and close the mouth to varying degrees and observe how you know where it is and what it is doing. What systems are monitoring that behavior?

2. Bring the teeth together. Put the lower lip up against the cutting edges of the upper teeth. Lift the tongue apex to the gingiva of the maxilla (alveolar ridge). What systems inform your brain of the action?

3. Concerning the craniomandibular muscles, explain why there are three primary muscles related to mandible bone elevation and only one primary muscle of mandible depression.

4. Which muscle of facial expression would you consider the primary one as you produce a [p] sound? What biological purposes would that muscle serve?

5. Which muscles in the mouth might be involved in the formation of the [t] sound?

6. Lower your soft palate while saying "*Ah,*" so the sound becomes more and more nasal. Which muscles were contracting at the outset? Which ones then had to relax and which had to contract to lower the velum?

7. Identify the nerves that would carry the signals for the behaviors described in question 6.

8. Which muscles in the oral region might be considered to reverse their origins and insertions, depending upon the task and the circumstances?

9. Why is mucous membrane important during speech?

10. Lift and then depress the tongue while producing a vocal sound; observe the effect on that sound. Observe mandible bone movement, feel tongue changes, and notice lip positions.

Chapter 4
The Pharynges

GENERAL INTRODUCTION

The *pharynges* are three contiguous walled spaces in the vocal tract (Fig. 4.1). They are suspended from the base of the skull and are attached to the upper vertebrae, to the bones of the nose and the palate, and to oral and laryngeal structures. The pharynges, lined with mucous membrane, are muscular tubes that generally contain air. During respiration, inhaled air from the nose enters the upper pharynx, continues through the middle division, and enters the lower pharynx before continuing through the opening into the respiratory tract. Food from the mouth enters the middle pharyngeal space (where it is restricted from moving upward into the nasal regions) and is squeezed inferiorly into the lower pharynx and thereafter into the digestive tract via the esophagus.

These functions of the pharyngeal cavities and their walls utilize few movements that are not among those required for the speaking act. Changes in the boundary walls of the pharynges create changes in the size, shape, and texture of the resonating cavities. The vocal (laryngeal) tone that is introduced into the pharynges is modified (filtered) by these chambers. This modification is an important determinant of the characteristic voice of the individual, and it contributes to the formation (articulation) of some speech sounds in some languages.

Clinical Note

The pharynges are not the only resonators of the voice, but some of the resonance disorders that occur can be associated with structural conditions within or affecting these spaces. The child with adenoids and tonsils that partially occupy the resonating chambers may have an unusual vocal quality. The individual of any age with a severe cold has a similar resonance change caused by the space-filling swollen mucous membranes. The person whose velopharyngeal closure system fails to separate nasal regions from lower ones has a hypernasal resonance quality. Clinical assessment of the contributions of the pharynges in disordered speech is often very important to understanding the nature of overall problems.

DIVISIONS OF THE PHARYNX

The pharyngeal divisions are continuous with one another, each division receiving its name from its relationship to adjacent areas.

The uppermost pharyngeal division is the *nasopharynx,* so named because it is intimately associated with the nasal passages via the *posterior nasal nares (choanae).* The nasopharynx is essentially a part of the respiratory tract. On each lateral wall of this space is found an entrance to the *auditory (Eustachian) tube.* This tube is responsible for the exchange of air between the nasopharynx and the middle ear, as well as providing for some drainage of fluids from the middle ear. The opening framework of the auditory tube forms a prominence *(torus tubarius)* on each lateral wall; below this prominence is a small fold of mucous membrane (the *salpingopharyngeal fold)* enclosing the salpingopharyngeal muscle. Other muscles associated with the auditory tube are the tensor (veli) palatine and the levator (veli) palatine muscles. The mucous membrane of the nasopharynx is continuous with that of the nose anteriorly and with that of the other pharyngeal cavities inferiorly.

The boundaries of the nasopharynx (also termed the *epipharynx)* start at its "roof," the sloping or angulated joining of the body of the sphenoid bone and the basilar portion of the occipital bone, the *spheno-occipital angle* or *clivus.* Lateral boundaries are the muscles and auditory tube, covered with mucous membrane. Anteriorly are found the posterior (nasal) nares, the midline vomer bone, and the medial plates of the pterygoid processes. Inferiorly, the sloping nasal surface of the soft palate and the opening *(isthmus)* into the oropharynx are found. Posteriorly, the mucous-membrane and muscle covered cervical vertebrae are found; there are also several potential spaces in and around this region. *Adenoids (pharyngeal tonsils)* sometimes found here will be discussed later.

The *oropharynx* (or *mesopharynx)* continues the pharyngeal tube inferiorly from about the level of the soft palate to that of the hyoid bone below. This division derives its name from the fact that it is a continuation of the oral cavity; it is a major portion of the digestive tract, while also serving the upper respiratory tract.

The oropharynx is bounded, very generally, by the *velopharyngeal port (isthmus),* the nasopharynx above, the oral cavity anteriorly, the cervical vertebrae posteriorly, and the laryngopharynx inferiorly. More specifically, the anterior boundary consists of the faucial isthmus into the oral cavity, the two sets of pillars and tonsils, and the pharyngeal portion of the tongue. Also anteriorly, the upstanding epiglottis protrudes variously into the spaces. Superiorly, boundaries are made by the sloping oral surface of the velum and the velopharyngeal isthmus into the nasopharynx. With the continuation of the lateral walls lined with mucous membrane, some signs of the salpingopharyngeal folds and the posterior faucial pillar are evident. Inferiorly, there is no outstanding division between the oropharynx and laryngopharynx.

The *laryngopharynx,* sometimes known as the *hypopharynx,* continues the pharyngeal tube inferiorly, narrowing to the smallest pharyngeal cross-section at the entrance to the esophagus. The boundaries are the oropharynx superiorly, the cervical vertebrae posteriorly, the esophagus inferiorly, and anteriorly the entrance to and dorsal surfaces of the structures of the larynx. Alongside the epiglottis and the entrance to the larynx is found a groove in the mucous membrane called the *pyriform recess (sinus),* for drainage of fluids past the laryngeal entrance into the digestive tract below.

CONNECTIVE TISSUES

There are few connective tissues in the pharynges although a few ligaments, considerable fascia and areolar tissue, and some cartilage connections are found in one area alone, the laryngopharynx. The superiorly located sphenoid and occipital bones are closely associated with the nasopharynx. To these, the most cephalad and broad portions of the pharynx are attached. The bony tissues of the nasal cavities provide further support for some parts of the pharynx, as do the cervical vertebrae. Another important cartilage is the auditory tube, which opens into the nasopharynx. The epiglottis, in the lower pharynges, is a cartilaginous structure, as is the laryngeal skeleton adjacent to the lowermost pharynx.

MUSCULATURE

Basically, the muscles of the pharynges are designed to change the shape of the tube in the swallowing act, constricting the tube in such a way as to squeeze

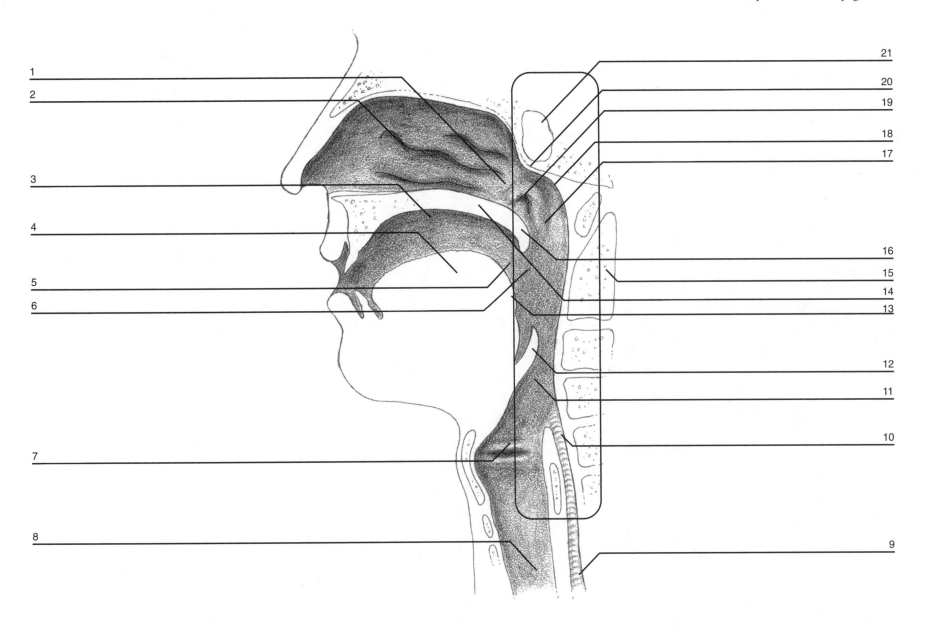

Figure 4.1 Vocal Tract: Pharynges (Sagittal View)

Table 4.1. Muscles of the Pharynx

Muscle	Origin	Insertion	Action	Nerve
Pharyngeal constrictor				
Superior constrictor	Lower posterior border of medial pterygoid plate, pterygomandibular ligament and raphe, mylohyoid ridge of mandible, sides of tongue	Posterior median raphe of pharynx	Narrows pharynx in peristalsis	Cranial X (pharyngeal plexus)
Middle constrictor	Both cornua of hyoid bone, stylohyoid ligament	Posterior median raphe of pharynx	Narrows pharynx in peristalsis	Cranial X (pharyngeal plexus)
Inferior constrictor	Inferior side of cricoid cartilage, oblique line of thyroid cartilage	Posterior median raphe of pharynx	Narrows pharynx in peristalsis	Cranial X (pharyngeal plexus)
Velopharyngeal sphincter	Midline of soft palate	Posterior median raphe of pharynx	Narrows velopharyngeal port, moving lateral walls medially and posterior walls anteriorly; retracts and spreads velum	Cranial X (pharyngeal plexus)
Cricopharyngeal	Sides of cricoid cartilage	Posterior median raphe of pharynx	Maintains closure of pharyngoesophageal entrance	Cranial X (pharyngeal plexus)
Pharyngeal levator				
Stylopharyngeal	Base of styloid process of temporal bone	Mucous membrane of pharynx and thyroid cartilage	Elevates and widens pharynx and larynx	Cranial IX
Salpingopharyngeal	Lower edge of auditory cartilage	Mucous membrane of pharynx	Elevates pharynx, opens the auditory tube	Cranial X (pharyngeal plexus)

the bolus of food down into the esophagus. Swallowing is commenced at the oral phase with musculature that is closely associated with that of the pharyngeal phase. In both instances, oral and pharyngeal phases of swallowing, there is close anatomic relationship between the biological function and the speech functions.

Five muscles are generally considered to be pharyngeal muscles: the superior pharyngeal constrictor, the middle pharyngeal constrictor, the inferior pharyngeal constrictor, the stylopharyngeal, and the salpingopharyngeal (Table 4.1, Fig. 4.2). Another two muscles, the glossopalatine (palatoglossus) and the pharyngopalatine (palatopharyngeal), have some association with the pharynges in structure and function. Still another two muscles, the velopharyngeal sphincter and the cricopharyngeal (both considered by some to be subdivisions of larger muscles), bring the total to nine muscles in this region.

Pharyngeal Constrictors

The *superior pharyngeal constrictor muscle* has its origins in several locations, from a superior to an inferior direction. Fibers originate from the lower border of the medial pterygoid plate of the sphenoid bone, from the pterygomandibular ligament and raphe, from the mylohyoid ridge of the mandible, and possibly from the sides of the tongue. These origins are all anterior to the body of the muscle, to its insertion, and to the cavity of the pharynx. An origin in the velum at the palatal aponeurosis gives rise to the velopharyngeal sphincter muscle, which is here arbitrarily related to the constrictor.

The fibers of the superior constrictor muscle arch nearly horizontally backward and form a thin quadrilateral muscle around the sides of the nasopharynx and part of the oropharynx. They insert into the fibrous posterior medial raphe, where they meet with similar fibers from the opposite side. At the superior border are found the pharyngeal opening to the auditory tube, the levator (veli) palatine muscle, and the pharyngeal aponeurosis. The action of the superior pharyngeal constrictor is to narrow the lumen of the pharynx by constriction and thus aid in the movement of the bolus of food inferiorly (*peristalsis*). Its nerve supply comes from the pharyngeal plexus of the vagus nerve (Cranial X).

The *middle pharyngeal constrictor muscle* is fan-shaped, with its narrow portion anterolaterally partially overlapping the superior constrictor muscle. It originates from the whole border of the greater cornu of the hyoid bone, from the lesser cornu of the hyoid, and from the stylohyoid ligament. The muscle fibers fan out from this origin, the lower ones passing beneath the inferior pharyngeal constrictor, the middle ones passing nearly horizontally back, and the superior fibers passing up-

ward and external to the superior pharyngeal constrictor muscle. All of these fibers insert at the midline posteriorly into the fibrous raphe. When contracted, the middle pharyngeal constrictor continues the squeezing action of the pharynx, forcing the bolus of food farther inferiorly toward the esophagus. Its innervation is the same as that of the superior constrictor, the pharyngeal plexus from Cranial X.

The *inferior pharyngeal constrictor muscle* is perhaps the thickest and widest of the constrictor group, with a somewhat narrow origin but a rather extensive insertion. Its fibers originate along the sides of the laryngeal cartilages, the cricoid inferiorly, and the thyroid at its oblique line. Its most inferior fibers pass nearly horizontally back; its upper fibers ascend around the sides of the pharynx. Both groups of fibers insert along with the same fibers from the opposite side into the fibrous posterior median raphe of the pharynx. Its action is to continue the previously described peristaltic effect upon the bolus of food in deglutition, forcing it inferiorly into the esophagus. The pharyngeal plexus furnishes the nerve supply to this muscle also.

The posterior pharyngeal raphe, here identified as being the insertion of the three constrictor muscles, is a structure of questionable status for the muscle fibers from each side may simply interdigitate with each other at the midline of the wall with little discernible "fibrous raphe" present.

Two highly variable muscles are also considered by some authorities to be important pharyngeal muscles. The first is the *palatopharyngeal sphincter (of Whillis)*, or the *velopharyngeal sphincter muscle*. The muscle may be a division of either the superior pharyngeal constrictor or the palatopharyngeal, probably of the first. Its fibers originate along the midline of the soft palate about midway on its anteroposterior axis. They pass as a muscle bundle horizontally back around the sides of the pharynx and insert into the posterior median raphe. Upon contraction three effects can be noted: (1) the posterior wall of the pharynx protrudes as an ele-

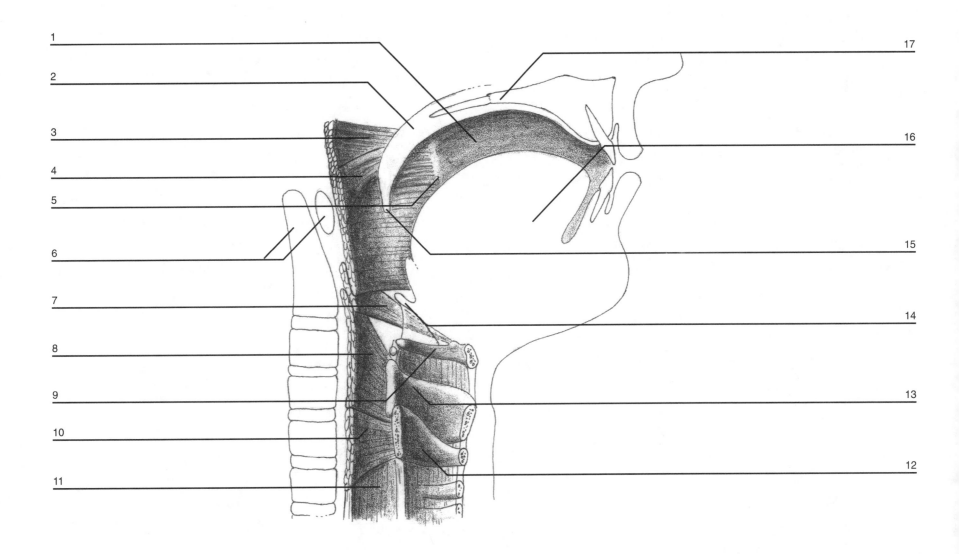

1

2

3

4

5

6

7

8

9

10

11

17

16

15

14

13

12

Figure 4.2 Pharygeal Constrictor Muscles (Sagittal View)

vated horizontal fold, producing what is often called *Passavant's pad*, or *cushion*; (2) the tissues of the soft palate are pulled posteriorly; and (3) the lateral pharyngeal walls move medially, completing a somewhat sphincteric closure of the isthmus. These actions occur during deglutition and during velopharyngeal closure accompanying the speaking act. The muscle is undoubtedly important for speech, as well as for effective separation between the nasal and oral pharynges. It shares the pharyngeal plexus nerve supply also.

The second important pharyngeal muscle is the *cricopharyngeal muscle*, the most caudal portion of the inferior constrictor muscle. Its bilateral origin is along the sides of the cricoid cartilage. Its fibers pass horizontally back around the sides of the most inferior portion of the laryngopharynx and insert into the posterior midline raphe. This muscle is of considerable importance in forming pharyngoesophageal closure and is a true sphincter. It relaxes as the food bolus approaches, allowing it to pass into the esophagus, whereupon it contracts to prevent reflux of food. It also receives neural innervation from the pharyngeal plexus, from Cranial X (vagus) and possibly Cranial IX (glossopharyngeal) and a subdivision of the parasympathetic nervous system.

Clinical Note

The usefulness of the muscles of the pharynx is evident when biological functions are considered. Speech, too, requires these muscles. The resonance system for the voice is importantly associated with the chambers of the pharynx. In some pathologies, speech disorders are frequent, and speech therapy is frequently the major rehabilitative procedure. The patient with a repaired cleft palate, for example, is one who needs pharyngeal muscle study and training. Loss of the attachments of some of these muscles may cause speech disorders (e.g., loss of attachment of the velopharyngeal sphincter muscle may preclude efficient velopharyngeal closure, causing both resonance and articulatory speech problems). When a person has a laryngectomy for laryngeal cancer, the surgeon usually tends to retain the cricopharyngeal muscle so that it can be used by the speech clinician in the development of adequate compensatory speech production (esophageal speech). Cancerous lesions elsewhere in the upper vocal tract can lead to pharyngeal dysfunction; neuromotor disorders can also lead to unusual and abnormal speaking patterns.

Pharyngeal Elevators

The pharyngeal levator muscles (Table 4.1, Fig. 4.3) are the stylopharyngeal and the salpingopharyngeal muscles, along with the palatopharyngeal (pharyngopalatine) muscle already discussed. The *stylopharyngeal muscle* is a slender group of fibers that, when considered bilaterally have broadly divergent origins and that pass to a much more medial insertion in the pharyngeal wall. Its origin is the base of the styloid process of the temporal bone; its fibers pass downward and medially, spreading out as they pass between the superior and middle pharyngeal constrictor muscles. The insertion of this muscle is within the mucous membrane lining of the pharynx, where it blends with the other soft tissues of the pharynx, and on the thyroid cartilage, along with the fibers from the palatopharyngeal muscle. From its orientation, it can be seen that its action is to elevate the entire pharynx and to widen it superiorly, an action occurring during deglutition to facilitate reception of the bolus of food within the pharynx. The nerve supply is derived from the glossopharyngeal nerve (Cranial IX).

The *salpingopharyngeal muscle* is similar to the stylopharyngeal muscle in that its fibers begin superiorly and insert inferiorly in the side walls of the pharynx. The origin is along the posterior lower border of the cartilage of the auditory tube, and the fibers pass directly downward, forming the mucous membrane-covered salpingopharyngeal fold. They insert into the walls of the pharynx inferiorly along with other muscle fibers at midpharynx or lower levels. Its action is twofold: to elevate the pharynx in deglutition and to distort the torus tubarius of the auditory tube in ventilating the middle ear. Innervation is provided by the pharyngeal plexus from the vagus nerve (Cranial X), possibly with other nerves contributing.

The general actions of the muscles of the pharynges in swallowing are basic to life support. Actions in speech production are refinements of those basic acts. It is apparent that synergic action of the constrictors is required to accomplish the squeezing function in a smoothly continuous act from superior to inferior, forcing the bolus of food from the oropharynx into the laryngopharynx and then into the esophagus. In the esophagus, a contiguous and continuous squeezing action of the smooth muscle tissues of the alimentary canal carries on this important function of peristalsis.

SWALLOWING

Of course, it is truly "vital" for the organism to acquire nutritional elements to sustain life. The food we use for that purpose enters the system through the effective use of the lips and teeth, initially. Once it has entered the oral cavity proper, the food is sliced, broken, and pulverized while being mixed with saliva to form a *bolus* to be swallowed. The *preparatory phase* of swallowing requires that the rima oris be closed (by lips and teeth) to prevent the extrusion of food. The tongue sweeps up the food and the lingual apex is elevated to approach the alveolar ridge. The *oral phase* is thus commenced. It continues as the dorsum of the tongue, carrying the bolus, sequentially is elevated against the oral surface of the palate. This squeezes the bolus posteriorly toward the faucial isthmus. As the food moves, taking about a second in time in all, sensory feedback monitors signal ahead for velopharyngeal closure and pharyngeal elevation. The food is thrust past

the faucial isthmus into the oropharynx and the isthmus then partially closes against the possible return of the food as it is pressured by pharyngeal constriction. The oral phase is largely voluntary neurologically.

Swallowing now is centered in the subject of this chapter, the pharynges, and we identify the *pharyngeal phase* of swallowing. The sequential narrowing of the pharynx has started with the most superior musculature creating velopharyngeal closure, thus preventing any food material from entering the nasopharynx or the nasal passages (and especially threatening the entrance to the auditory tube). That protective function is accomplished by the uppermost portion of the superior constrictor muscle; the pharyngeal constrictor musculature below contracts to narrow the pharyngeal space and literally pushes the bolus down the tube. This sequential narrowing of the digestive tube is called *peristalsis* and continues throughout the digestive tract. Although the musculature is striated or so-called voluntary, the pharyngeal phase of swallowing is involuntary neurologically under the control of brainstem centers.

Clinical Note

The speech activities occurring in these regions utilize similar muscular activities. Velopharyngeal closure is necessary for most American English speech, otherwise the laryngeal tone as well as the airflow passes into the nasopharynx and nasal passages; this weakens the supply of available air for consonant production and adds an overly nasal (hypernasality) component to the vocal quality.

As the bolus passes down through the pharynx, signals sent to the larynx below cause its musculature to elevate the entire structure. In the process, the entrance to the larynx is closed, it is hoped, and the food is rapidly propelled past that opening down the laryngopharynx. Again, signals sent ahead to the cri-

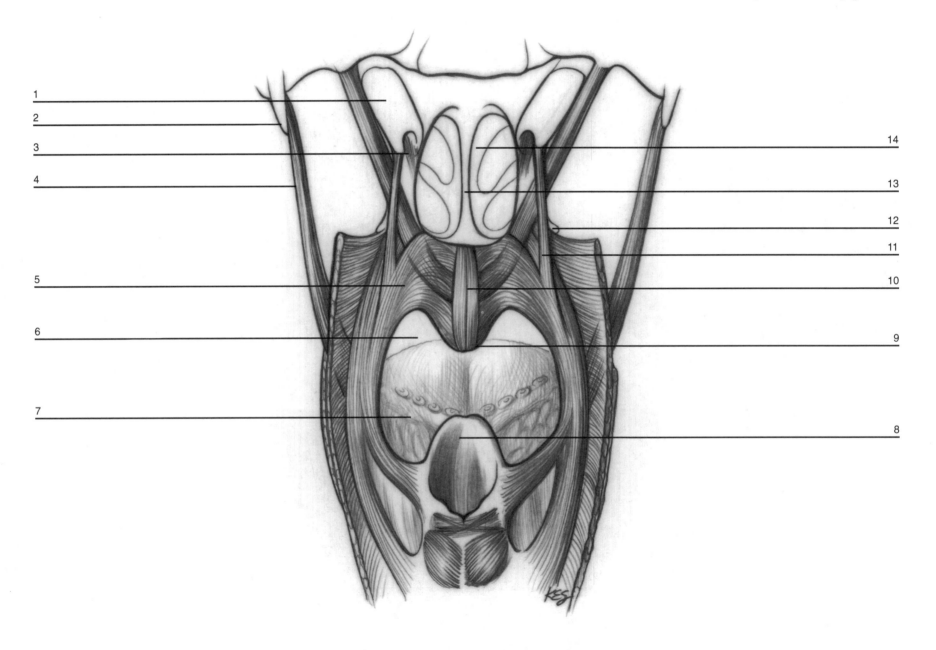

Figure 4.3   Pharygeal Levator Muscles

copharyngeal muscle, a true sphincter (being in constant contraction until signaled to relax), opens the entrance to the esophagus. The bolus passes this sphincter to enter the esophagus and starts the *esophageal phase* of swallowing. The mixed striated and smooth musculature at the upper end of the esophagus continues the peristaltic contractions and the bolus is pushed downward toward the stomach. As it approaches the stomach, signals cause another sphincter (the cardiac) to relax and the food enters the stomach. Both the pharyngoesophageal and cardiac sphincters close behind the bolus to prevent reflux (return) of food upward. All of these muscle activities are under involuntary control from the brainstem centers controlling them.

Clinical Note

The swallowing act, or deglutition, is the product of an extremely complicated series of muscular contractions. The muscles and muscle groups involved contract in controlled sequences that are directed both by the inherent demands of swallowing and by the effects of learned neuromuscular patterns. Structural factors also influence deglutition. The role of the speech clinician faced with a speech aberration is to program appropriate therapeutic procedures that consider the relative importance of all these factors. Swallowing disorders (*dysphagia*) are vital concerns and the role speech pathologists play in assessing and treating patients with such problems, often as part of a special team, is an important contribution to the health and welfare of such patients.

NERVOUS TISSUES

The *pharyngeal plexus* plays an important role in both efferent and afferent functions of the pharynx. This network of nerves probably comes from both Cranial X (vagus nerve) and Cranial IX (glossopharyngeal nerve), with other possibilities as well. It supplies a large number of structures in the head and neck, but most importantly for the present discussion the pharyngeal constrictors and their subdivisions. The same nerve source also supplies the salpingopharyngeal muscle. However, the stylopharyngeal muscle receives its innervation from the glossopharyngeal nerve only.

Some variation in nerve supply is thought to occur. Such variation can be especially apparent when one is considering the inferior constrictor muscle, some fibers of which may be innervated through the external laryngeal and the recurrent laryngeal nerves (from the vagus). This is understandable in light of the intimate relationship between the laryngopharynx and the larynx.

The sensory nerve supply to the pharyngeal and oral regions was touched on in Chapter 3. Taste, temperature, and other senses operate in this region. In the mouth, the anterior two-thirds of the tongue is supplied for taste sensation by the facial nerve (Cranial VII) through the chorda tympani nerve. The posterior third of the tongue, as well as the pharynx and other sites where taste buds are found, is served by the sensory fibers from the glossopharyngeal nerve (Cranial IX). Most taste buds are found on the surface of the tongue, but some are found on the soft palate and on the epiglottis. Few are found on the walls of the pharynx.

Other sensory functions of the pharynges have been only incompletely described. Some awareness of the status of the pharynges might be possible, but which aspects of the nervous system might serve this ability is unclear. Some sensory systems must be present to account for common sensations and reactions (e.g., touch is involved in learning pharyngeal sounds as well as reflexive behaviors as in gagging). The extent of involvement of the sensory systems in the pharynges is a worthy subject for future study.

STRUCTURES AND FUNCTIONS OF THE PHARYNX

In life-sustaining activities, control of the actions of the pharynges is largely reflexive. As swallowing takes place, velopharyngeal closure is an involuntary accompaniment. In breathing, the velopharyngeal aperture must be patent (open) so that air can pass from the nose and nasopharynx through the pharynges and into the lower respiratory tract. Of course, the air destined for the lungs may enter the body through the mouth and thence pass into the pharynges and lower respiratory tract. Both nasal and oral entranceways are used to some extent by most persons at some times.

The presence of environmental air in the nasopharynx is of considerable importance for other purposes as well. The pharyngeal terminus of the auditory tube in the lateral pharyngeal wall exchanges environmental air with that of the middle ear, maintaining a balance of air pressure on both sides of the tympanic membrane. Although the opening to the auditory tube is not always patent, it opens frequently during the actions of the palatal and pharyngeal muscles attached to the cartilaginous tube. The dilator tubae muscle is attached to this structure. This muscle, along with the salpingopharyngeal muscle (when it is of sufficient magnitude), contracts during swallowing, yawning, and other such activities and exerts a twisting pull on the cartilaginous end of the tube. This is sufficient to cause the entire tube to open, thus providing for the important air exchange. The levator (veli) palatine muscle, either by direct attachment or juxtaposition, might also be part of this system.

Clearly, the function of the pharynges in dealing with environmental air is to channel the air from the nose or the mouth downward to the lower respiratory tract. In respiratory activities, the pharynges are generally patent; associated structures, such as the velum, epiglottis, and tongue, have an effect on the direction of air flow. Obvious, too, is the pharyngeal activity in swallowing food; once it has passed from the oral cavity the bolus is propelled by peristalsis down into the esophagus.

In speaking, control of the pharynges might be a combination of reflexive and voluntary control. It is clear that humans can control movements of the pharyngeal structures to some extent; in fast-moving speech, however, it appears that the habitual patterning must be coordinated too rapidly for detailed voluntary control over each structure and movement to be possible. A well-developed programmed feedback system appears to be responsible for controlling such movements.

The pharynges are part of the resonance system of the vocal tract. This means that the pharynges modify the sound delivered to them from the tone-producing apparatus (the larynx). The size, shape, and status of the pharyngeal walls are importantly related to the nature of the voice. Changes in any of these factors change the nature of the sound. Such modification of sound (resonance) is volitional in some instances; in others, it occurs with changes in health and emotional condition and with age.

In the case of resonance changes that occur with age, changes in status that are due to changes in muscle, fat, or mucous membrane are thought to create the voice characteristics of the older person. Other changes, such as in size and shape, are largely due to the velopharyngeal apparatus. Here the pharynges can be separated at the level of the palate or can be made continuous. As a result of such manipulations, speech sounds may be produced in an acceptable fashion or may become unacceptably hypernasal. In English it is acceptable to nasalize only three consonants, no other; these are [M], [N], and [NG].

A Note on the Tonsils

The *tonsils* are space-filling structures and can thus impact upon the vocal tract and its functions. The term *tonsil* has several meanings. Probably most common is its use to refer to the visible structures in the posterior oral cavity, between the two bilateral faucial pillars. There are, however, several tonsils, all associated with the pharynges.

These several tonsils form a near-circle known as *Waldeyer's ring.* They encircle the two major entryways into the body at the head end, the nasal and the oral. This ring is composed of lymphoid tissue, important to body functions. The fluid (lymph) within helps defend the body against foreign particles, especially microorganisms. The lymph also serves to transport waste products and other materials to various regions of the body, where they ultimately drain into the system of venous blood vessels. The various tonsils are found as large structures in the child, sometimes larger than they would be in the adult, for tonsillar tissues tend to atrophy after puberty.

The different portions of Waldeyer's ring are named in various ways. The mass of lymphoid tissue found on the posterior-superior wall of the nasopharynx is the *pharyngeal tonsil,* more commonly known as the *adenoids.* A projection of this tonsillar material may be found around the auditory tube entryway or beyond. This mass of tissue, the adenoids, can fill the nasopharynx, closing both the posterior nares and the auditory tubes. In such cases speech might be affected so that nonnasal (hyponasal) vowel production, as well as interference with nasal consonant production, can occur.

The *palatine tonsil,* colloquially the *tonsil,* protrudes from between the faucial pillars on both sides, extending toward the midline. It can be observed at varying medial extensions, sometimes nearly meeting its opposite member at midline. The *lingual tonsil* might be found across the posterior (pharyngeal) tongue surface, completing the lymphoid ring.

SUMMARY

The pharynges, three contiguous walled spaces in the vocal tract, perform vital functions in both respiration and food ingestion. These walls behave in similar manners for speech production so that the pharynges function as resonance cavities.

The divisions of the pharynges, from uppermost to lowermost, are the nasopharynx, the oropharynx, and the laryngopharynx. They are so named because of their structural and functional relationships to the nose, oral cavity, and larynx. There is also an extremely important air exchange tube (auditory, or Eustachian) connecting to the ear.

Connective tissues make up little of the pharynx. Certain bones and cartilaginous structures play a supporting role.

The muscles of the pharynges are designed to move the tube in such a way as to effect swallowing (peristalsis) and speech production. They are divided into the pharyngeal constrictors and the pharyngeal elevators.

The nerve supply to the pharynges comes mainly from the pharyngeal plexus largely derived from vagus (Cranial X) nerve, but with possible contributions from Cranial IX and even Cranial XI. The sensory functions of the pharynx are not completely known.

The pharynx must deal with environmental air during respiration and during speech. Changes in the pharynges (e.g., with age) can cause changes in the resonance of the voice.

Tonsils, composed of lymphoid tissues, are of several types. They all form a near-circle known as Waldeyer's ring. They serve a protective function in the child and may be related to speech disorders in some cases, both child and adult.

Clinical Implications

At least two aspects of oral communication relate to normal pharyngeal structure and function. One is the resonance of the voice and the second is the health (and function) of the ear. Other pathologies may stem from failure in velopharyngeal closure, causing speech disorders in both consonant and vowel productions.

An individual, child or adult, with an extremely nasal voice (*hypernasality*), may demonstrate this problem because of incompetence of the velopharyngeal closure system. If the tone produced by the vocal folds is allowed to enter the nasopharynx and even the nasal passages, the effect is a disorder of resonance. Normal speech, of course, makes but little use (in the English language) of the nasal resonators. We examine the structures and the spaces associated with velopharyngeal closure when we hear such a resonance problem.

The same velopharyngeal closure deficiency, whether because the function is disturbed (as in a paralysis of the muscles involved) or the structures are lacking (as in cleft palate or surgical removal of important structures), may be responsible for disturbance in the necessary flow of air through the oral cavity to form important consonant sounds. The abnormal shunting of the airflow and air pressure to produce consonants such as [k] or [s], for example, so that some amount of the required air flows nasally, will also produce insufficient oral aerodynamic support for those consonant sounds. As a result they are "weakened," distorted, or even omitted insofar as a listener is concerned.

Occasionally, a person is found demonstrating too little nasal resonance in his/her vocal quality. This *hyponasality* may stem from a number of different causes, but one cause relates to the pharyngeal tonsils (the adenoids). At times, these are *hypertrophied* (enlarged) to the extent that they occlude the nasopharynx. Of course, the individual is an obligatory mouth breather, a problem in itself.

Of importance to normal hearing is the opening to the *auditory* (Eustachian) *tube*. This tube provides an exchange of air into the (middle) ear so that air pressure within is equalized with that of external environmental air pressure; this allows for normal functioning of the auditory system (especially the *tympanic membrane*) and, thus, normal hearing. The normal air exchange is often obvious to any person as a popping or other sound or sensation when we go up or down in an elevator or over a mountain pass, when environmental air pressure changes. The auditory tube also provides for a drainage of mucus from the (middle) ear. If the muscles that open the auditory tube fail to function appropriately or the pharyngeal tonsils or other sources fail to allow the tube to open, then problems may arise in the (middle) ear, and hearing could be negatively impacted.

In general, although frequently overlooked, the pharyngeal chambers are of considerable importance to speech and hearing and thus to normal oral communication. They are of great importance to normal respiration and swallowing, functions that may be assessed and served by the speech pathologist and audiologist.

Study Questions

1. *Monitor your own resonance system by changing the vocal tract: produce an "Ah" sound orally, then give it a nasal quality. What sensations, other than auditory, can you observe?*

2. *Attempt to yawn, especially with the mouth closed; can you observe auditory tube muscle function by ear sensations (other than auditory)?*

3. *What structures and what movements can you monitor while swallowing as slowly and deliberately as possible?*

4. *Change the pharyngeal resonance system by attempting to will your voice placement up behind the nose or deep in the throat. Such a "tonal focus" approach can change the quality of character of the voice.*

5. *Does your pharynx sense hot and cold liquids? Can it feel touch?*

Chapter 5
The Larynx

GENERAL INTRODUCTION

The lowermost point of the vocal tract is the *larynx*, known colloquially as the *voice box*. Here is generated a sound that subsequently is modified by the vocal tract above into the characteristic voice of the individual, as well as formed (articulated) into the speech sounds of our language. Voice production, *phonation*, is the communicative function of the larynx, but it has other, more vital, functions to perform.

First, it serves as a part of the airway for both inhaled and exhaled air. Second, it provides valves within that airway that can close to prevent the passage of a foreign object, such as a piece of food or a flying dust particle. Such an object must be prevented from penetrating the respiratory tract beyond this (laryngeal) point for there are few defenses against it thereafter. Third, the valves can stem the flow of air from the lungs so as to increase air pressure from the lungs; the abrupt release of this air results in a cough to dislodge foreign objects that might have entered the upper respiratory tract. Fourth, the valve can entrap air in the lungs to assist in fixing (anchoring) thoracic structures to facilitate other physical activities, such as lifting, defecation, and childbirth. Fifth, the movement of the larynx up and down within the neck during swallowing is important in preventing the entrance of food.

SPACES OF THE LARYNX

It is important to identify the spaces within the larynx where this airborne sound is created and resonated. Spaces have boundaries, and in the larynx the boundaries are extremely mobile. When these structures are mobile, their movements are the result of muscle contraction, external forces, and elasticity.

A rather generalized description of the spaces of the larynx (Fig. 5.1; see Fig. 5.3A) starts with a somewhat wide upper region narrowly constricted inferiorly, to open again as a lower space. The last is then continuous with the airway to and from the lungs. The upper laryngeal space is called the *vestibule*, while the lower one is the *atrium (infraglottal cavity)*. The narrow constriction is the *glottis (rima glottidis)*.

The vestibule opens into the posterior laryngopharynx via a doorway that is called the *aditus ad laryngis*. Further down the vestibule, just above the glottis, another narrowing occurs, beneath which there is a bilateral opening in the side walls, the *laryngeal ventricles (of Morgagni)*. The lowermost space (the atrium) is not closed; it opens into the permanently patent *trachea* (windpipe), which carries air to and from the lungs in the thorax below. The atrium narrows upward into the glottis; the shape of the space has been compared to a mobile cone, the *elastic cone*.

The walls and boundaries of the spaces of the larynx are several. The entranceway to the larynx from the laryngopharynx, the aditus ad laryngis, is formed by the *collar* of the larynx. This collar has several components, all covered by mucous membrane, as is most of the vocal tract. Anteriorly, the collar is formed by the *epiglottis,* a highly elastic cartilage that extends above the larynx to behind the pharyngeal portion of the tongue. From the sides of the epiglottis, a rounded and thickened bundle curves around the sides of the laryngeal entrance; this bundle, the *aryepiglottic fold,* is so named because it attaches the epiglottis anteriorly to the arytenoid cartilages posteriorly. Near the posterior-inferior end of the aryepiglottic fold is a prominence on each side formed by the underlying *cuneiform cartilage,* a stiffening and elastic structure that maintains the openness of the larynx in this region. At the posterior end of the aryepiglottic fold there is a slight *notch* between the two bulging *arytenoid cartilages.*

Beneath, the aditus opens into the vestibule, the side walls of which are formed by mucous membrane, the *quadrangular membrane.* As the vestibule narrows, the first shelf-like structure running from front to back on either side is the *ventricular fold* (or *false vocal fold*). It is a moderately bulbous fold overhanging a space, the ventricle. Both the vestibular folds and the walls of the ventricle provide mucus for lubricating the mobile structures.

The walls of the lateral ventricles, however deep into the sides of the larynx they may be, slope downward and then abruptly toward the midline of the larynx, thus narrowing the laryngeal spaces. This is the upper surface of the *true vocal fold.* From each side, then, a vocal fold extends into the larynx, ending in a rather thin edge, or lip, that runs from front to back. At the front, just internal to the Adam's apple, the mucous membrane covering the two vocal folds comes together at a point called the *midline anterior commissure.* This same covering tissue continues posteriorly over the vocal fold, covering the muscles and cartilage of the vocal fold, until it reaches the posterior end of the vocal folds; from there, the mucous membranes of the two folds again join each other to form the *posterior commis-*

sure. The vocal folds can adjust in length, tension, thickness, and cross-sectional mass. Such adjustments are essential in producing changes of pitch during phonation.

The undersurface of the vocal fold curves downward and laterally to bound the atrium. This curved surface is also adjustable and has the deserved name *elastic cone.* As the vocal folds above come together and separate (called *adduction* and *abduction*), the elastic cone has the function of a variable nozzle for the flowing air exhaled from the lungs below. From the elastic cone inferiorly, the mucous membrane of the airway continues and lines the trachea below.

Clinical Note

Voice disorders—that is, dysphonias—may be caused by changes in the vocal folds, especially their surface coverings. A bad cold or other upper respirator disorders, a tumor (whether from unknown causes or from strong and violent collisions of the vocal fold edges), ulcers, and other pathologies associated with the vocal fold structures can cause the tissues to swell. Of course, dysphonia can have other causes (etiologies), but the clinician cannot ignore the possibility of organic damage during differential diagnosis. Appropriate medical consultation is essential, of course.

CONNECTIVE TISSUES

The larynx (Fig. 5.2) is supported by one major bone and formed by five major cartilages. There are at least four and perhaps as many as six minor cartilages that act as supporting tissues. These vary in size and occurrence from individual to individual.

The bone is the *hyoid,* a horseshoe-shaped bone providing basic support for various muscles of the tongue and for the majority of the laryngeal tissues. (See the earlier discussion of the hyoid bone in the

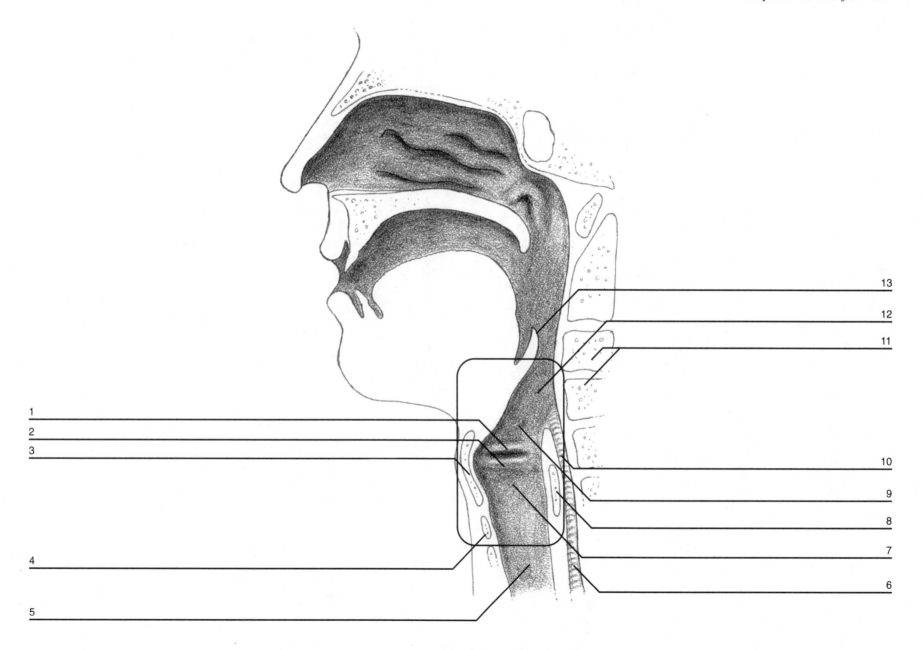

Figure 5.1   Vocal Tract: Larynx (Sagittal View)

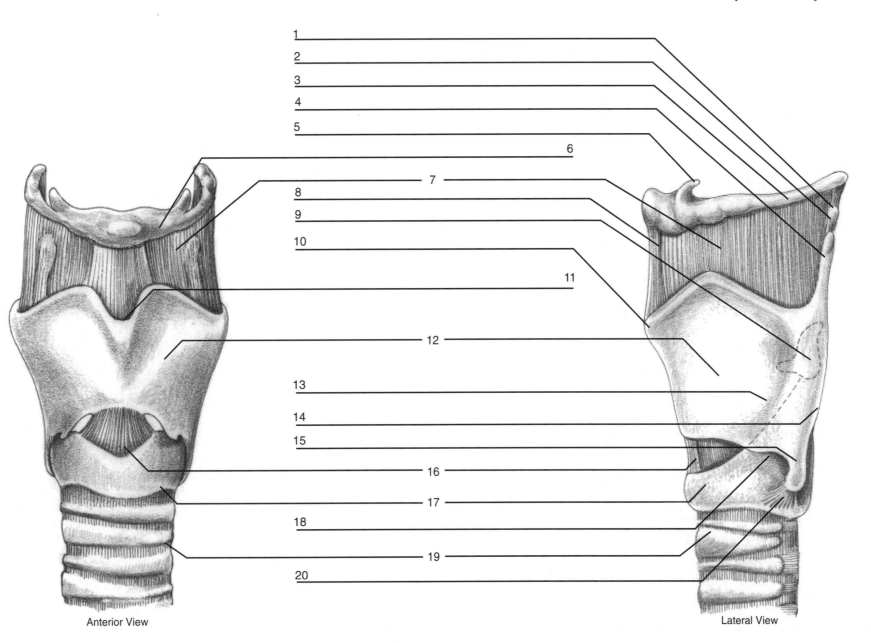

1

2

3

4

5

6

7

8

9

10

11

12

13

14

15

16

17

18

19

20

Anterior View

Lateral View

section "The Facial Skeleton" in Chapter 2.) It is supported in the neck by muscular and ligamentous tissues running superiorly to the mandible and the skull. The hyoid bone is oriented with its open end directed posteriorly; its large body extends anteriorly. Extending backward from the body on either side is the greater horn of the hyoid. At about the point of juncture between the body and the greater horn is a smaller, upward projecting lesser horn. These parts— the body, greater horn, and lesser horn—serve as points of attachment for muscles and ligaments of the larynx and of other structures.

The largest and most prominent of the laryngeal cartilages is the *thyroid cartilage.* This is actually a two-walled cartilage, the thin sheets (lamina) meeting at the anterior aspect of the larynx and neck and forming the *laryngeal prominence,* or *Adam's apple.* These laminae form a V shape, with the angle being rather narrow in the adult male and somewhat broader in the female. Posteriorly, the laminae terminate in a border on each side. To this free border are attached muscles and membranes of the laryngopharynx posteriorly.

Inside the walls of the thyroid cartilage, extending from the angle formed by the two laminae, are housed the vocal folds, as well as the other internal tissues of the larynx. Each of the two posterior borders of the thyroid cartilage have two projections, one upward and one downward; these are the *superior* and *inferior thyroid horns (cornua).* The superior horn is connected through ligaments with the end of the greater horn of the hyoid bone, above. The inferior thyroid horn is in contact through a true, diarthrodial joint with the cricoid cartilage, below. This is the *cricothyroid joint.* The external surface of the lamina of the thyroid cartilage has an *oblique line,* a ridge of slight prominence extending from near the superior cornu down across the lamina toward the anterior medial aspect. This oblique line separates the points of attachment of muscles running to the larynx from above and below

and provides a part of the origin for the inferior pharyngeal constrictor muscle. The superior thyroid notch is that space just above the angle of the thyroid cartilage and just below the hyoid bone; it can be palpated with a finger rather easily by finding the prominence and moving slightly above it to the soft area.

The second largest cartilage of the larynx is the *cricoid* (Fig. 5.2; see Figs. 5.4 and 5.6B through E), a ring-like cartilage encircling the larynx immediately beneath the thyroid cartilage. It has its narrowest part (the *arch*) in the front, and it expands upward posteriorly into a tall and broad *lamina,* or *signet.* This posterior lamina stands high in the space between the open ends of the thyroid cartilage. The superior surface of the lamina of the cricoid is broad and somewhat concave and supports the paired arytenoid cartilages, which further fill the posterior space between the two laminae of the thyroid cartilage. The cricoid cartilage is attached to the thyroid through ligaments at the cricothyroid joint and to the first of the cartilaginous rings of the trachea below by the same means. The muscles attached to this cartilage pass from its sides and lamina to the thyroid and arytenoid cartilages and have a definite effect upon the vocal folds; another important muscle attachment is the cricopharyngeal muscle on either side.

The *cricothyroid joint* (Fig. 5.2). a true joint, is formed on each side by the adjoining of the inferior cornu of the thyroid cartilage with the side of the cricoid cartilage and is held together by ligaments that stretch little. The general opinion is that when appropriate muscle contraction takes place, this joint allows the cricoid cartilage to rotate. Rotation around the cricothyroid joint causes the arch of the cricoid cartilage to elevate toward the lower aspect of the angle of the thyroid cartilage. More importantly, the lamina of the cricoid cartilage, posteriorly, is depressed or is lowered in an arc-like motion. This movement increases the distance between the internal aspect of the thyroid cartilage angle and the top of the cricoid cartilage lamina. The increase of this distance results in lengthening of the interposed vocal fold.

The paired *arytenoid cartilages* (Figs. 5.3B and 5.4; see Fig. 5.6) are located on and articulate with the lamina of the cricoid cartilage in the larynx. These cartilages are small pyramids somewhat irregular in their angles and sides. The arytenoids are so formed that there is a broad surface facing backward and another facing anteriorly and laterally. A forward-projecting angle is called the *vocal process,* for it is part of the vocal fold. The laterally projecting angle is the *vocal muscular process,* which serves as the point of attachment for several important muscles that act to move the arytenoid. The anterolateral surface serves as the attachment point for muscles and ligaments running anteriorly from the arytenoid to the internal angle of the thyroid; these make up a large portion of the vocal fold.

The third angle of the arytenoid cartilage, the *apex,* is thin and bent medially and posteriorly. From its summit runs the thickened aryepiglottic fold, which connects with the epiglottis. Running across or near the summit are muscle fibers from below, connecting the apex with the epiglottis. These muscle and membranous tissues assist in vigorous closing of the aditus in swallowing and coughing. The medial surface of the arytenoid is lined with mucous membrane and bounds the intercartilaginous one-third of the glottis. The medial surfaces can approximate each other and thus effect closure of that part of the glottis. Such approximation is made possible by the *cricoarytenoid joint* (Fig. 5.3B and 5.4; see Fig. 5.6A, B, and C), a true joint. Each of the arytenoid cartilages can move (articulate) on the upper aspect of the cricoid lamina in two manners, gliding from side to side and rocking. Considered in isolation, in the first movement the two arytenoid cartilages are separated (*abducted*). In the second movement, the vocal processes (with vocal folds attached) are brought forward, depressed, and probably brought together (*adducted*). These two movements, isolated or

combined, affect the status and relationship of the vocal folds.

The forward-projecting angle, the vocal process, of the arytenoid cartilages is of considerable importance in laryngeal structure and function. To this process and to the anterolateral surface are attached mucous membrane lining, the vocal ligament, and the muscle of the vocal fold. These pass directly forward and slightly caudad and attach into the angle of the thyroid cartilage internally. Movement of the vocal process causes changes in the vocal fold. Movement of the cricoid, and thus of the arytenoids sitting on the cricoid lamina, also causes a change in the vocal folds. It is very important to remember that changes in the vocal folds may change phonation. Bringing the vocal folds together (adductory movements), taking the vocal folds apart (abductory movements), lengthening (and thus thinning and tensing) the folds, and shortening (and thus thickening and relaxing) the folds, whether alone or in combination, have great effects on the manner in which the folds will vibrate, and thus on how the phonatory product will sound.

Clinical Note

Voice therapists are often called upon to serve persons having voice problems that result from cartilage defects. These defects may result from injury (as from a blow or a penetrating object) or from an abnormal growth (such as cancer or other neoplasm) which affects the operation of the larynx. Therapists are also called upon when the muscular tissues operating the structures of the larynx are injured or paralyzed—for instance, as a result of poliomyelitis, cerebral vascular accidents (strokes), or localized nerve damage.

Another of the cartilages of the larynx is the *epiglottis* (Figs. 5.1, 5.3A, and 5.4). The epiglottis is

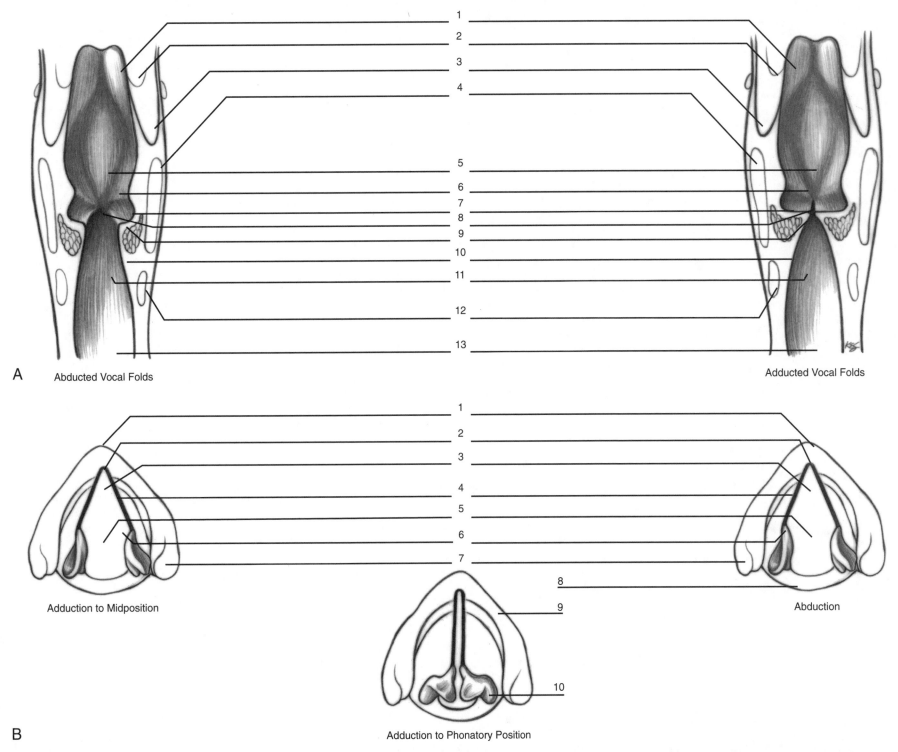

A Abducted Vocal Folds

Adducted Vocal Folds

Adduction to Midposition

Adduction to Phonatory Position

Abduction

B

Figure 5.3A   Larynx (Coronal Views)

Figure 5.3B   Vocal Fold Movements (Superior Views)

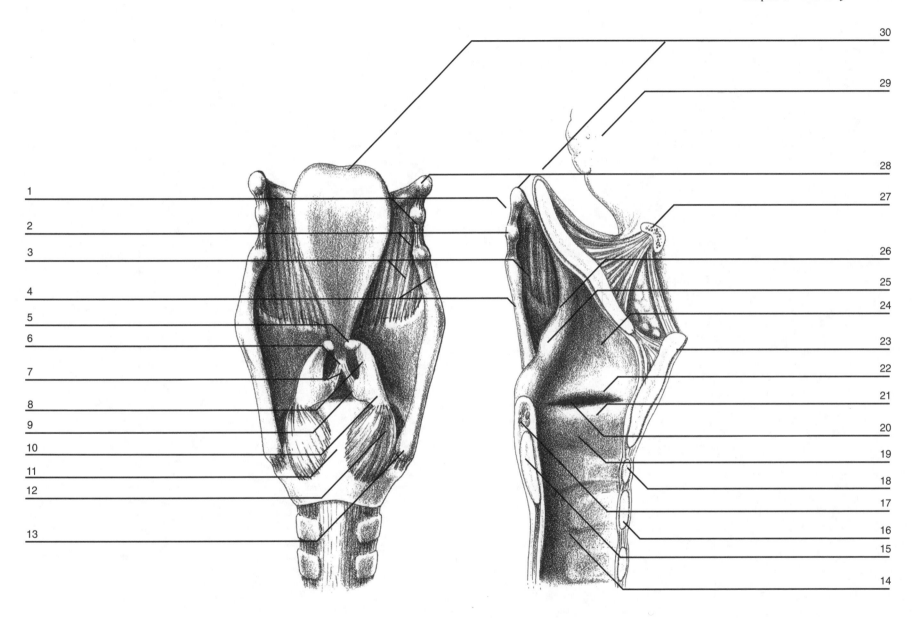

Figure 5.4   Larynx (Posterior and Sagittal Views)

the relatively large, unpaired cartilage at the superior terminus of the larynx, having its broad end cephalad and its narrow, stem-like petiole attached at the angle of the thyroid, internally. This attachment is provided through the *thyroepiglottic ligament,* a ligamentous membrane. The epiglottic cartilage itself is described as being concave-convex, as having a rather undulating appearance and action, and as having many indentations over its surface for the accommodation of mucous glands. As part of the collar of the larynx, the epiglottis can serve to close the opening to the larynx. Although humans can swallow food without an epiglottis, it is considered to be helpful in preventing foreign materials from entering the laryngeal vestibule.

The first of the minor cartilages of the larynx are the *corniculate cartilages* (Fig. 5.4; see Fig. 5.6A, B, C, and D). These paired cartilages cap the arytenoids, serving to continue the length of the apexes. In some individuals, the corniculate cartilages are fused with the larger structures and cannot be seen as separate. Another pair of minor cartilages are the *cuneiform cartilages* (Fig. 5.4). This extremely variable pair of cartilages is found in the aryepiglottic fold; they serve to stiffen and provide elasticity to that fold. A third minor cartilage pair is the *triticeal cartilage,* which is found within the ligaments, or membranes, connecting the superior horns of the thyroid cartilage with the greater horns of the hyoid bone (the hyothyroid ligament). A fourth minor cartilage is the *sesamoid cartilage,* infrequently found in man on the lateral borders of the arytenoid cartilages and connected with the corniculates by elastic ligaments.

The various cartilages vary in composition. The thyroid, cricoid, and arytenoid cartilages are made up of hyaline tissue; the epiglottis, the corniculate cartilage, the cuneiform cartilage, and the apexes of the arytenoids are made up of elastic tissue. Hyaline tissues tend to ossify with age, commencing to do so in early adulthood; by age 65 these cartilages may be entirely ossified.

Connective tissue includes not only bone and cartilage, but ligaments and membranes as well. The ligaments of the larynx are important in supporting the cartilages and the actions of the soft tissues in both respiration and phonation. There are two types of ligaments: (1) the extrinsic, which connect the hyoid bone with the thyroid and epiglottic cartilages and which connect the tracheal rings with the cricoid cartilage (Figs. 5.2 and 5.4), and (2) the intrinsic, which interconnect the laryngeal cartilages (Figs. 5.2, 5.3B, and 5.4).

Of the extrinsic ligaments, the uppermost is the *hyoepiglottic,* internally connecting the body of the hyoid bone with the anterior surface of the epiglottis. Running from the end of the greater cornu of the hyoid bone down to the tip of the superior thyroid cornu is the *hyothyroid ligament* (often termed the lateral hyothyroid ligament, to distinguish it from the middle hyothyroid ligament). Extending from this ligament is the *hyothyroid membrane,* which runs from the inferior border of the hyoid bone to the superior border of the thyroid cartilage. At the anterior midline, this membrane thickens to become the *middle hyothyroid ligament.* The last of the extrinsic ligaments is the *cricotracheal ligament,* which connects the ring of the cricoid with the ring of the first tracheal cartilage.

The intrinsic ligaments of the larynx connect the movable smaller cartilages of the larynx. The *middle cricothyroid ligament* is found anteriorly at the midline, fanning up to the thyroid cartilage from the arch of the cricoid. It is continued laterally by the *cricothyroid membrane,* which is the major structure of the elastic cone of the atrium of the larynx. There is a *posterior* (or *lateral*) *cricothyroid ligament* interconnecting the cricoid cartilage and inferior horn of the thyroid cartilage at the joint. The middle of the posterior surface of the arytenoid cartilage is attached to the lamina of the cricoid below by the *posterior cricoarytenoid ligament.* The epiglottis is attached to the thyroid cartilage by a thin ligament running from the stem to the angle of the

Table 5.1. Extrinsic Muscles of the Larynx

Muscle	Origin	Insertion	Action	Nerve
Suprahyoid				
Stylohyoid	Styloid process of temporal bone	Body of hyoid bone	Elevates and retracts hyoid bone	Cranial VII
Digastric	Anterior belly arises from internal aspect of mandible close to midline; posterior belly arises on medial side of mastoid process of temporal bone	Intermediate tendon and hyoid bone via fascial loop	Elevates hyoid, depresses mandible; separate bellies may move hyoid bone forward or dorsal	Cranial V (anterior belly), Cranial VII (posterior belly)
Mylohyoid	Mylohyoid ridge of mandible	Hyoid bone and median raphe	Raises and projects hyoid bone and tongue	Cranial V
Geniohyoid	Internal surface of mandible at the inferior mental spine	Anterior surface of hyoid bone	Draws hyoid bone forward	Cranial XII
Infrahyoid				
Sternohyoid	Medial extremity of clavicle, superior and posterior portion of sternum, sternoclavicular ligament	Body of hyoid bone, inferior surface	Depresses hyoid bone	Cranial XII
Sternothyroid	Superior and posterior portion of sternum and first costal cartilage	Oblique line of thyroid cartilage	Depresses thyroid cartilage	Cranial XII
Thyrohyoid	Oblique line of thyroid cartilage	Body and greater cornu of hyoid bone	Depresses hyoid bone or elevates thyroid cartilage	Cranial XII
Omohyoid	Superior margin of scapula	Inferior border of body of hyoid bone	Depresses hyoid bone	Cranial XII

thyroid, just above the attachment of the ventricular ligaments, the *thyroepiglottic ligament*.

Other ligaments of the larynx include those of the vocal folds, which are discussed later.

The membranes of the laryngeal skeleton serve important connective tissue functions. The *hyothyroid* (or *thyrohyoid*) membrane is a sheet of thin tissue extending around the upper region anteriorly-posteriorly between hyoid bone and superior border of thyroid cartilage; it is penetrated by nerves and blood vessels serving internal structures. There is also a *cricothyroid*

membrane, mentioned earlier, among the several scattered membranes of the laryngeal region.

Structural differences are found in the laryngeal cartilages. Some are due to growth. As the male child approaches puberty, his laryngeal structures grow larger. The thyroid angle, as a result, becomes more acute. Consequently, the vocal folds are lengthened as well as enlarged in the growth process. The female larynx also grows but, more commonly, does not attain the degree of growth of that of the male. The angle of the thyroid is not acute, giving a rounded impression of the prominence in the neck. The vocal effects are obvious in the male with a fundamental frequency decrease of about an octave, while in the female it is but a note or two.

Clinical Note

Because it is an important part of the vital airway, a damaged larynx can be a threat to life. Accidents (automobile, for example) that crush the larynx can occlude the airway, threatening suffocation. A similar threat may develop when an object (a large piece of food or a toy) may be caught in the glottis between the two vocal folds, again interfering with the passage of air. A person with dysphagia and associated failure of laryngeal closure may aspirate fluids, with the possible result of aspiration pneumonia.

MUSCULATURE

The classic procedure of dividing the laryngeal muscles into two groups, extrinsic and intrinsic, is followed here.

Extrinsic Muscles

By definition, the muscles of the extrinsic group are those attached to the cartilages of the larynx from nonlaryngeal structures—in general, the thorax, the mandible, and the cranium. In viewing the origins in this way, it is not difficult to see the vertical, sling-like arrangement nor to understand that contraction of certain groups affects the position of the larynx in the throat. During the actions of these muscles, gravity is an important antagonist, along with elasticity and the forces produced by other, noncontractile tissues attached to the laryngeal cartilages. In speech production, the extrinsic muscles change the larynx enough to be identified as at least secondary mechanisms in the control of the pitch of the voice.

The extrinsic muscles are further divided into those that are above the hyoid (the suprahyoids) and those that are below the hyoid (infrahyoids). Both groups affect the position of the hyoid bone, which is basically the foundation of the larynx; movement of the hyoid is translated almost directly into movement of all the laryngeal structures.

The *suprahyoid muscle group* consists of muscles passing from the mandible and cranium downward and inserting somewhere upon the hyoid bone. The principal suprahyoid muscles are the stylohyoid, digastric, mylohyoid, and geniohyoid (Table 5.1). Also related are the palatopharyngeal, the stylopharyngeal, and the two lower constrictor muscles of the pharynx, because of their possible insertions upon the hyoid and upon the thyroid cartilage. The hyoglossus muscle, which was discussed earlier as an extrinsic muscle of the tongue, may also be considered a suprahyoid muscle.

The Suprahyoids

The four main paired suprahyoid muscles form a hammock-like arrangement, with the hyoid bone acting as the hammock itself (Fig. 5.5). Thus, the hyoid bone might be pulled upward by anterior and posterior contraction of all muscles or it might be pulled upward and backward or upward and forward by contraction of one or the other end of the supporting muscles. There is also some provision for lateral movement because of the unique arrangement of some of the suprahyoid muscles. These muscles have a close anatomic and functional relationship with both the mandible and the tongue.

The *stylohyoid muscle* originates at the base of the skull at the styloid process. Its fibers pass downward and forward and insert into the body of the hyoid bone at its juncture with the greater cornu. Just before this attachment, the muscle is penetrated by the tendon of the digastric muscle. The nerve supplying the stylohyoid is a branch of the facial nerve (Cranial VII). This muscle retracts and elevates the hyoid bone, with similar effects upon the larynx in general.

The *digastric muscle* is a sling-like muscle with a belly at each end; each belly has its own origin, but the two have a common insertion at their shared tendinous attachment. The anterior belly originates on the internal aspect of the mandible, close to the midline (symphysis menti); its fibers pass backward toward the hyoid bone, ending in the intermediate tendon, located just superior to the hyoid. The posterior belly originates on the medial side of the mastoid process of the temporal bone; its fibers pass downward and forward and terminate in the same intermediate tendon. This tendon, connecting the two bellies of the digastric muscle, is invested with a fibrous loop that continues inferiorly to the hyoid and attaches to its body and part of the greater cornu. Combined action elevates the hyoid bone or depresses the mandible. Individual action of the anterior belly would pull the hyoid bone forward, while the posterior belly would move the bone in the opposite direction. The nerve supply to the two bellies is thought to differ, with the anterior belly receiving its innervation from the trigeminal nerve (Cranial V) and the posterior belly from the facial nerve (Cranial VII).

The *mylohyoid muscle* is a muscle sheet forming the floor of the mouth, upon which rests the tongue. It is oriented between the two sides of the mandible, laterally, and attaches to the hyoid bone centrally. Its origin is generally given as the mylohyoid line of the internal aspect of the mandible, running from the symphysis to the level of the last molar tooth. Its most posterior fibers pass medially and downward and insert into the body of the hyoid bone; the fibers anterior to this meet those fibers from the opposite side at the midline raphe, a thickened line of fibrous tissue extending from the symphysis menti to the hyoid bone. Its action is to elevate the hyoid and thus the laryngeal structures in general, as well as the tongue. Its nerve supply is from the trigeminal nerve (Cranial V).

The *geniohyoid muscle* is a paired muscle, with both members lying close to the midline, originating from the internal surface of the mandibular *genu* at the inferior mental spine. The muscle bundle is fairly compact and thin, running posteriorly and slightly downward and inserting into the anterior surface of the body of the hyoid bone slightly away from its midline. The geniohyoid muscle acts to draw forward the hyoid bone. This muscle is innervated by the hypoglossal nerve (Cranial XII), with some fibers supplied from the first cervical nerve.

Group actions of the suprahyoid muscles require some consideration at this point. Both the tongue and the hyoid bone are recipients of the energies of these muscles, especially in the process of deglutition. Movement of the bolus of food toward the pharynx and protection of the laryngeal entrance are partially effected by suprahyoid muscles. During the first stages of deglutition, the hyoid bone is elevated, forcing the tongue cephalad. The bone also is moved anteriorly. Involved in these actions are the anterior belly of digastric, mylohyoid, and geniohyoid muscles. As the bolus of food enters the pharynx, the stylohyoid and the posterior belly of the digastric contract to pull the hyoid bone and the larynx posterior and upward; this contraction assists in closing the oropharyngeal isthmus and occludes the entrance to the larynx against food particles. Relaxation of these muscles, along with elastic forces and contraction of the infrahyoid muscles, returns the hyoid bone (and consequently the larynx) to its original position.

Clinical Note

Vertical movement of the hyoid bone and thus of the suspended larynx is critical to healthy swallowing. In cases of failure of this movement, as in the case of some stroke victims or of surgical damage to the suprahyoid muscles, may cause the aditus ad laryngis to remain open and available to the penetration of liquids or solids in

1

2

3

4

5

6

7

8

9

19

18

17

16

15

14

13

12

11

10

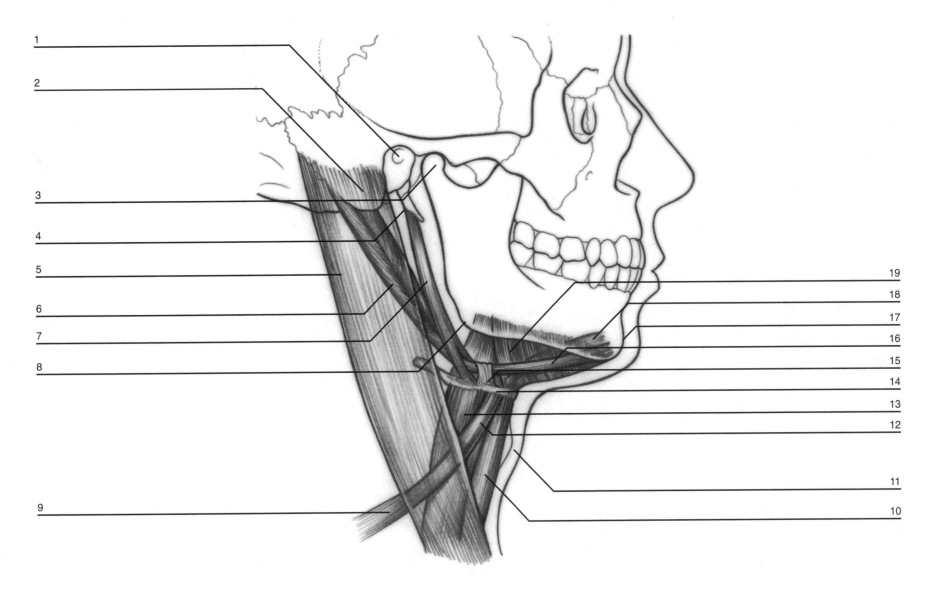

Figure 5.5   Extrinsic Laryngeal Muscles

swallowing. This, in turn, may prove to be life threatening.

The Infrahyoids

The paired *infrahyoid muscle group* is below the hyoid bone, generally running between the larynx and the thorax. The four muscles of this group form a large part of the anterior portion of the neck, immediately alongside the larynx and the trachea. They are the sternohyoid, sternothyroid, thyrohyoid, and omohyoid muscles (Table 5.1, Fig. 5.5). Because of their length and thinness, they are sometimes called the *ribbon* or *strap* muscles of the larynx.

The *sternohyoid muscle* has its origin in the most superior surface of the thorax, at the clavicle bone (posterior surface of the medial end), the sternoclavicular ligament, and the internal surface of the sternum near the midline. From this origin, the thin band of muscle passes upward and slightly medially, finally running in close approximation to its opposite fellow and inserting into the hyoid bone on its inferior surface. Sternohyoid muscle action depresses the hyoid bone, especially in the recovery from the first stages of deglutition. Its nerve supply comes from the hypoglossal nerve (Cranial XII).

The *sternothyroid muscle* is close to the midline of the neck, as is the sternohyoid muscle. It originates at the internal surface of the sternum and from the costal cartilage of the first rib. It is a shorter and wider muscle band than is the sternohyoid muscle, and it runs upward and somewhat laterally to insert into the thyroid cartilage of the larynx at its oblique line. Its action is to depress the thyroid cartilage. It receives its nerve supply from the hypoglossal nerve (Cranial XII).

The *thyrohyoid muscle* appears to be a continuation of the sternothyroid muscle, traveling from the thyroid cartilage to the hyoid bone. Its origin is from the oblique line of the thyroid cartilage. It inserts into the body and lower border of the greater cornu of the hyoid

bone. The action of this muscle is to depress the hyoid bone if the larynx is fixed or to elevate the larynx if the hyoid bone is fixed. The nerve supply to the thyrohyoid muscle comes from the hypoglossal nerve (Cranial XII).

The *omohyoid muscle* is a two-bellied, two-directional muscle with a relatively fixed central tendon. Its course is from the superior margin of the scapula bone in the shoulder region to the hyoid bone. From the scapula, the inferior belly of the omohyoid muscle continues as a flat and narrow band across the lower part of the neck, passing behind the sternocleidomastoid muscle. At this point, it forms a tendon that is ensheathed by a fibrous expansion; this fibrous material is firmly attached to the clavicle, as well as to the deep cervical fascia. The omohyoid muscle then changes its direction, rising nearly vertically and inserting into the lower border of the body of the hyoid bone, just lateral to the insertion of the sternohyoid muscle, which it parallels. Its action is to depress the hyoid bone, to retract it, or to pull it to one side or the other. It receives its nerve supply from the hypoglossal nerve (Cranial XII).

The infrahyoid musculature does have the neural innervation as just indicated. However, there is a more accurate and more detailed nerve supply that might be of interest. Cranial nerve XII (hypoglossal) remains the neural source for this group (as well as for other important muscles of the vocal tract). However, to supply the infrahyoid muscles the main nerve has an offshoot that is joined by branches of the upper two or three cervical (spinal) nerves. These form nerve branches that course down either side of the neck as ansa cervicalis and ansa hypoglossus. Together, these two branches join below the infrahyoids so that a loop (ansa) is formed. From this larger loop, smaller nerve branches travel to each of the infrahyoid muscles.

Group actions of the infrahyoid muscles appear to be restricted to returning the hyoid, and thus the larynx, to its normal position following swallowing. This, then, re-opens the airway for normal breathing.

Table 5.2. Intrinsic Muscles of the Larynx

Muscle	Origin	Insertion	Action	Nerve
Cricothyroid	Caudal border and anterior surface of lower cornu of thyroid cartilage	Anterior and lateral surfaces of arch of cricoid cartilage	Elevates cricoid arch, depressing cricoid lamina; lengthens and tenses vocal folds	Cranial X (superior laryngeal nerve)
Lateral cricoarytenoid	Superior borders of cricoid cartilage	Anterior surface of muscular process	Draws arytenoids forward and medially, aids in rocking arytenoids, adducts vocal folds	Cranial X (inferior laryngeal nerve)
Posterior cricoarytenoid	Posterior surface of cricoid cartilage	Muscular process of arytenoid cartilage	Rocks arytenoid dorsally, abducting vocal processes and folds	Cranial X (inferior laryngeal nerve)
Thyroarytenoid	Internal and inferior surface of the angle of thyroid cartilage	Vocal process and anterior lateral surface of arytenoid cartilages	Draws arytenoids forward, shortens and thickens vocal folds	Cranial X (inferior laryngeal nerve)
Vocalis	Inferior surface of angle of thyroid cartilage at one end and vocal process of arytenoid cartilage at other	Vocal ligament along its length	Differentially tenses vocal folds	Cranial X (inferior laryngeal nerve)
Interarytenoids Transverse	Posterior surface of arytenoid cartilage	Posterior surface of opposite arytenoid	Draws together arytenoid cartilages, adducts vocal folds	Cranial X (inferior laryngeal nerve)
Oblique	Base of one arytenoid cartilage at muscular process	Apex of opposite arytenoid	Draws arytenoid cartilages together, narrows aditus	Cranial X (inferior laryngeal nerve)

The suprahyoids have already elevated the hyoid and drawn it forward and then dorsally in early stages of deglutition. This creates changes to close the laryngeal entrance against the invasion of food or drink during the swallowing act. After the bolus has passed the laryngeal entrance, the infrahyoids contract to return the structures. It is also believed that the omohyoids contract during deep inspiration to stiffen the cervical tissues; this is thought to prevent constriction of the neck blood vessels during the inspiratory action. The extrinsic muscles probably have some effect upon phonation, largely in pitch variation.

Intrinsic Muscles

The intrinsic muscles of the larynx (Table 5.2, Fig. 5.6) are generally felt to be responsible for changes in the condition and position of the vocal folds in various functions of the larynx, including phonation. The extrinsic muscles of the larynx—the suprahyoids

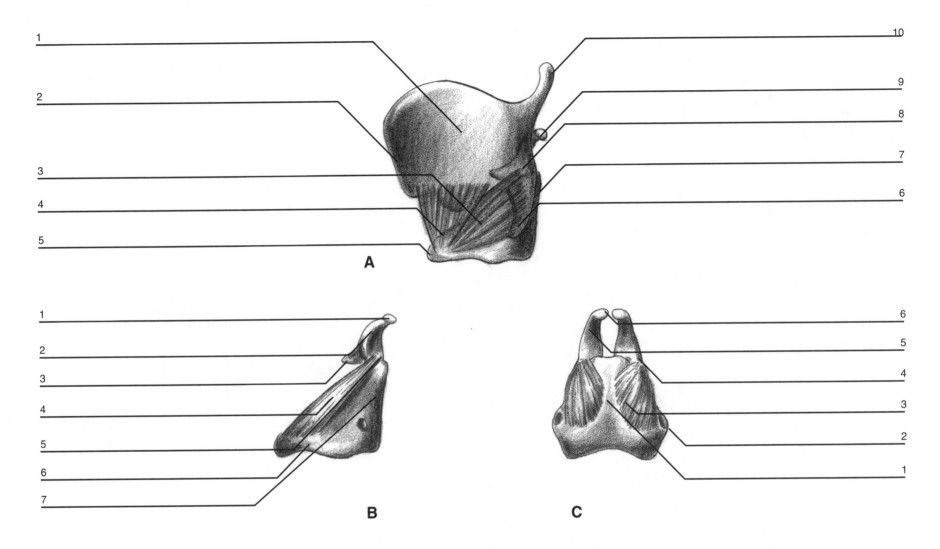

1
2
3
4
5

A

10
9
8
7
6

1
2
3
4
5
6
7

B

6
5
4
3
2
1

C

Figure 5.6A   Intrinsic Laryngeal Muscles: Superficial (Lateral View)

Figure 5.6B   Intrinsic Laryngeal Muscles: Lateral Cricoarytenoid

Figure 5.6C   Intrinsic Laryngeal Muscles: Posterior Cricoarytenoid

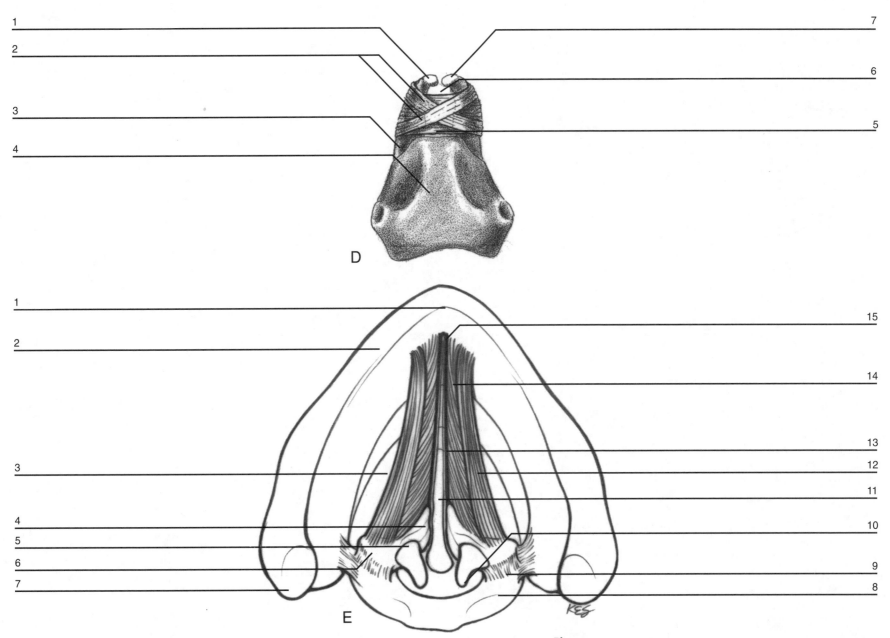

D

E

Figure 5.6D   Intrinsic Laryngeal Muscles: Interarytenoid

Figure 5.6E   Intrinsic Laryngeal Muscles: Thyroarytenoid

and infrahyoids—contribute to voice production to some extent, but the major consideration in the production of vocal sound is the role of the intrinsic musculature upon the structures more directly responsible for production of the laryngeal tone.

Five muscles constitute the group that provides for internal adjustments of the larynx during phonation and other functions. There are smaller divisions of these muscles that may be separate and thus named separately. The five larger muscles commonly recognized are the cricothyroid, lateral cricoarytenoid, posterior cricoarytenoid, interarytenoid, and thyroarytenoid.

The *cricothyroid muscle* is found on the outer surface of the larynx in two parts, one oblique and one erect (or vertical). The name of the muscles (origin first, insertion second) indicates the traditional view of the origin and insertion, but in recent years somewhat different views have resulted from careful studies. Because the action appears to be one of lowering of the cricoid lamina (rather than depression of the thyroid lamina), the origin is seen as the inferior border of the thyroid lamina and the anterior border of the inferior thyroid cornu for the erect and oblique bundles, respectively. The insertion of the cricothyroid muscle is the superior border of the arch of the cricoid cartilage anterolaterally. Upon contraction, the arch of the cricoid cartilage is elevated toward the thyroid cartilage as the entire cartilage rotates at the cricothyroid joint. As the cricoid arch elevates, the lamina lowers. With the vocal folds attached to the arytenoid cartilages atop the cricoid lamina, the posterior-inferior arcing lengthens the distance from the internal aspect of the thyroid angle, and the vocal folds are lengthened and tensed and thinned. Uniquely, the *superior laryngeal nerve* from the vagus nerve (Cranial X) innervates this muscle.

The *lateral cricoarytenoid muscle* on either side connects the cricoid with the arytenoid cartilages. Its origin is the upper lateral border of the arch of the cricoid cartilage, and its fibers pass upward and backward. They insert into the anterior surface of the muscular process of the arytenoid cartilage. In many instances, differentiation of this muscle from the thyroarytenoid muscle is difficult or even impossible. The lateral cricoarytenoid muscle is a vocal fold adductor; upon contraction, it pulls the muscular processes of the arytenoid cartilages anteriorly, and the vocal processes move medially to approximate and slightly tense the vocal folds. This action results in medial compression of the vocal folds, adduction that partially establishes a phonatory posture. The nerve supply comes from the anterior branch of the *inferior laryngeal nerve,* a division of the vagus nerve (Cranial X).

The *posterior cricoarytenoid muscle,* the "safety" muscle of the larynx, runs from the external surface of the cricoid lamina to the posterior surface of the arytenoid's muscular process (Figs. 5.4 and 5.7C). Its origin is oriented vertically alongside the midline of the cricoid lamina, so that the uppermost fibers of this muscle run nearly horizontally and the lower fibers nearly vertically. They insert onto the dorsal surface and tip of the muscular process of the arytenoid cartilage. The action of the posterior cricoarytenoid muscle is to abduct the vocal folds by retracting the muscular processes, contributing to a rocking, rotating movement of the arytenoid cartilage. This muscle is the only abductor of the larynx (thus the name "safety" muscle). It is the antagonist of the lateral cricoarytenoid muscle. The nerve supply is from the posterior branch of the inferior laryngeal nerve (Cranial X).

The *interarytenoid (arytenoid) muscle* is a posterior midline muscle consisting of two portions, one of which is not paired (Fig. 5.6D). These two are the transverse portion and the oblique portion. The transverse part is unpaired and runs from the posterior concave surface of one arytenoid cartilage to the same region of the opposite cartilage. The oblique and outermost portion originates dorsally near the tip of the muscular process of each arytenoid cartilage. Its fibers rise toward the apex of the opposite arytenoid, crossing the fibers of the other of the pair at the midline. At the apex, some fibers insert and terminate; others continue on around the apex, joining the thyroarytenoid muscle; some fibers run into the aryepiglottic fold to become the *aryepiglottic muscle.* The interarytenoid muscle, especially the transverse portion, contracts to adduct the arytenoid cartilages thus completing the glottal closure partially accomplished by the lateral cricoarytenoid muscle. This is important as a valve against the invasion of foreign materials and basic to establishing a phonatory posture. This muscle also closes the laryngeal opening by approximating the apexes of the two arytenoid cartilages; at the same time, the laryngeal vestibule is narrowed and the vocal folds are approximated. The nerve supply of both parts of the interarytenoid muscle is the anterior branch of the inferior laryngeal nerve from the vagus nerve (Cranial X).

The *thyroarytenoid muscle,* the fifth of the larger intrinsic laryngeal muscles, forms a large part of the vocal fold and the lateral walls bounding the fold. It arises internally from the lower portion of the angle of the thyroid cartilage, and its fibers pass posteriorly as a triangular band. The broad horizontal part of the triangle forms a part of the lateral wall of the larynx and of the ventricular fold. The narrow medial band of fibers runs parallel to the vocal ligament, with approximately the same anterior and posterior attachments. The thyroarytenoid muscle inserts into the vocal process and the anterolateral surface of the arytenoid cartilage. This muscle contracts to move the arytenoid cartilage anteriorly, thus shortening and thickening the vocal fold. This muscle may be antagonistic to the cricothyroid muscle as it lengthens, tenses, and thins the vocal fold. The nerve supplying this muscle is the anterior branch of the inferior laryngeal nerve from the vagus nerve (Cranial X).

The *vocalis muscle* is generally considered to be a part of the thyroarytenoid muscle, and thus may be called the *internal thyroarytenoid muscle.* However, its fibers exit from the larger muscle along the length of the thyroarytenoid (vocal) ligament to insert along that

ligament. The action may be rather complex and certainly is not well understood. Upon contraction of this muscle, the arytenoid cartilage is pulled anteriorly, thickening and shortening the vocal fold. Also considered as part of its action is a contraction that provides for differential tensing of the vocal fold, which may account for fine control during phonation. Earlier investigators had considered this an important function of this muscle and termed the fibers so identified the *pitch fibers* of the thyroarytenoid muscle. The nerve supply is thought to be identical with that of the main muscle, the anterior branch of the inferior laryngeal nerve.

Noted earlier is another lesser muscle, the *aryepiglottic.* This probably is derived from the oblique fibers of the interarytenoid muscle, but passes from the arytenoid apex through the aryepiglottic fold to insert into the midlateral border of the epiglottic cartilage. It probably serves during closure of the aditus and laryngis (laryngeal opening) to depress the epiglottis and narrow the opening to prevent the entrance of foreign (food) materials. It is an inconstant and "wispy" muscle and may prove to be less than essential, as the epiglottis itself may be. Its nerve supply is probably the same as that for the interarytenoid muscle, the anterior branch of the inferior laryngeal nerve (Cranial X).

An even more inconstant muscle is the *thyroepiglottic,* a muscle originating above the petiole of the epiglottis at the internal aspect of the thyroid cartilage angle. Its fibers pass dorsally and superiorly to insert into the midregion of the anterior surface of the epiglottic cartilage. If present, its action is likely to assist the epiglottis to return to its rest position, by elevation, after it has been depressed during deglutition. It too is probably not an essential muscle and joins the other structures of the epiglottic complex in that sense. Its nerve supply is probably the inferior laryngeal nerve (Cranial X).

Studies of the actions of the vocal fold and of the prime movers of the fold indicate that simple adduction or simple tensing rarely occurs. It should also be clear that the descriptions given above are simply of the primary functions of each of the muscles. Researchers have demonstrated that the contraction of individual muscle groups that produces either rotation or gliding of the arytenoids to effect changes in the vocal folds is not so simple. For example, the normal resting position of the arytenoids is posteriorly over the crest of the lamina of the cricoid dorsally, and group muscular contraction causes the arytenoids to mount this crest. The effect is that the vocal processes of the arytenoids seem to approximate, first by rocking and then by gliding of the bodies of the arytenoids. Bringing the vocal folds into and sustaining a phonatory posture is a delicate and elegant maneuver, far more so than the gross glottal closure required for protective valving. It is likely that both intrinsic and extrinsic muscle serve various phonatory behaviors, a most sophisticated activity.

GROUP ACTIONS

Although actions of the various muscles have been described somewhat in the earlier sections, a restatement and slight expansion might clarify some of the details of laryngeal activities. It must be remembered that the larynx is (1) a protective valve against accidents in the respiratory tract, (2) an active participant in swallowing in part because it is a protective valve, and (3) an important generator of the laryngeal tone in speech production. Of course, it serves other functions as well; for example, as a valve to fix thoracic air for an anchor against which to lift heavy weights and eliminate abdominal contents.

As a protective valve, the vocal folds adduct rapidly at such times that a foreign object (a food crumb, a drop of saliva) enters the laryngeal vestibule and stimulates the sensory system within. With air pressure increasing from exhaled air below the vocal folds, sudden release (by abducting the folds) causes a rush of air carrying the foreign material from the larynx: a cough. Naturally, this maneuver (coughing) is a life-protecting one.

In swallowing, the protective function is the product of a widespread activity involving both the pharynges and the larynx. As the bolus of food being swallowed enters the pharynx, signals direct the laryngeal structures to elevate in the neck. This causes, among other things, the opening of the larynx (aditus) to be pressured nearly closed. It may be that the epiglottis is bent backward and downward to cover the entrance and that the aryepiglottic fold is brought toward midline in this activity. However it happens, there is less of an opening for the food to enter the larynx to threaten the airway below. One can easily palpate (feel) laryngeal excursion as one swallows. In a similar maneuver, the larynx has a vertical excursion during pitch changes in the voice. Singing up and down the scale is often mirrored by elevation and depression of the larynx in the neck.

In the preceding eventuality, laryngeal excursion during pitch changes, one can conjure similar maneuvers during nonsinging speech activities. Pitch changes occur in regular speech (melody, intonation), and movement of the larynx may be observable during that activity. One also could imagine that not only are the extrinsic laryngeal muscles changing the position of the larynx in the neck, but at the same time intrinsic muscles are creating vocal fold changes to create pitch changes. It is not difficult to conclude that both extrinsic and intrinsic musculature can be working together in the complex speech act.

The third major function of the larynx is to create phonation itself. This important physiologic behavior generates the laryngeal tone. That sound is essential for normal vowel production and for an important component (voicing) in many consonant sounds. The complex activity in phonation demands coordination of more than one of the activities described above. All of the respiratory mechanisms must be involved, for we speak on exhaled air. The vocal folds then must be adducted to provide a narrow constriction against the exhaled air. The folds might be shortened or lengthened, depending upon the pitch to be generated. So, there must be a finely coordinated muscle activity of adduction-abduction, exhaled air, lengthening-shortening (thinning-tensing), and elevation or depression of the entire laryngeal structure. The complexity of the system is truly wondrous.

NERVOUS TISSUES

The primary cranial nerve supplying the laryngeal region (Fig. 5.7) is the vagus nerve (Cranial X). Two branches of this nerve are of import to the muscles of the larynx. After it leaves its protective cranial vault to course down the neck, the vagus nerve gives off a branch called the *superior laryngeal nerve*. This nerve runs along the side of the larynx and innervates the cricothyroid muscle, and only that muscle. The superior laryngeal nerve has an extremely important sensory branch; it serves to communicate to the central nervous system the condition of (e.g., dryness and pain) and the presence of foreign objects in the vestibule. Other afferent laryngeal systems include those of proprioception in the musculature and joints and touch-pressure systems in the mucosal lining.

Later in its course the vagus nerve gives off a larger branch, which travels caudally below major blood vessels in the upper thoracic region (the arch of the aorta on the left side and the subclavian artery on the right) and then reverses its direction. Hence, its name is the *recurrent laryngeal nerve* (or the *inferior laryngeal nerve*), and it ultimately supplies all of the intrinsic muscles of the larynx except the cricothyroid muscle.

Clinical Note

Of considerable interest to the clinician are neural lesions producing phonatory defects. Such lesions are frequently irreversible, and treatment is complex and difficult. Among the types of dysphonias that may be produced are those caused by lesions developing in the region of the brain's nucleus ambiguus; this type of lesion causes difficulties similar to those caused by paralytic influences of the bulbar type. Phonation may be destroyed or seriously disturbed in such cases, and voice therapy becomes a major procedure in the rehabilitation process. Another type of defect, infrequently encountered by the speech pathologist, is a lesion or disturbance of the peripheral nerve. Thyroid gland problems, surgery, accidents, tumors, and pressures produced by edemas or foreign matter may well produce phonatory defects. The extent of the lesion determines the extent of the phonatory defect; it is possible that only a small portion of the muscles will be affected, and the vocal sound may only be disturbed, not absent.

The muscles of phonation in the larynx are closely related to those of swallowing. Both the glossopharyngeal and the vagus nerves, which are in very close approximation, contribute to the pharyngeal plexus. The pharyngeal plexus, in turn, is largely responsible for nerve supply to the muscles of the pharynx and mouth, except for the tensor (veli) palatine. The vagus nerve (with possible added fibers from Cranial XI, the accessory nerve) gives off the superior laryngeal and recurrent laryngeal nerves, serving the laryngeal musculature. The constrictors of the pharynx, lying as they do in close proximity to the cartilages of the larynx and even finding origin in those cartilages, are closely related to the muscles of the larynx through the common neural origins.

The extrinsic (strap) muscles of the larynx (see Table 5.1) receive a somewhat complex neural innervation. For example, although the table indicates that Cranial XII serves the infrahyoid musculature, it is more likely that several nerves provide that innervation.

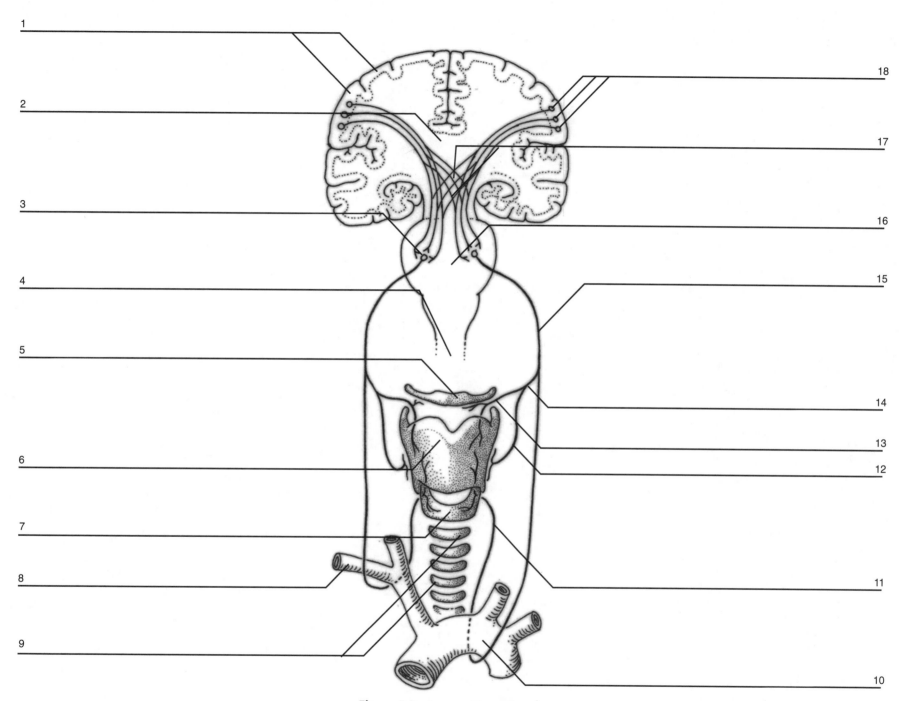

Figure 5.7   Larynx Nerve Supply

Agreement does not seem to exist on the exact structure of the nerves in this region; contributions to these muscles are said to come from Cranial X, Cranial XI, and Cranial XII, as well as from the top two or three cervical nerves of the spinal cord. Apparently, these cranial nerves act as sources of some fibers that contribute to a long, looping nerve network sometimes called the *ansa hypoglossi*. From this network come the various nerve fibers that serve to stimulate the musculature of the infrahyoid group. In contrast, the suprahyoid group does not present quite as complicated a picture, although there is considerable variation in the innervation of this group. This innervation can be associated with embryonic development and with functional relationships. Cranial VII (the facial nerve) serves both the stylohyoid muscle and the posterior belly of the digastric muscle, which are associated with similar actions. Cranial V innervates the anterior belly of the digastric and the mylohyoid, both being superior and anterior to the larynx in origin and having somewhat similar effects upon the laryngeal region. The hypoglossal nerve (Cranial XII) serves the geniohyoid muscle and the genioglossus muscle, which are closely related in location and perhaps in actions.

THEORY OF PHONATION

A simple theory of phonation has the vocal folds opening and closing during exhalation. This gives rise to puffs of air that set up a vibratory activity in the air above the glottis. Since sound is vibration in a medium, this *puff theory* is plausible. It is a simple theory and probably incomplete; it does not concern itself with information that adds considerable detail to the description of phonation.

Another somewhat widely held explanation of phonation is called the *neurochronaxic theory*. In simple terms, this theory associates the vibratory rate of the vocal folds with the rate that nerve impulses reach the laryngeal musculature. This theory caused a flurry of research, which resulted in a theory more acceptable to many specialists, the *aerodynamic-myoelastic theory*.

The aerodynamic-myoelastic theory of phonation describes the phonatory act as follows. First, the laryngeal musculature contracts to adduct the vocal folds, thus constricting the glottis. Second, the exhaled air flowing up from the lungs meets the folds and the narrowed opening; the pressure and the rate of flow increase. The air rapidly streaming past the lips of the vocal folds gives rise to a negative pressure, and the folds are further adducted. Third, the exhaled air is met with increased resistance from the closing glottis (i.e., the adducting vocal folds) until the air pressure from below literally blows apart the vocal folds, and a puff of air is emitted. This lowers the air pressure from below, and the elastic and muscular conditions of the folds cause them to adduct again. Thus, the event repeats in a periodic, regular manner. The laryngeal tone results when the puffs of air create a pressure wave of disturbances (sound) in the airway above.

Different sounds are produced at the larynx in a number of ways. The subglottal air pressure changes along with air flow changes. The adherent mucous membrane covering of the vocal folds plays a role, as do the activities of the various centers of elasticity in the larynx and the length, tension, and cross-sectional mass of the vocal folds. Other variable factors also are considered important.

In the name *aerodynamic-myoelastic theory*, *aero-* refers to air (both pressure and flow); *-dynamic* refers to movement and change (during exhalation and phonation); *myo-* refers to the muscular forces establishing the posture of the vocal folds (adduction); and *-elastic* refers to the ability of an object to return to its original state.

The aerodynamic-myoelastic theory provides some explanation of phonation, particularly of changes in pitch and loudness. However, other phonatory phenomena and laryngeal behaviors are still in need of explanation.

VOICE CHARACTERISTICS

The vocal folds produce laryngeal tones that differ among us as much as the anatomy of the vocal system differs among us. Add to those latter differences those differences in our individual utilization of the vocal mechanisms and we find even more disparities. So, we do not expect all voices to sound alike

First, we expect there to be a difference between the voices of prepubertal children and adults. One difference lies in the *fundamental frequencies* characteristic of the two groups. The fundamental frequency refers to the lowest acoustic element of the phonatory product; it is the product of the vibration of the vocal folds themselves. Because the child's vocal mechanisms are still relatively small and the vocal fold vibration is result of the size and configuration of those folds, the fundamental frequency is approximately 250 Hertz (or cycles per second). There is little difference between male and female children's voices. It must be remembered that this figure is definitely an approximation; it is close to middle C on the piano scale.

Second, we know there are phonatory differences between the adult male and the adult female voices. At puberty, the larynges of both sexes grow. The cartilages, and thus the vocal folds, of the male grow considerably with the thyroid angle becoming rather acute while that of the female becomes more obtuse. Thus, the male vocal folds are longer and larger than those of the female. The resulting fundamental frequencies differ considerably. The adult male changes about an octave, dropping to around 125 Hertz (cycles per second). The adult female to slightly more than 200 Hertz, a musical note or two.

Third, pitch ranges vary considerably from person to person. The extreme comparison might be between highly trained singers and the individual who has no musical experience. One might expect the nonsinger to have a range of one and a half to two octaves. This could be exceeded greatly by the singer. The range is complicated by its two ends. At the upper (highest pitch) end, we find the falsetto. At the lower end (lowest pitch), the glottal fry occurs. The question arises as to the inclusion or exclusion of these extreme pitch levels in calculating the pitch range.

Phonation is the result of physical and physiologic conditions. Underlying is the anatomic nature of the sound generator. What the structures are, in terms of size and shape and ballistic abilities, the nature of the muscles in terms of their use, the aerodynamics and the auditory feedback are all aspects of phonation to be considered.

SUMMARY

The vocal tract begins inferiorly at the larynx, which functions importantly in phonation and as part of the respiratory tract. The larynx is shaped somewhat like an hourglass. The upper space is the vestibule; the lower space is the atrium, and the narrow opening between them is the glottis. The doorway between the vestibule and the posterior laryngopharynx above is the aditus ad laryngis. The atrium opens into the trachea.

The aditus ad laryngis is formed by the collar of the larynx, which is composed of the epiglottis, the aryepiglottic fold, the cuneiform cartilage, and the arytenoid cartilage.

The vestibule contains the ventricular folds. The (true) vocal folds are found at the glottis, with their undersurface bounding the atrium. As the vocal folds adduct and abduct, the undersurface (the elastic cone) acts as a nozzle for the flow of exhaled air.

The connective tissues of the larynx consist of the hyoid bone, five major cartilages, four minor cartilages, and various ligaments.

The musculature of the larynx is divided into the extrinsic muscles (consisting of the suprahyoids and the infrahyoids) and the intrinsic muscles. The extrinsic muscles function mainly in deglutition and secondarily in phonation. The intrinsic muscles mainly effect changes in the position of the vocal folds.

The nervous tissues of the larynx consist of the vagus (Cranial X) nerve and its subdivisions, the superior laryngeal and the recurrent laryngeal nerves, serving the intrinsic musculature, while branches of the hypoglossal (XII) nerve serves the infrahyoids and other cranial nerves innervate the suprahyoid muscles.

The theory of phonation is still incomplete. The so-called puff theory and the neurochronaxic theory have been supplanted by the more sophisticated aerodynamic-myoelastic theory. Broadly speaking, phonation arises when puffs of air emerge from the glottis and set up vibrations in the spaces above. However, further research of how such puffs of air arise and are controlled continues.

Clinical Implications

Voice disorders may be fairly common in our social world. They may stem from abuse that negatively affects the anatomic structures. Thus, when the vocal folds are severely adducted (as in yelling or constant loud vocalizations), the overlying mucous membranes may have tissue changes that could be deleterious to normal phonation. Such changes as vocal nodules or contact ulcers occur in the persons with voice disorders. Obviously, the vibratory behavior of the folds might be disturbed by such changes, and the voice affected.

We might find that the nerve supply, via the recurrent laryngeal nerve, to the intrinsic muscles of the larynx do not serve those muscles adequately. The resulting phonatory disorder may stem from vibratory abnormalities of the vocal folds. Examples of underlying pathologies include stroke and damage to the nerves in the neck region.

At times, transitory health problems are causally related to abnormalities of vocal fold function, and thus of voice disorders. A severe cold or other upper respiratory tract condition might create swollen vocal folds. This change in the size and the regularity of the vocal fold margins can result in vibratory patterns that yield abnormal phonation.

Moving from phonation to other clinical implications, we examine the functions of the vocal folds and the larynx as a whole in other body disorders. Here, for instance, we find swallowing problems. Perhaps as a result of a brain injury or stroke, the patient's swallowing functions are disturbed. Some of this is associated with failure of the laryngeal spaces to close during swallowing to protect the lower respiratory tract from foreign materials. As a result, aspiration pneumonias may occur in such patients. Examination of the larynx and its behavior is usually a part of a swallowing assessment by the speech pathologist.

Laryngeal functioning in phonation is an important part of human life. It serves many other animals as well, for we find food calls and mating calls and threatening calls important to the lives of such creatures. The human adds more "social" purposes, of course, to his/her reason for talking, which is the most important human function, and is heavily dependent upon phonation.

Study Questions

1. *With your mouth open, hold your breath, then abruptly release it with a vocal tone. What physiologic events occur at the glottis?*

2. *To contract your abdominal muscles efficiently, the glottis should be closed. Can you monitor this laryngeal action?*

3. *Produce an [h] sound alone. What is the status of the glottis? How did it get there?*

4. *Produce an [h] sound, then slide into phonation. What muscles are contracting to affect what conditions in the glottis?*

5. *Phonate an [Ah] sound at a low pitch. With your fingertip on your laryngeal prominence, elevate the pitch rapidly as high as you can. What happens to the larynx? After stopping phonation, what happens to the larynx? Why do these actions occur?*

6. *Place one finger on the laryngeal prominence and an adjacent finger just behind the symphysis menti. Observe what happens as you swallow. What muscle groups and muscles are involved?*

7. *With your finger on the laryngeal prominence, alternate between a very high pitched tone and a low one. Can you identify a change in position of the larynx and describe the prime movers?*

8. *Observe all of the body actions occurring during a cough.*

9. *What seems to be occurring during throat clearing? Can this be performed easily without phonation?*

10. *Can you phonate while inhaling? What are the physiologic differences?*

Chapter 6
The Respiratory System

GENERAL INTRODUCTION

One speaks with air as it is exhaled from the lungs. Although the speaking act is the focus here, the primary purpose of breathing is to support life by supplying oxygen for the body cells and removing from the body the waste, carbon dioxide. These gases (oxygen and carbon dioxide), which are transported into and out of the lungs via the respiratory tract, are carried to and from the cells of the body by the blood in the circulatory system. The lungs serve the blood by providing for this life-supporting exchange of gases.

There are three aspects of respiration. The first is *ventilation*, the movement of air back and forth between the outside atmosphere and the internal spaces of the lungs. The second is *external respiration*, the exchange of gases between the walls of the lung spaces and the transporting blood. The third is *internal respiration*, in which gases are exchanged between the blood and the cells of the body.

In the speaking act, the structures of the respiratory tract develop the forces (in the form of pressures) required to generate the sounds of spoken language. The respiratory system functions as a pump that produces air pressures (e.g., subglottal air pressure) that move structures, such as the vocal folds. The flowing, pressurized air is set into vibration by the folds, and sound is produced. The air under pressure also flows past constrictions (e.g., tongue, lips, and teeth) in the upper vocal tract, and sound is produced by the turbulent air flow. The respiratory tract produces the energizing flows and pressures essential for the production of the acoustic events called speech.

Clinical Note

Some normal but highly skilled individuals expend considerable time and effort in training their respiratory systems; public speakers and especially singers often do this to improve performance. Persons with nervous system damage (for example, those with cerebral palsy) may demonstrate important communication problems stemming from breath support difficulties. Speech clinicians may be required to attend to this weakness, as well as providing techniques for the person to use in improving the speaking act. Observation of the functioning of the respiratory support system for speech is commonly part of a total evaluation of a client.

The thorax houses the *pulmonary system*, a large part of the respiratory tract. This system includes the trachea, the bronchi, and the lung structures themselves. It lies within a bony and muscular rib cage anatomically and functionally associated with the abdomen. This enclosure is called the *chest wall*. The tract lies above the abdomen and its contents, but the two regions are importantly associated in the act of breathing. The connective tissues (i.e., the bones and cartilaginous structures in the thorax) serve to protect the respiratory tract within. More importantly, they serve to produce many of the changes in that tract that ultimately result in the passage of air into and out of the body from the surrounding atmosphere.

THE RESPIRATORY TRACT

Anatomically, the respiratory tract is extensive; it also is subject to individual and sex differences. The tract starts superiorly with the two nasal passages; the mouth is also used occasionally to conduct atmospheric air into (and out of) the pharynx. The air then passes into and through the larynx and thence into the *trachea* (or windpipe). Within the thorax (the bone-encased upper region of the trunk), the trachea divides into two *bronchi*. Each of these penetrates and becomes part of the right or left lung, where it further divides. Over 20 such divisions take place, producing at the blind ends of the tubular tract over a million tiny alveoli, minuscule pouches whose walls are in intimate relationship with the walls of the vessels of the blood (vascular) system.

The spaces, or volumes, of the respiratory tract are formed by walled tubes and chambers. The nature of these walls may affect the volume and pressure of air.

The *trachea* (Fig. 6.1) is a tube lined with mucous membrane and supported by cartilaginous rings and musculomembranous portions. It extends downward from the lower border of the cricoid cartilage of the larynx, which is at about the level of the sixth cervical vertebra. The trachea descends nearly vertically downward until it bifurcates (divides) at about the level of the fifth thoracic vertebra. The 16 to 20 tracheal rings are incomplete circles of hyaline cartilage and are irregular in width and thickness. The incomplete portion of the cartilaginous rings is dorsal, where the musculomembranous portion completes the circle. This dorsal portion is adjacent to the similarly descending esophagus, which carries food to the stomach.

From the point of bifurcation of the trachea, the two bronchi pass laterally to the lungs. The right and left bronchi differ from each other in angulation, diameter, and length. Entering the lung through its *hilus*, each bronchus subdivides into *pulmonary bronchi;* each bronchus serves a *pulmonary lobe.* Further subdividing takes place until the blind ends of the last division are reached. Each such end is a *pulmonary alveolus.*

Each alveolus shares a wall one cell thick with the vascular capillaries. Through this wall external respiration takes place. The oxygen-carbon dioxide exchange occurs *via* diffusion: the red blood cells give up carbon dioxide across the membrane barrier into the alveoli and the cells then take up oxygen that has diffused through the barrier.

A lung is a highly elastic, cone-like structure; it is easily collapsible because of the large amount of air held within the alveoli. A lung has a *base,* an *apex,* and two *surfaces.* The base is large and concave, the right lung's being larger and more concave than that of the left. The concavity accommodates the convexity of the diaphragm muscle and the lobe of the liver beneath. As the diaphragm elevates or depresses, the base of the lung follows that movement. The apex of the lung is a small, rounded projection, usually extending up into the root of the neck above the clavicle bone.

The two surfaces of the lung are the *costal (rib) surface* and the *mediastinal (medial) surface.* The former is quite extensive, being formed in part by the extent and shape of the ribs. This costal surface is smooth and convex and sometimes demonstrates the position of the individual ribs by appropriate indentations. The mediastinal surface is concave and irregular and faces medially toward the mediastinum, the middle space of the thorax that contains the heart, its vessels and its coverings, major portions of the trachea and bronchi, and the esophagus. The surface facing this region is indented to accommodate the pericardium of the heart. It has a further depression, the hilus, which carries the bronchus, the pulmonary blood vessels, and nerves into and out of the lung.

Lungs are divided into *lobes.* The difference in the

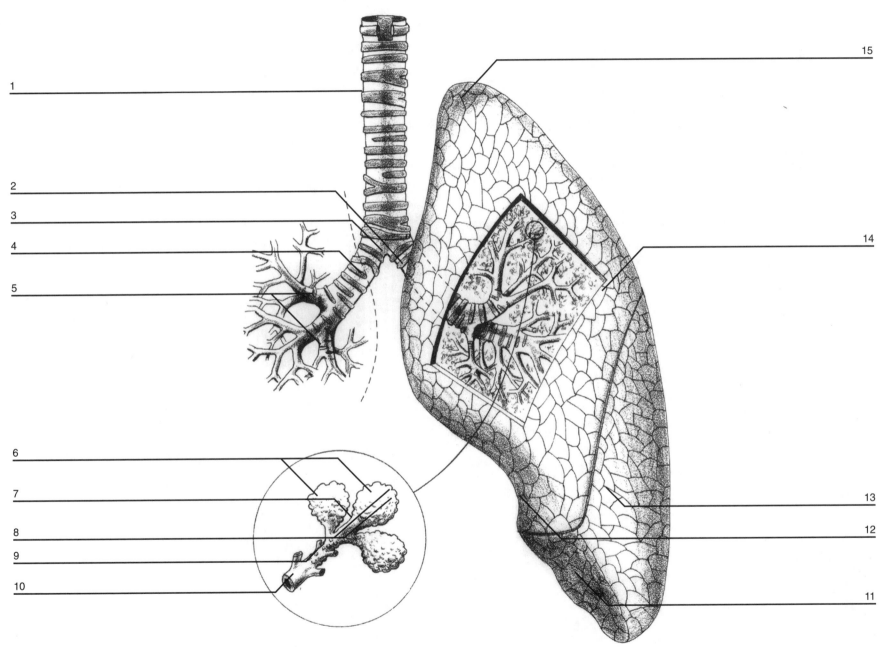

Figure 6.1   Lower Respiratory Tract

number of lobes in the two lungs is because of the placement of the heart and other mediastinal contents. The three right pulmonary lobes are called the superior, middle, and inferior; the two left lobes are the superior and inferior.

Adherent to each of the lungs is a serous (fluid-producing) membrane, the *pleura*. The *pulmonary (visceral) pleura* covers the outer surface of the lungs and extends deep into the fissures between the lobes. The outermost membrane layer is the *parietal pleura,* which lines the inner surface of the thorax and covers the diaphragm. The two pleurae are fused together at the hilus. There may be a potential space between the two layers, the *pleural cavity.* In healthy individuals the two layers are linked together via a fluid interface that also provides for smooth, lubricated movements of the lungs in respiration. The framework for the system, the ribs and floor of the thorax, is moved by muscles, enlarging the thoracic volume.

To breathe, one must expand the thorax and increase its volume. This is accomplished in part by movements of bones to which muscles are attached. This discussion of respiration begins with the bones of the vertebral column, partly because the ribs articulate with them and muscles are attached to them; the spinal cord found within them will be discussed later.

CONNECTIVE TISSUES

There are numerous bones of interest in the thoracic region. At the dorsal aspect of the thorax are found the vertebrae (Fig. 6.2), which join to form the "backbone" and through which passes the spinal cord. From the vertebrae, passing around the sides of the chest and oriented medially thereafter, are the flat ribs, which are interconnected by muscles and attached by cartilages ventrally to the sternum bone. Surmounting the entire structure are the clavicles and the scapulas of the shoulder region, protecting the thorax superiorly. Abdominal structures relate to respiration, and the hip bones of the pelvic girdle provide abdominal muscle and other attachments of some importance in respiratory activities.

The typical unpaired *vertebra* (Figs. 6.2 to 6.4) is formed by a *body* and three *processes,* which extend from the lamina. The body is the largest portion of the vertebra and is nearly cylindrical. It has a large, spongy bone centrum and the usual compact bone cortex. It is the most anterior portion of the vertebrae, facing the belly wall. From its more dorsal extremity project the two *lamina* that form the *arches* of the vertebra. These, along with the body, enclose the *central canal,* which houses the spinal cord. The two lamina are fused posteriorly and extend farther as a single *spinous process* at the midline. Projecting somewhat laterally from the lamina on either side are the paired *transverse processes,* of importance for the articulation of ribs. On the transverse processes and body are the *articulating facets,* two inferior and two superior, which permit movement of the head and neck of the ribs. Adjacent vertebrae articulate with each other via *superior* and *inferior* articulating processes. There is a cartilaginous disc between adjacent vertebrae.

The typical vertebral column is a flexible structure composed of groups of vertebrae. The superior *cervical vertebrae* are seven in number; the first, supporting the cranium, is named the *atlas,* and the second is the *axis.* Below the seven cervical vertebrae are the 12 *thoracic vertebrae,* which receive the 12 ribs and therefore serve as parts of the respiratory system. Beneath the thoracic vertebrae and continuing the vertebral column caudad are the five *lumbar vertebrae.* Subsequent to these are the five fused *sacral vertebrae* and the four or five fused *coccygeal vertebrae* (Fig. 6.2; see Fig. 6.6). The vertebrae increase in size and mass as one examines them from above and travels inferiorly. This might be expected because of the increase in pressure and stress as one compares lower with upper vertebrae. Also, the vertebral column has increasingly larger *intervertebral discs* to form joints, permit vertebral column movements, and absorb vertical shock. Spinal nerves enter and exit the spinal cord via foramina between the vertebrae.

The *clavicle* is the paired *collar bone,* forming a large part of the anterior portion of the shoulder girdle. It is located immediately superior to the first rib, articulating ventrally with the manubrium of the sternum bone. From this point it extends laterally and then curves backward to the acromion process of the scapula bone. Muscles that originate or insert along the clavicle's length may be involved in respiration (e.g., the sternocleidomastoid, pectoralis major, and some of the laryngeal strap muscles).

The *costae,* or *ribs* (Figs. 6.4 and 6.5; see Fig. 6.7) are paired flat bones twisted in two planes. They form the highly mobile, yet protective thoracic cage surrounding the lungs. There are usually 12 ribs, although supernumerary ribs in the cervical region are not uncommon. They articulate dorsally with the body and transverse process of the thoracic vertebrae. Somewhat lateral to the articulating *head* of the rib is the straight *neck,* with its *articulating tubercle* moving upon the transverse process of the vertebra immediately above.

Beyond its neck, the rib passes toward the lateral portion of the back of the human body until it makes a rather abrupt change in direction at the *angle* of the rib. Here it turns to curve anteriorly and then medially toward the ventral midline of the thorax. At the angle, too, occurs the twist of the rib that allows for an outward movement of the rib when it is elevated. The rib terminates in its own *costal cartilage.* In the case of the upper seven ribs, this hyaline cartilage continues independently to articulate with the sternum at a facet provided. The next three ribs have their costal cartilages attached to those of the rib above. The last two ribs are unattached; these are the so-called *floating ribs.* (These lower five are sometimes called *false ribs* because of their lack of direct medial attachment to the sternum.)

Muscle sheets interconnect the ribs, and there are muscles serving to attach the ribs to the vertebrae and to the sternum; such muscles are found internally and externally on the thorax. Another group of muscles are extrathoracic, serving to attach the ribs as a group to structures above the thorax (such as the arms, neck, and cranium), as well as to structures below the thorax (such as the pelvic girdle).

At the midline of the thorax is found the unpaired *sternum bone,* a segmented bone that serves to fix the ventral ends of the costal cartilages, as well as to protect the contents of the thorax. The sternum (sometimes called the breast bone) is composed of three easily identified portions: the uppermost is the manubrium, the large middle portion is the body, and the highly variable inferior portion is the xiphoid process.

The *manubrium sterni* is an irregular octagon, and its free and concave cephalad side is termed the *jugular notch,* or *sternal notch.* Its most lateral side is also concave for articulation of the first costal cartilage. Between the jugular notch and the costal cartilage is the slanting surface that receives the clavicle. The single caudal surface articulates with the body of the sternum at the *sternal angle.*

The *body (corpus, gladiolus)* frequently demonstrates obvious segmentation, with concavities designed for articulation with the costal cartilages. At the sternal angle itself, the second rib has its facet. Ribs three, four, five, and six are generally located inferiorly along the sides of the body until rib seven is reached, with its facet usually intermediate between the body and the xiphoid process. The costosternal articulations take place as synovial joints.

The *xiphoid process* is highly variable from individual to individual, although in general it is a long and thin cartilaginous process that usually ossifies in older age. It serves as the attachment for the ligamentous linea alba of the abdomen, as well as for the rectus abdominis muscle. There are no costal cartilage attachments.

The paired *scapula bones,* otherwise known as the *shoulder blades,* combine with the clavicle bones to form

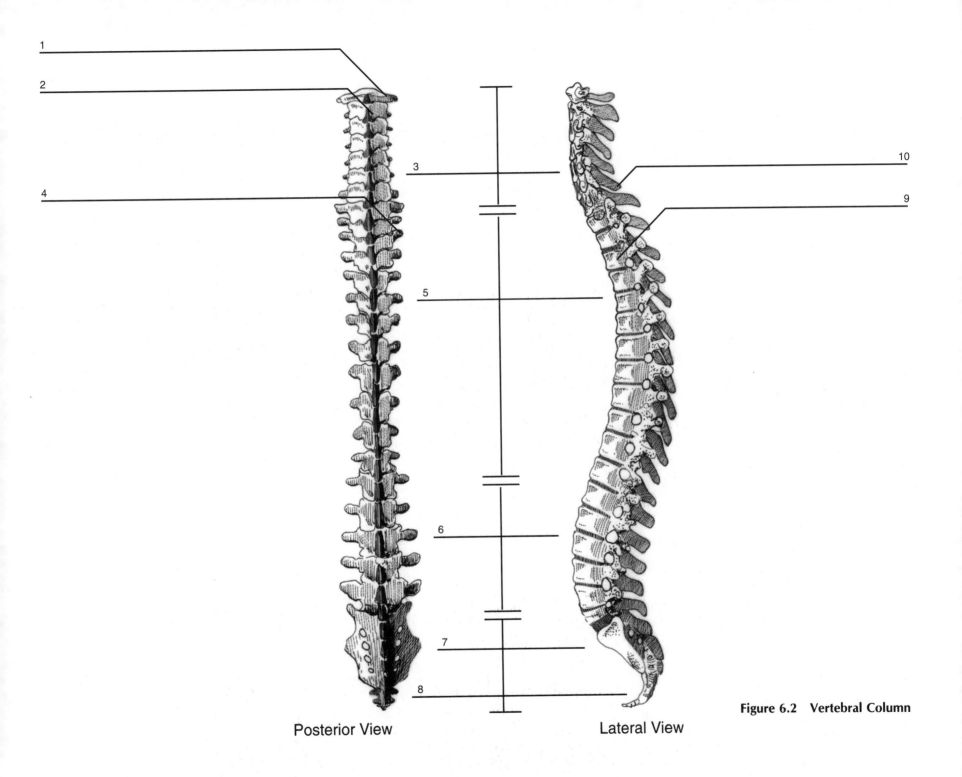

1

2

3

4

5

6

7

8

9

10

Posterior View

Lateral View

Figure 6.2   Vertebral Column

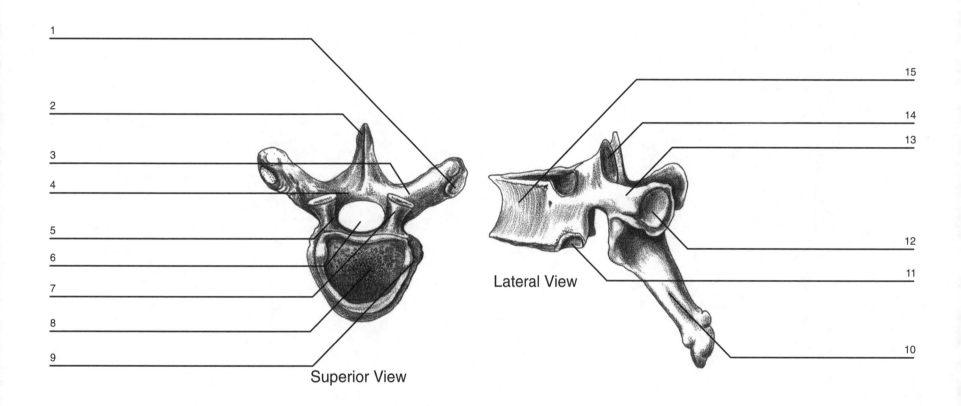

1

2

3

4

5

6

7

8

9

Superior View

15

14

13

12

11

10

Lateral View

Figure 6.3   Thoracic Vertebra: Superior and Lateral Views

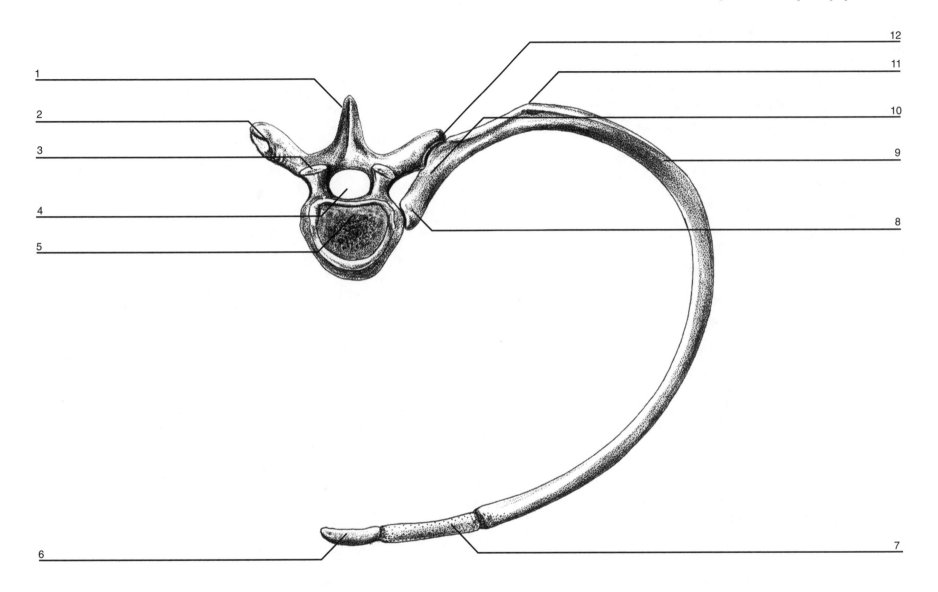

Figure 6.4   Vertebrosternal Rib

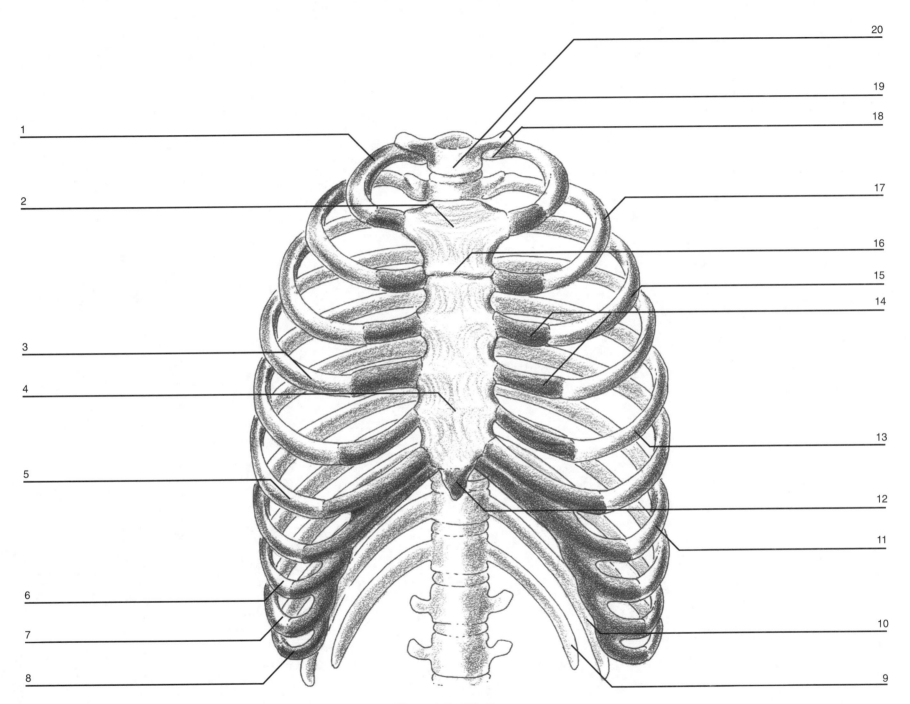

Figure 6.5   Rib Cage

the shoulder girdle. The scapula rests upon the clavicle in part and provides an articulation via its glenoid fossa with the upper arm bone, the *humerus*. The scapula has several important muscle attachments, largely for the humerus bone, but the omohyoid muscle originates here as well. The body of the scapula covers the upper seven ribs in the main; the *acromion process* articulates with the clavicle bone; and the *coracoid process* serves the omohyoid muscle. Other important landmarks relate to postural and arm muscles and attachments (see Fig. 6.8).

The *ilium* is one of the three divisions of the paired *hip bone,* which forms a large part of the pelvic girdle (Fig. 6.6). The other two bones are the *ischium* and the *pubis*. The ilium presents attachments for abdominal muscles of respiration and comprises the upper and outer sides of the hip region. To the outermost edge, the *crest,* are attached some of the muscles mentioned. The fan-shaped ilium narrows at the cup-shaped *acetabulum,* the joint socket for the upper leg bone (*femur*). From the acetabulum, the two other parts of the hip bone diverge. The ischium portion passes downward and then curves medially to fuse with the pubis portion. This latter part extends medially from the acetabulum, forming the anteroinferior wall of the pelvis until it meets with its fellow from the opposite side. Here, there is a fibrocartilaginous plate adjoining the two so that the pubic symphysis is formed at the midline. Running from the *pubic symphysis* to the iliac crest is the *inguinal ligament,* which is in part of the lower margin of the abdominal muscles. Dorsally, the two hip bones articulate with the sacrum as the latter completes the pelvic girdle.

MUSCULATURE

Respiration is the result of a pumping action. The number of muscles involved in the pumping varies considerably, depending upon the demand the body is placing upon the pump. In *quiet inhalation* relatively few muscles are used. When more oxygen for body tissues or more air for certain phonatory activities is required, the number of muscles used increases (*forced inhalation*). In either case, the muscles act to enlarge the volume of and decrease the pressure within the thorax so that air will flow into the lungs from the environment (Table 6.1). Such suction contrasts with the compressive pumping action of exhalation, in which the decreasing volume of the thorax increases the pressure on the air within, which is forced from the lungs.

To increase the thoracic volume, and thus to decrease the thoracic air pressure, we utilize a combination of approaches. One approach, in its simplest form, can be described as thoracic (chest wall) enlargement, by elevating the ribs through muscular action. The other is to increase the vertical dimension of the thorax by contracting and thus flattening the diaphragm muscle. Anyone, of course, may also have some combination of these actions. The muscles used in respiration may be separated into major and minor groups, the latter being auxiliary or stabilizing as they are not capable of being sole initiators of thoracic enlargements. The major muscles of respiration are the diaphragm, external intercostals, and the internal intercostals. These will be discussed, followed by a sampling of the minor muscle group.

Major Muscles

The *diaphragm muscle* (Fig. 6.7) is a musculotendinous septum that has its origin around the entire internal circumference of the lower bony thorax. Included are the lumbar vertebrae and the lumbocostal fascia dorsally, the cartilages and bony portions of the lower six or seven ribs, and the xiphoid process ventrally. The muscle fibers fan centrally, developing two central tendons that support the lungs (and heart) above. When at physiologic rest, the diaphragm is elevated and forms two semicircular domes, upon which rest the bases of the lungs. Upon contraction, the domes are flattened because of the low origins of the muscle fibers; a potential space is created between the diaphragm and the bases of the lungs. The decreased pressure within the lungs causes them to inflate as the atmospheric pressure outside the body forces air through the respiratory tract into the lungs. The depressed domes of the diaphragm muscle encroach upon the abdominal viscera; upon controlled relaxation of the muscle, abdominal pressure (among other forces) causes the domes to return to express air from the lungs. Nervous stimulation to the diaphragm muscle is derived from the phrenic nerve from cervical nerves 3, 4, and 5.

The *external intercostal muscles* (Fig. 6.8) are found along the borders of the ribs, running from one rib to the next in an oblique direction. There are 11 pairs of such muscles, extending from the tubercles of the ribs dorsally around the thorax to the costal cartilages. These are superficially located; the origin is on the outer lip of the lower border of a rib, and the insertion is on the outer lip of the upper border of the rib below. It is generally agreed that the external intercostal muscles contract to elevate the ribs, thus acting as thoracic cavity enlargers in inhalation. This action is dependent upon fixation of the first rib by the scalene muscles. The intercostals are innervated by the intercostal nerves, supplied through thoracic nerves 1 to 11.

The *internal intercostal muscles,* also 11 in number, are found on the upper borders of the ribs, more internal than the external intercostal group. The fibers are also oblique, but their course is nearly at right angles to that of the external muscle, running from below, upward, and laterally from the front of the thorax and angling medially at the dorsal aspect of the thorax. These fibers start ventrally, near the sternum, so that they pass between the costal cartilages and continue along the rib until they pass the angle. They originate on the upper border and inner surface of the rib and on the costal cartilage, and they insert into the lower border and inner surface of the rib and into the costal

cartilage, immediately above. These muscles are generally considered to be muscles of exhalation, since they lower the ribs. The nerve supply to the internal intercostal group is from the intercostal nerves, supplied through thoracic nerves 1 to 11.

Minor Muscles

The lateral vertebral group is composed of the three highly variable *scalene muscles*. All originate upon the cervical vertebrae (C-3 to 7), at the transverse processes. They pass downward and slightly laterally, internal to other muscles (especially the sternocleidomastoid). The *anterior scalene muscle* inserts into the first rib, just anterior to the tubercle; the *medial scalene muscle* inserts into nearly the same place, but somewhat more toward the midline of the thorax. The *posterior scalene muscle* is even deeper than the other two and inserts into the second rib, at about its tubercle. The action is said to elevate the ribs, and it is fairly certain that they are fixators of the first and second ribs for the inspiratory act. Cervical nerves 4 to 8 provide the innervation for these muscles.

The *transverse thoracic muscle,* also variable, is generally found with its origin internally at the midline of the thorax, at the body and xiphoid process of the sternum. Its fibers pass in bundles, some upward in a nearly vertical fashion, some upward obliquely, and some nearly horizontally; they insert into the costal cartilages and the bony ends of ribs 2 to 6. Its action is said to depend upon the fixation of the 12th rib by the quadratus lumborum muscle; generally it depresses the ribs and thus is a muscle of expiration. Its nerve supply comes from the branches of the intercostal nerves (thus from thoracic nerves 2 to 6).

The *quadratus lumborum muscle,* the fixator of the lower ribs, originates from the posterior portion of the crest of the ilium bone, the ligamentous and fibrous tissues of the posterior lumbar region, and the transverse processes of the lumbar vertebrae. Its fibers pass upward

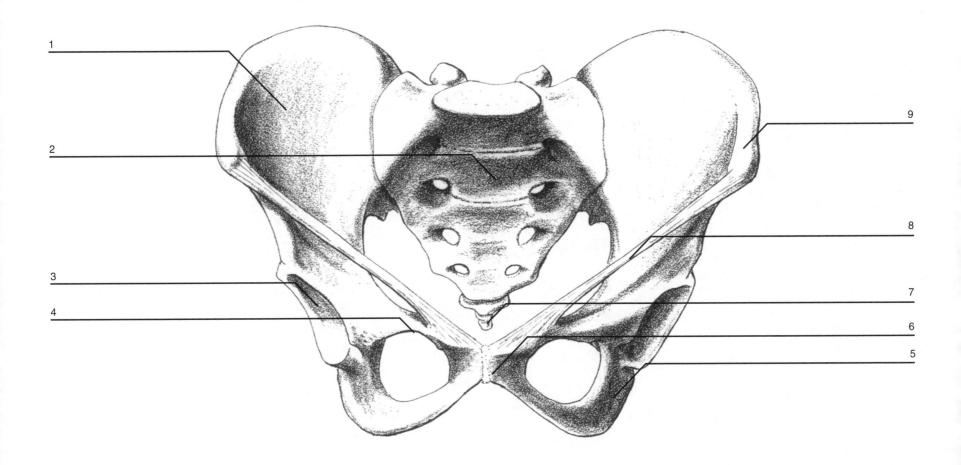

Figure 6.6   Pelvic Girdle

Table 6.1. Thoracic Muscles of Respiration

Muscle	Origin	Insertion	Action	Nerve
Diaphragm	Entire internal circumference of lower thorax; xiphoid cartilage anteriorly; cartilages and bony portion of 6 or 7 lower ribs laterally; upper lumbar vertebrae posteriorly	Central tendons	Chief muscle of respiration; elevates ribs and draws down upon central tendon; increases vertical dimension of thorax	Phrenic (from C-3, 4, 5)
External intercostals	Outer lip of lower border of each rib from tubercle to costal cartilages	Outer lip of upper border of rib below	Elevates ribs in inhalation	Intercostal (from T-1 to 11)
Internal intercostals	Inner edge of upper border of rib and costal cartilage	Inner lip of lower border of each rib from angle to sternum	Aids in depression of ribs in exhalation	Intercostal (from T-1 to 11)
Scalenes	Connected variously to cervical vertebrae 3 to 7 at transverse processes	Upper surface of ribs 1 and 2 or outer surface of rib 2	Elevates or fixates ribs	C-4 to 8
Transverse thoracic	Internal surfaces of sternum and xiphoid process	Costal cartilages and bony end of ribs 2 to 6	Depresses ribs	Intercostal (from T-2 to 6)
Quadratus lumborum	Posterior portion of iliac crest; transverse processes of lumbar vertebrae 3, 4, and 5; iliolumbar ligament	Lower border of rib 12; tendons of abdominal muscles	Draws down rib 12; aids in fixing origin of diaphragm	T-12, L-1 to 2
Pectoralis major	Head of humerus bone	Ventral end of clavicle, sternum, costal cartilages 2 to 6	Elevates ribs	Lower cervical and first thoracic
Pectoralis minor	Coracoid process of scapula	Bony ends of ribs 2 to 5	Elevates ribs	C-7 to 8

and insert into the tendons on the abdominal muscles and into the 12th rib. Its action is mainly to bend the vertebral column, but it also assists in fixating the lowermost rib and in depressing the rib cage in exhalation. In inhalation, it fixates lower ribs to provide purchase for the diaphragm muscle. Its nerve supply comes from lumbar spinal nerves 1 and 2 and from thoracic spinal nerve 12.

The larger muscles of the thorax are the pectoralis major and minor. The *pectoralis major muscle* is a large fan-shaped muscle with several divisions. The attachments are generally described as of thoracic origin, the insertion then being on a single tubercle of the humerus bone (Fig. 6.8). However, it is important here to consider this muscle as one of respiration; therefore, the usual origin and insertion are reversed. The origin, then, is the head of the humerus bone, and the insertion, broad and fan-shaped, runs from the ventral end of the clavicle, the sternum, and the costal cartilages of ribs 2 to 6. The aponeurosis from the external abdominal oblique muscle is also involved in this insertion. Its action, when the humerus bone is fixed, is to elevate the ribs and thus actively participate in enlarging the thorax in inhalation. Its nerve supply comes from the lowermost cervical and the first thoracic spinal nerves.

The *pectoralis minor muscle* originates from the scapula at its coracoid process. Its fibers radiate downward beneath the pectoralis major to the bony ends of ribs 2 to 5. Its action, as here considered (with basic origin-insertion reversal), is to elevate the ribs in inhalation. It is innervated by cervical nerves 7 and 8.

The *levatores costarum* is actually a series of fan-shaped muscles that arise from the transverse processes of the vertebrae, from C-7 to T-11. The fibers pass downward and slightly laterally and insert into the next inferior rib, from the head to the tubercle; lower in the thorax, some fibers pass to the second rib below. This muscle group serves to elevate the ribs in inhalation. Its innervation comes from the intercostal nerves, from thoracic 1 to 11.

Superiorly in the thorax is the *serratus* group, including the serratus posterior superior and posterior inferior, as well as the serratus anterior muscle. The *posterior superior* and *posterior inferior* arise from the spines of the vertebrae; in the case of the superior group it is the cervical vertebrae, and for the inferior group it is the lower thoracic and upper lumbar vertebrae. Serratus posterior superior fibers then pass downward and slightly laterally and insert into the upper borders of ribs 2 to 5, dorsal to the angle. Serratus posterior inferior fibers rise to fan out and insert into the inferior borders of the lower four ribs, 9 to 12. The two muscles oppose each other in action, with the upper assisting in elevation of the rib cage in inhalation and the lower depressing the lower ribs in exhalation. The lower group also fixes the lowermost ribs during contraction of the diaphragm muscle. Nerve supply to the superior group comes from the upper thoracic spinal nerves and for the inferior group from the lower thoracic spinal nerves.

The *serratus anterior muscle* is a large series of bundles connecting the lower border of the scapula with the majority of the ribs (the upper eight or nine). This muscle arises from the angle of the scapula; its bundles pass anteriorly around the rib cage and insert into the ribs. Its action in respiration is to elevate the ribs in forced inhalation. The nerve supply is provided by the long thoracic nerve from the lowermost cervical spinal nerves.

The exact roles of many of the muscles of respiration are uncertain. Among these are the subcostal, paralleling the internal intercostals, and the sternocleidomastoid, which is the large muscle bundle running from the sternum to the mastoid process of the temporal bone across the side of the neck.

Abdominal Muscles

The *abdominal muscles* (Fig. 6.9, Table 6.2) are four in number and primarily operate on the abdominal contents, or viscera. Changes in the position or density of the viscera change the pressure on the thoracic cavity from below and thus decrease the volume of the thorax. The muscles to be considered in this category are the rectus abdominis, external abdominal oblique, internal abdominal oblique, and transverse abdominis. Together with the tendinous aponeuroses, these form the major portion of the belly wall. Characteristic of the wall are the adhesive portions of the tendons, in some areas forming distinct lines extending in a superior-inferior direction. At the midline of the ventral belly wall is the *linea alba,* a thickened tendinous portion that extends from the xiphoid process down to the symphysis pubis.

The *rectus abdominis muscle* is a paired, near-midline muscle, extending from the thorax to the symphysis. It originates along the crest and the symphysis of the pubis and inserts at the xiphoid process and costal cartilages of ribs 5, 6, and 7. It passes directly superiorly alongside the midline of the belly as a thick regular bundle that has characteristic tendinous inscriptions. This muscle contracts to compress the abdominal

1

2

3

4

5

6

7

8

16

15

14

13

12

11

10

9

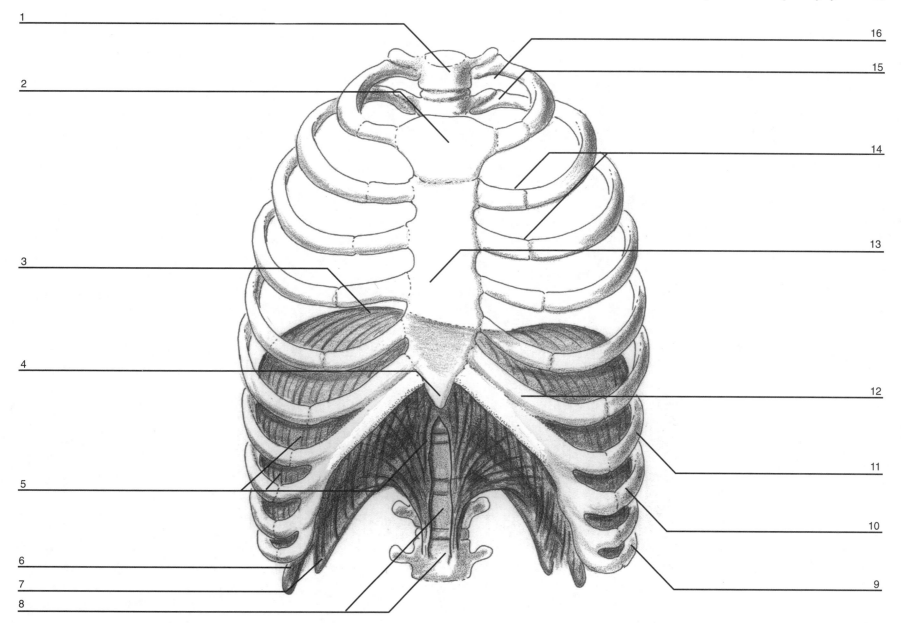

Figure 6.7   Diaphragm Muscle

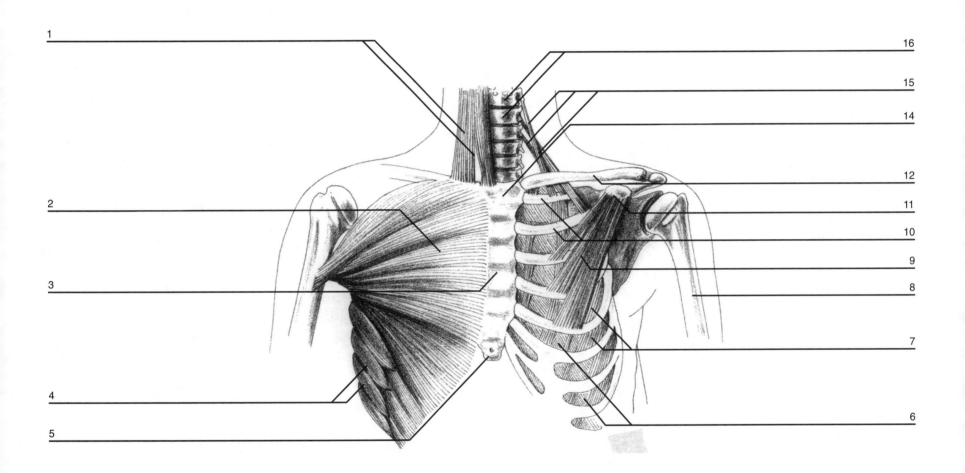

Figure 6.8   Thoracic Respiratory Muscles

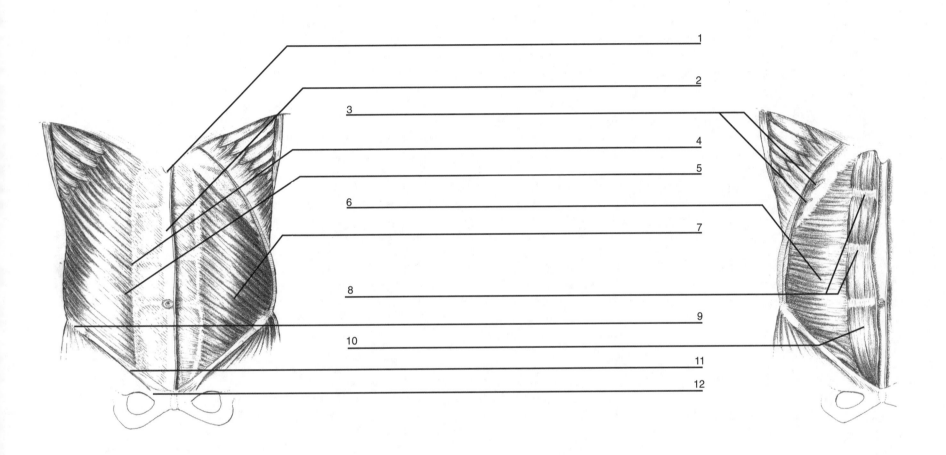

Figure 6.9   Abdominal Muscles

Table 6.2. Abdominal Muscles of Respiration

Muscle	Origin	Insertion	Action	Nerve
Rectus abdominis	Crest and symphysis of pubis	Xiphoid process; costal cartilages 5, 6, and 7	Supports and compresses viscera	Lower intercostals (T-7 to 12)
External oblique	External borders of ribs 5 to 12	Crest of pubis, front half of iliac crest, linea alba, inguinal ligament	Supports and compresses viscera, depresses thorax	Lower intercostals (T-8 to 12, L-1)
Internal oblique	Anterior half of iliac crest, lumbar fascia, inguinal ligament	Linea alba; cartilages of ribs 8, 9, and 10; abdominal aponeurosis	Supports and compresses viscera	Lower intercostals (T-9 to 12, L-1)
Transverse abdominis	Inguinal ligament, iliac crest, lower borders of ribs 6 to 12, lumbar fascia	Xiphoid process, linea alba, crest of pubis	Supports and compresses viscera	Lower intercostals (T-7 to 12, L-1)

viscera; during respiration it becomes a muscle of forced exhalation. Its nerve supply comes from the last intercostal nerves (thoracic 5 to 12 and lumbar 1).

The *external abdominal oblique muscle* is a muscle of the lateral abdominal wall that is continued ventrally by its aponeurosis. It originates on the external borders of the lower eight ribs as well as from the aponeurosis of the belly wall. Its fibers pass downward and forward and insert on the crest of the pubis, the anterior portion of the iliac crest, the linea alba, and part of the inguinal ligament. Its action, as far as respiration is concerned, is to depress the thorax and compress the abdominal viscera in forced exhalation. Its nerve supply comes from the last intercostal nerves (thoracic 5 to 12 and lumbar 1).

The *internal abdominal oblique muscle* originates in the lower dorsal regions of the abdomen, particularly from the iliac crest, the inguinal ligament, and the lumbodorsal fascia. Its fibers pass medially and superiorly; the more dorsal fibers end on the lower three ribs, and the lower-originating fibers pass nearly horizontally toward the midline and terminate in the linea alba, the abdominal aponeurosis, and the cartilages of ribs 8, 9, and 10. This tendinous sheath splits as it approaches the rectus abdominis muscle, part of the tendon passing beneath and part outer to the rectus. The internal oblique acts along with the external oblique to compress the abdominal viscera in forced exhalation. Its nerve supply comes form the last intercostal nerves (thoracic 9 to 12 and lumbar 1).

The *transverse abdominis muscle* is the innermost of the layered abdominal muscles. It arises from a rather broad origin, from the iliac crest and the inguinal ligament inferiorly, along the lumbodorsal fascia, and from the innermost portions of the lower six ribs. This origin blends with part of the costal origin of the diaphragm muscle. The fibers of the transverse pass nearly horizontally forward until they terminate as a tendon in the linea alba at the midline of the abdomen, from the xiphoid process to the crest of the pubis. Its action is to support and compress the abdominal viscera in exhalation. It is innervated by the lower intercostal nerves, thoracic 7 to 12.

Physiology

The respiratory pump must be considered as a two-way pump. In quiet inhalation, an active musculature expands thoracic volume to decrease internal air pressure, and air enters the lungs. Passive relaxation of inspiratory muscles allows for elastic recoil of the chest wall, which decreases lung volume, increasing air pressure and forcing air externally. In forced exhalation, expiratory muscles join the recoil forces to greatly increase the air pressure.

The primary active muscle in quiet inhalation is the diaphragm, which is joined by the external intercostal muscle. Quiet exhalation results from relaxation of the muscles of inhalation, the result being that the ribs and/or the diaphragm muscle return to their rest positions, decreasing thoracic volume and increasing thoracic pressure. Prolonged exhalation during speech and singing is in part the result of controlled relaxation of inspiratory muscles, that is, checking of the impetus of elastic recoil, the nonmuscular force that returns the thorax and lungs to their resting postures.

In more active inhalation, the three scalene muscles and the sternocleidomastoid muscle can help elevate the thorax. Under special circumstances, the pectoralis major and pectoralis minor can further elevate the sternum and upper ribs. Such muscles as the levatores costarum, subclavius, and serratus posterior superior might also participate in active inhalation.

In forced exhalation, the internal intercostal muscles of the rib cage probably depress the ribs to decrease thoracic volume. Smaller muscles of the thorax, such as the subcostals and the transverse thoracic, would also come into play, along with the serratus posterior inferior and quadratus lumborum of the lower abdominal area. Perhaps most active in strong forced exhalation would be the four muscles of the abdomen: the rectus abdominis, external abdominal oblique, internal abdominal oblique, and transverse abdominis. Upon contraction of these muscles, there is an increase of pressure upon the abdominal viscera, forcing upward the diaphragm muscle; this creates a lowered thoracic volume and an increased thoracic air pressure and the air within the lungs is "squeezed" out in exhalation.

NERVOUS TISSUES

The two functions of the respiratory system (breathing and speaking) require a somewhat complicated nerve supply comprising both sensory and motor elements.

In voluntary breathing a twofold feedback apparatus is involved. One aspect consists of proprioception served by stretch (inflation) receptors located in the walls of the alveoli. As the alveoli are inflated by air, the walls expand and the stretch receptors are stimulated. The sensory nerve impulse is carried by the vagus nerve (Cranial X) to the medulla oblongata and to the expiratory center located therein. From there, messages are sent to inspiratory centers nearby, which send out inhibitory messages to the muscles of inhalation, stopping their activity. Thereafter, at least in quiet breathing, exhalation occurs by means of elastic recoil forces that cause the thoracic structures to return to their resting positions. The cycle of respiration then continues, with inspiratory center stimuli initiating muscle contractions that again enlarge the thorax.

Chemical-sensitive nerve centers (chemoreceptors) located within the walls of some of the arteries constitute a second sensory system associated with involuntary breathing. These centers indirectly monitor the carbon dioxide concentration in the blood, comparing that with body cell requirements for oxygen and sending appropriate messages to the reticular formation in the lower portion of the brain. As the body suffers depletion of oxygen (hypoxia), necessary adjustments are made to increase the oxygen supply through an increase in the rate or depth of inhalation.

To some extent, both of these sensory feedback control systems can be voluntarily overridden. It would be extremely difficult for voluntary systems to maintain such antagonistic control, however, for long enough to seriously damage body cells. The involuntary control system would assume command at some point, perhaps at the point of unconsciousness.

The voluntary motor control system, originating in the motor centers of the cerebral cortex, is primarily made up of spinal nerve effectors. The various spinal nerves mainly serve the muscles related to quiet inhalation, with the phrenic nerve (stemming from the cervical spinal nerve group) to the diaphragm muscle being the primary effector. Other spinal nerves serve other muscles during inhalation. Muscles associated with exhalation are used when forced exhalation or other conscious control of the respiratory system is required. Inhibition of certain muscles and muscle groups to achieve controlled relaxation, as well as active stimulation of other muscle groups to effect a smoothly flowing breathing pattern, is the product of a fairly complex, highly integrated nervous function centered in the cerebrum, the pons, the reticular formation, the medulla, and elsewhere.

RESPIRATORY QUANTITIES

The rate and depth of breathing obviously vary tremendously, depending upon a number of factors such as age, sex, health, training, demand for oxygen at the moment of measuring, and so on. Certain broad standards have been developed for measuring respiration at different stages of breathing (Tables 6.3 and 6.4).

First, a healthy young adult bearing no physical demands at the moment should breathe between 12 and 18 times per minute. This figure is much higher in infants and when the body cells are in need of oxygen. Second, the pulmonary system has a maximum capacity; in a healthy young adult male total lung capacity is as great as 6000 ml, while in a healthy young adult female it is as great as 4200 ml.

The *total lung capacity* is the amount of gas (i.e.,

Table 6.3. Respiratory Quantities (in milliliters)

Quantity	Males 20–30 Years[a]	Kaplan[b]	Hixon[c]	Zemlin[d]	Males 50–60 Years[a]	Females 20–30 Years[a]
Inspiratory capacity	3600	2000–3000	3000		2600	2400
Expiratory reserve capacity	1200		2000		1000	800
Vital capacity	1200	3500	5000	3500–5000	3600	3200
Residual volume	2400	1500	2000	1000–1500	2400	1000
Functional residual capacity	6000	3000	4000		3400	1800
Total lung capacity		5000	7000		6000	4200
Tidal volume	400–500	500	500	750		
Inspiratory reserve volume		1500–3000	2500	1500		
Expiratory reserve volume		1500		1500		

[a]Adapted from Comroe JH, Jr. Physiology of respiration. Chicago: Year Book Medical Publishers, 1965.
[b]Kaplan HM. Anatomy and physiology of speech, 2nd ed. New York: McGraw-Hill, 1971.
[c]Hixon TJ. Respiratory function in speech. In: Minifie F, Hixon TJ, Williams F, Normal aspects of speech, hearing and language. Englewood Cliffs, NJ: Prentice-Hall, 1973.
[d]Zemlin WR. Speech and hearing science: Anatomy and physiology. Englewood Cliffs, NJ: Prentice-Hall, 1968.

Table 6.4. Respiratory Quantities: Definitions

Volume	Definition
Tidal	The total volume of each breath, that which is inspired or expired during each respiratory cycle.
Inspiratory reserve	The maximal volume of gas that can be inspired from the end-inspiratory position (i.e., the amount in excess of tidal air volume).
Expiratory reserve	The maximal volume of gas that can be expired from the end-expiratory position (i.e., the amount in excess of the tidal air exhaled).
Residual	The volume of gas remaining in the lungs at the end of a maximal expiration.

Capacity	Definition
Total lung	The amount of gas contained in the lungs at the end of a maximal inspiration.
Vital	The maximal volume of gas that can be expelled by forceful effort following a maximal inspiration.
Inspiratory	The maximal volume of gas that can be inspired from the resting expiratory level (i.e., after a quiet expiration).
Functional residual	The volume of gas remaining in the lungs at resting expiration level (i.e., at the end of a normal expiration).

air) that is contained in the lungs at the end of a maximal inhalation, which amounts to the total volume of air the lungs can hold. If all of the inhaled air were exhaled with force and if the amount of exhaled air were measured, the measurement would be of the *vital capacity*. The averages for this quantity run from 4800 ml in the young male to 3200 ml in the female. These figures differ from total lung capacity because one cannot exhale all the air contained in the respiratory tract; some 1000 to 1200 ml of residual air remain.

Another interesting question concerns the amount of air taken in and out during nonmaximal efforts. A useful measurement is *tidal volume,* the amount of air used during a quiet respiratory cycle, an inhalation followed by an exhalation. Because this is not a maximal volume, the volume that remains available to be filled with air is the *inspiratory reserve volume,* varying from 1500 to 3000 ml. After a quiet exhalation, the air remaining in the lungs is called the *expiratory reserve volume,* an amount around 1500 ml. Two residual quantities are also useful. The *functional residual capacity* is

that volume of air that remains in the lungs at the end of a quiet expiration; the *residual volume* is the volume of gas remaining in the lungs after a maximal expiration. The first ranges between 1800 and 4000 ml in young adults; the second ranges between 1000 and 1200 ml in the same population.

SUMMARY

The respiratory system functions importantly in speech but primarily in breathing for vital oxygen-carbon dioxide exchange with the blood. The three aspects of respiration are ventilation, external respiration, and internal respiration.

The respiratory tract consists of the nasal passages and the mouth, the pharynx, the larynx, the trachea, the bronchi, which divide into the alveoli, and ultimately the lungs.

The connective tissues of the respiratory system are mainly the bones. The vertebrae, clavicle, ribs, sternum, and shoulder blades all serve to support the respiratory system and attach many of the muscles that function in respiration. Costal cartilages serve also as connective and elastic sources.

The number of muscles involved in respiration varies considerably, depending upon whether respiration is quiet or active. Some of the principal respiratory muscles are the diaphragm, the external and internal intercostals, the scalene muscles, the transverse thoracic muscle, the quadratus lumborum, the pectoralis major and minor, the levatores costarum, the serratus group, and a few others. Four abdominal muscles (the rectus abdominis, external abdominal oblique, internal abdominal oblique, and transverse abdominis) also can play a role in respiration, especially forced exhalation.

The nervous tissues that function in respiration consist of both sensory and motor elements to control both voluntary and involuntary activities.

Various respiratory quantities are used to evaluate respiration. Some of these are total lung capacity, vital capacity, tidal volume, inspiratory and expiratory reserve volume, and two residual quantities.

Clinical Implications

Exhaled air supplies the energy for vocal fold vibration to produce the laryngeal tone and air flow and pressure in the oral cavity to produce certain consonant sounds. Insufficient air supply that impacts speech production may develop from several clinical pathologies. A form of myesthenia, emphysema, poliomyelitis, and amyotrophic lateral sclerosis are among the several neurologic disorders affecting air supply, among other aspects of speech production. Motor control problems as found in some individuals with cerebral palsy create breath support abnormalities ranging from insufficient air supply to lack of normal control of respiratory cycles in speaking. Voice problems frequently are associated with decreased efficiency of breath support; many voice specialists concern themselves first with breath support activities in dealing with such patients. Breath support to normal phonation and articulation is a basic requirement and usually is one of the first behaviors assessed in speech disorders.

Study Questions

1. Observe the movement of your rib cage as you inhale and then exhale. Do you regard the amount of movement as considerable? Do your clavicles and general shoulder area move concurrently? Change from quiet breathing to deep breathing and note any changes in chest wall movement.

2. Observe your abdominal wall movement during quiet and deep breathing, especially inhalation. Compare the movement you feel with that of the chest wall. Is one region more mobile than the other? Which, and why?

3. What structures do you feel moving in the abdominal wall during inhalation? Can you palpate the diaphragm muscle?

4. Distort the body trunk and note changes in your breathing pattern; for example, bend over and breathe in that posture, or rotate the trunk. What changes occur? Are anatomic relationships changed to accommodate breathing changes?

5. Observe breathing patterns in others. Watch athletes breathe while engaged in strenuous activities; watch singers, public speakers, or persons breathing quietly. Do the variations observed relate strictly to demand or are some constitutional?

Chapter 7
The Ear

GENERAL INTRODUCTION

In many animals, including humans, the vocal tract is used to produce sounds that function in communication; but communication through sound cannot take place unless the sounds produced are received. The sense of hearing (audition) allows such reception to happen. The ear, a remarkable and complex structure, is the primary anatomic structure involved in hearing.

Hearing is basic to most human communication. We learn to talk as children in the language we hear around us. We maintain and embellish our means of expression through hearing. We increase our knowledge with a major input through the auditory sense. We establish social bonds and we develop personality characteristics in large part with the help of our hearing. Its diminution or loss is more than the loss of sensation. It is a loss of a means of relating to the world around us.

The anatomy of the auditory system includes a number of different types of tissues in the ear: mucous and fibrous membranes, bones, ligaments, muscles, canals filled with fluids, nerve fibers, and various types of supporting tissues. These tissues are closely integrated in structure and function, so that the auditory stimulus is transferred from the environment through the various anatomic transducing devices until it reaches the brain. There it becomes meaningful.

Specifically, the environmental air vibrates with sound. Entering the ear, the vibration is transferred to a taut membrane. The membrane passes the vibration on to a trio of closely articulated bones (ossicles), which amplify and pass on the vibration through a window in the petrous portion of the temporal bone. This window communicates with a series of fluid-filled canals, in which the sound continues as waves of pressure. These wave disturbances are picked up by sensitive hairs and hair cells that act as triggers to set up nerve impulses. The neural impulses travel along nerve fibers to nerve pathways and centers until they are received and perceived in the cerebral cortex of the brain.

The *auditory system* is here considered to have four parts (Fig. 7.1). The first three parts, in the order in which the stimulus passes, are the external ear, consisting of those structures providing a sound-containing air channel into the skull (specifically, the temporal bone); the middle ear, consisting of those structures in which the sound-transforming chain of bones are found; and the inner ear, which is within the petrous portion of the temporal bone, and houses the fluid-filled canals that transport the sound waves to the sensory end organ of hearing. The neural ear, the fourth section of the system, consists of the sensory end organ and the nerve pathways that connect it to the cerebral cortex. Considering this neurologic component as a fourth division allows it to be highlighted anatomicly, functionally, and in its relationships.

The student should be aware that most texts make a three-division ear rather than the four-division described here. The last two are combined in those references and usually named the inner ear. This text highlights the four different means by which sound is carried in the total ear: airborne (external ear), bone articulation (middle ear), fluid borne (inner ear), and nerve impulse (neural ear).

Clinical Note

Disorders in hearing may be located in each of the divisions of the ear. External ear defects that can result in auditory problems may be illustrated by objects that occlude the canal; children sometimes insert tiny toys or bits of food, for example. The middle ear's very important chain of bones may be disturbed in function by an accumulation of fluid or by a rupture of the tympanic membrane. The fluids of the inner ear may be causally related to infectious processes or to powerful sound waves that lead to hearing impairments. The nerve impulses that serve sound transmission to the brain may be disturbed by neurologic problems anywhere along the neural train to and within the brain.

THE EXTERNAL EAR

The external auditory structures form a channel for air to enter the sides of the skull. Delicately formed and delicately arranged structures ultimately will respond to pressure waves in the air (i.e., sound).

The *pinna*, or *auricle* (Figs. 7.1 and 7.2), of the external ear is the so-called sound collector; it is composed of a thin plate of cartilage covered by skin. It has numerous ridges and indentations and a variable pendulous lobule. The ridges and indentations are unique in each individual and are expressions of the skin-covered cartilage, which funnels toward the centrally located depression, the *concha*. The upper portion of the concha is the *skiff*. A ridge, the *crus of the helix*, separates the concha from the larger *cave*, which leads into the external acoustic meatus (canal). The *helix* is the folded

rim of the auricle, extending from between the skiff and cave up and around the pinna until it blends below and behind with the *lobule*. From the upper midpoint of the lobule projects a slight cartilaginous elevation, the *antitragus*. The broad C-shaped ridge forming the posterior margin of the concha is termed the *antihelix (anthelix)*. Between it and the helix is the *scaphoid fossa* of the external ear. Projecting from the skin of the face outward over the entrance of the external acoustic meatus is the flap-like *tragus (buck)*. Other landmarks are the two *limbs of the antihelix*, the *internal notch, Darwin's tubercle*, the *anterior notch*, the *posterior sulcus*, and the landmarks found on the posterior surface of the auricle.

The *external acoustic meatus (canal)* is the air-filled canal entering the side of the head from the pinna. The overall length of the meatus is about 25 mm (about 1 inch). The canal has a complex bend as it enters the head; it is difficult to see its end by simply looking into it, for the pinna must be pulled up and back to straighten the canal. The outer third of the meatus is supported by cartilage lined with skin that houses both *hair follicles* and *ceruminous (wax) glands*. The other two-thirds of the meatus is supported by bone from the folds of the tympanic portion of the temporal bone. The cutaneous lining of the osseus portion of the meatus is very thin and very tightly adherent to the bone beneath and contains no hairs or glands. This skin lining continues to become the external and very delicate layer of the tympanic membrane.

Clinical Note

The external auditory mechanism contains the environmental air that conducts sound. The air, and the sound, has access to the first receptor mechanisms of the auditory system. Strictly speaking, the pinna cannot be considered a conductor of sound. It serves very little as an active participant in the hearing act; loss of the auricle itself produces a barely distinguishable auditory disorder. Loss of the external meatus is more signifi-

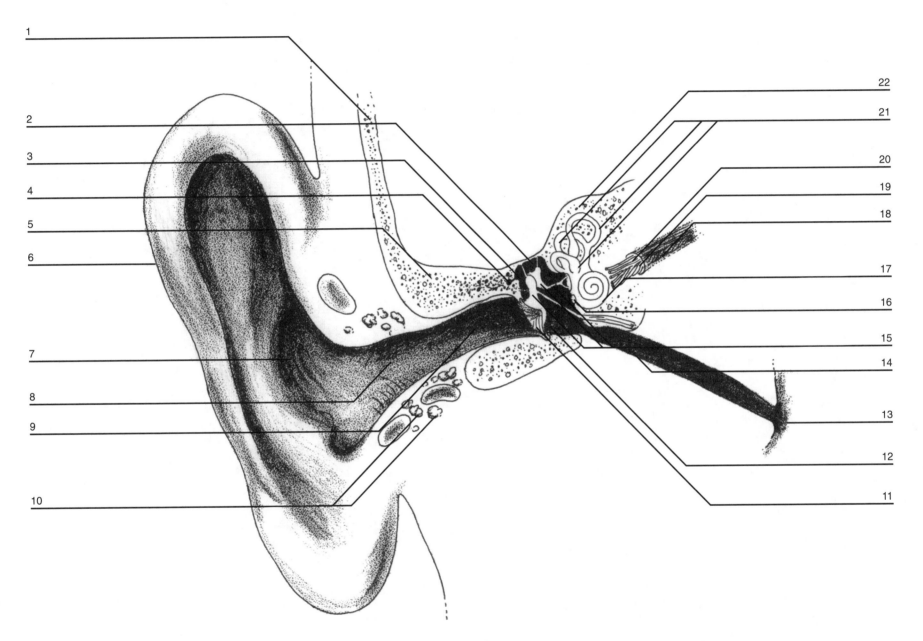

Figure 7.1 The Ear

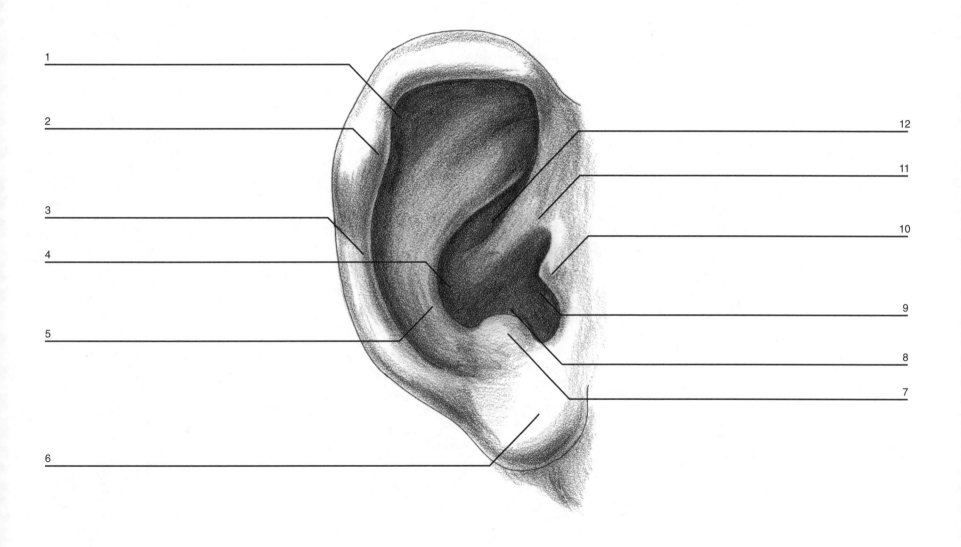

Figure 7.2   Pinna (Auricle)

cant, for then the airborne acoustic vibrations cannot reach the remainder of the system. The auditory disorders resulting from such loss are highly variable, depending upon the type and extent of the canal defect. More commonly, these are congenital disorders. Other problems result from impacted cerumen, from blockage by foreign bodies, and from injuries and infections of the canal. The loudspeaker of a hearing aid delivers sound into this canal; thus, defects of the canal anatomy count heavily in determining whether such an instrument can be used successfully.

THE MIDDLE EAR

The *middle ear* (the *tympanic cavity* or the *tympanum*) is an air-filled space lined with mucous membrane. It houses an articulating set of ossicles that transduces sound vibrations from the tympanic membrane to the inner ear. Air reaches the middle ear through the auditory (Eustachian) tube from the nasopharynx; the same tube provides for drainage of fluids from the ear. The cavity of this space is largely the *tympanum proper,* essentially the region medial to the tympanic membrane. The smaller space above is the *epitympanic recess,* or the *attic.* Portions of the ossicular chain and their ligaments are found in this space. In the upper posterior aspect of this region, a smaller opening *(aditus)* leads to the *antrum,* a slightly enlarged cavity. From the antrum, multitudinous *mastoid air cells* extend into the mastoid process of the temporal bone.

The first of the mechanically conducting vibrators is the *tympanic membrane* (Figs. 7.1, 7.3, and 7.4). This is a three-layered, disc-like structure that is exposed laterally to the external air. Further, it has as part of its structure a major portion of the first bone in the ossicular chain that transmits the acoustic stimulus.

The perimeter of the tympanic membrane is largely affixed into the *tympanic sulcus* of the temporal bone. Here, we find the *tympanic portion* of that bone. The membrane is oriented in a sloping plane downward,

forward, and medially. It is also deeply concave near its midpoint; the deepest part of the concavity is the *umbo,* corresponding to the end of the manubrium of the malleus bone. This attachment keeps the majority of the tympanic membrane under tension; this part of the membrane is thus labeled *pars tensa* (or *tense portion*). There is a loose portion, known as the *pars flaccida* (or *Shrapnell's membrane*), that extends from a V-shaped line (*malleolar fold*) across the upper portion of the tympanic membrane to its superior margin. The flaccid portion has no tympanic sulus for attachment.

The innermost and most medial layer is a continuation of the mucous membrane lining of the middle ear cavity. This mucous membrane lining produces fluids, of course, that ultimately drain to the nasopharynx via the auditory tube. The lining material partially encompasses the manubrium of the malleus bone; in this way, the first bone of the ossicular chain becomes a functional part of the tympanic membrane. Also found on the surface of the mucous membrane lining is the *chorda tympani nerve.* This is a division of the facial (Cranial VII) nerve, a mixed nerve. It provides motor innervation to the muscles of facial expression and, through the chorda tympani branch, to the salivary glands. Its sensory functions serve taste to the anterior third of the tongue.

The middle tissue of the tympanic membrane is a fibrous lamina in intimate contact with the manubrium of the malleus bone, which in turn is covered by the layer of mucous membrane. The middle layer is of utmost importance to audition, for it provides the thin, resilient connective tissue important for proper vibration of the entire structure. The fibers of this layer are both circularly and radially arranged within the tense portion; some authorities consider that this arrangement allows identification of two middle layers, one of circular and one of radial fibers. In the flaccid portion, only elastic fibers are found, a matter of some importance when it is considered that the major function of the upper part of the tympanic membrane is to provide for equalization of air pressure, at least to a minimal degree, between the middle ear and the atmospheric air of the external environment through the auditory tube.

The *auditory tube (Eustachian tube)* leaves the middle ear from its anterior-inferior region and passes through the temporal bone at the junction of the squamous and petrous portions. It continues beyond that point as a tube formed of cartilaginous plates until it terminates in the lateral walls of the nasopharynx, just above the level of the velum. At this point, the cartilage becomes thicker and vertically oriented and forms the torus tubarius. To this frame about the opening of the tube are attached at least two of the muscles of the nasopharynx and palate, the dilator tubae and salpingopharyngeal muscles. The auditory tube is generally horizontally oriented in infancy. As the head grows, the tube assumes a sloping angle until it is obliquely oriented downward, forward, and medially from the tympanum, reaching a length of about 35 mm.

Clinical Note

One of the most common causes of hearing loss in children is auditory tube dysfunction. If it is difficult to open the tube to ventilate the middle ear, the pressure difference between atmospheric and middle ear air can distort or even damage the middle ear. Fluids can build up and rupture the tympanic membrane. Adhesive materials can be laid down, interfering with the movement of the mechanisms of the middle ear. Such blockage can stem from adenoids occluding the opening or from other causes.

The tympanum (Figs. 7.1 and 7.4) is high in its vertical dimension, about 15 mm, or slightly over a half of an inch; its anterior-posterior dimension is about the same. Its lateral dimension is variable, being as small as 2 mm at the level of the tympanic membrane and as much as 6 mm at its uppermost region. Thus, its widest point is less than a quarter of an inch from

side to side. However, these figures vary greatly among individuals.

The roof over the middle ear, a very thin layer of the petrous portion of the temporal bone, is called the *tegmen tympani*. The posterior wall is called the *mastoid wall* because it communicates with the mastoid air cells. The *medial wall* is also called the *labyrinthine wall*, because it relates to the labyrinth of the inner ear. The floor of the middle ear is called the *jugular wall*, because of its association with the jugular (vein) bulb beneath. The *anterior wall* is called the *carotid wall* because of the proximity of the internal carotid artery within. The *lateral wall* is called the *membranous wall* because of the presence of the tympanic membrane thereon.

The labyrinthine wall presents important anatomic landmarks. There are two openings into the wall: the *oval (vestibular) window*, which is occluded by a portion of the last bone in the ossicular chain, and the *round (cochlear) window*, closed by a flexible membrane called the *secondary tympanic membrane*. Between the two windows is a bulging *promontory*, which corresponds to a canal within the bony wall, the basal turn of the cochlea. There is a plexus of nerve fibers across the surface of the promontory. Just to one side of the promontory is a slight projection, the *cochleariform process*, which is associated with a muscle of the middle ear. Above the oval window is a horizontally oriented *facial canal prominence*, containing the facial nerve (Cranial VII); this prominence makes a curve as it approaches the posterior wall, turns downward on that wall, and disappears in the lower regions of the tympanic cavity.

Clinical Note

In recent years, otologists and audiologists have followed the effectiveness of cochlear implants. For patients, commonly adults with profound hearing impairments, this amplification device requires surgical implantation of a magnetic receiver into the mastoid process. Sound is deliv-

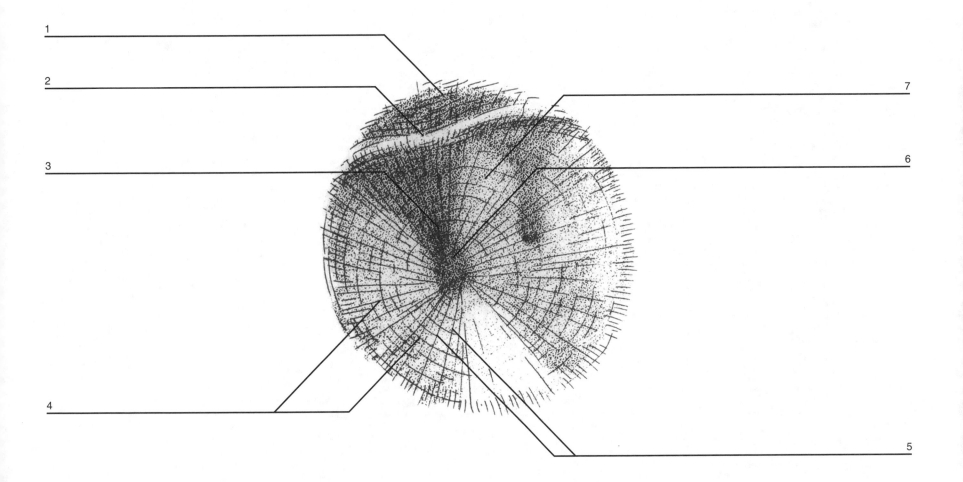

1

2

3

4

7

6

5

Figure 7.3 Tympanic Membrane

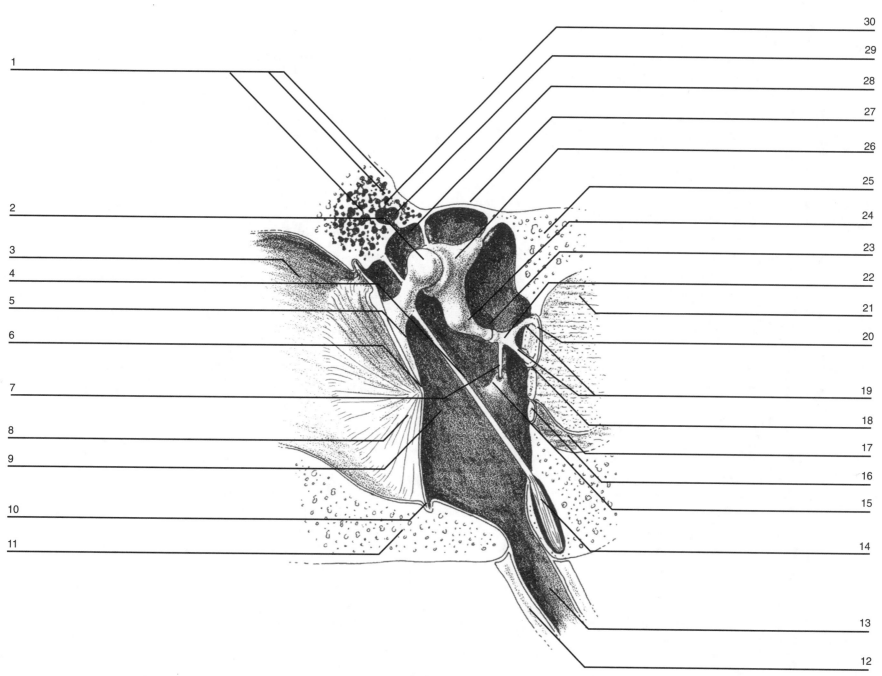

Figure 7.4   Middle Ear (Tympanum)

ered magnetically to this receiver from an externally worn instrument. The implanted device is connected via wire to up to 20 electrodes that have been inserted through the round window into the tympanic canal. The electrical stimulus is then received by the nerve fibers of the auditory system. Although somewhat limited in its application, the cochlear implant offers some promise of improved hearing for severely impaired persons.

The *epitympanic recess* is traversed by the *ossicular chain.* The overall distance covered by this bony chain is 2 to 6 mm. The first ossicle is the *malleus bone.* A part of this ossicle, the *manubrium,* may be considered to be a functional part of the tympanic membrane. The malleus also has a head, a neck, and two smaller processes, the anterior and the lateral. The large upper portion of the malleus bone, the *head,* is housed above the level of the tympanic membrane in the attic. It is oval, presenting on its posterior surface a large articular facet for the second ossicle, the incus bone. The malleus head and the manubrium are connected through the slightly constricted *neck,* immediately below which is a prominence to which the two processes are attached. The *anterior process* is a very tiny spicule that projects anteriorly. To this process is attached the *anterior ligament,* running to the fissure between the petrous and tympanic portions of the temporal bone. The *lateral process* of the malleus bone also arises just below the neck and projects laterally against the tympanic membrane at about the level of the malleolar fold. From this process also extends the *lateral ligament,* attaching the malleus bone to the tympanic portion of the temporal bone at the *tympanic fissure,* or *notch of Rivinus.* A third ligament, the *superior malleolar ligament,* supports the malleus bone and extends from the head to the tegmen tympani.

The manubrium is embedded within the layers of the tympanic membrane; thus, vibratory actions of that membrane are transmitted onward via the manubrium. Movement of the manubrium causes movement of the head of the malleus bone. This movement is transmitted through the articulation at the diarthrodial joint with the incus bone. At these joints of the middle ear bones, changes in the physical character of the sound (especially amplification) may take place.

The second ossicle, the *incus bone,* is shaped somewhat like an anvil. It projects the bulk of its body up into the epitympanic recess. It, too, has special landmarks and processes, in this case called *crura.* From the rather flattened and rounded *body,* with its anteriorly facing articular surface for the malleus bone, the *short crus* extends posteriorly. This is attached to the mastoid wall of the tympanum, just below the aditus ad antrum, by the *posterior incudal ligament.* There may be a *superior incudal ligament* that connects the body of the incus to the tegmen tympani; this ligament often appears as a simple fold of mucous membrane. The *long crus* of the incus bone is oriented at right angles to the short crus, being directed downward and medially toward the labyrinthine wall. At its extremity it thins and then expands into a rounded knob called the *lenticular process (of Sylvius).* This process articulates with the stapes bone, the last of the three ossicles. Here, too, a true joint is found.

The *stapes bone* presents, at the articulating end, a *head* and a *neck* from which diverge two *crura.* These crura are affixed into the two ends of an *oval footplate.* The neck extends slightly below the somewhat broad head and provides insertion for the stapedius muscle. The two crura are oriented with one rather straight crus directed anteriorly and a more curved second crus directed more posteriorly. The oval footplate is received into the oval (vestibular) window and attached thereto by the *anular ligament* around its circumference. The bone can move in a rocking fashion as it is held in place by this ligament.

Clinical Note

Pathologies involving the tympanic membrane or the ossicles are common among people having hearing losses, especially of the conductive type. A scarred or distorted tympanic membrane has limited sensitivity to vibratory stimuli (sound). The articulation of the ossicles is also limited under certain conditions: otosclerosis (growth of spongy bone at the stapes footplate), adhesions fixating or interfering with articulation, fluids in the middle ear, and auditory tube closure resulting in decreased air pressure and subsequent distortion or disturbance of the middle ear mechanisms. Tumor growth, mastoiditis, and other less common conditions also affect the auditory abilities of some individuals because these conditions interfere with the mechanical transmission of sound across the middle ear.

The two muscles of the middle ear are the stapedius and the tensor tympani (Table 7.1, Fig. 7.4). The *stapedius muscle* has its origin in a cavity on the mastoid wall of the tympanum; this cavity forms a small *pyramidal eminence* and presents a tiny hole at its apex. Through this aperture extends the minute tendon of the stapedius muscle, which then attaches to the posterior aspect of the neck of the stapes bone, along with blood vessels and other tissues. Its action is reflexive, moving the stapes laterally and thus tensing or immobilizing the parts within the oval window. The stapedius is probably a protective muscle in this action, especially against ossicular vibrations of great amplitude that might cause damage either at the articular joints or beyond the ossicles within the inner ear. It receives its nerve supply from a branch of the facial nerve (Cranial VII).

The *tensor tympani muscle* is somewhat similar to the stapedius muscle in that it, too, has its muscle fibers encased in a bony cavity, with only its tendon passing to the point of attachment. The tensor tympani's origin is from a deadend canal whose opening is near that of the auditory tube. The tendon of the muscle exits from this semicanal, makes a right-angle turn around the cochleariform process, and passes laterally.

It inserts into the upper part of the medial surface of the manubrium of the malleus bone. Its action is also thought to be reflexive, moving the malleus medially and tensing the tympanic membrane protectively during stimulations of great amplitude. Its nerve supply derives from the trigeminal nerve (Cranial V).

In summary, the tympanum is an air-filled space across which travels a chain of three articulated bones. These bones respond to the vibrations of the tympanic membrane, which in turn is sensitive to acoustic vibrations in the external air in the external acoustic canal. The ossicular chain is supported in space by various ligaments and is acted upon by two muscles. The tympanum surrounding the ossicles is in communication with the environment through the auditory tube, the nasopharynx, and the nose, and with the air cells of the mastoid portion of the temporal bone. It is also in indirect contact with other regions, including the convolutions of the brain (through the very thin tegmen tympani) and the mechanisms for equilibrium and for auditory reception in the inner ear.

Clinical Note

Certainly one of the more common sites of ear pathologies leading to hearing impairment, especially in children, is the middle ear. In the 1st year of life, it may not be completely airfilled and it is inadequately served for fluid drainage by the auditory tube, in part because of the latter's nearly horizontal orientation among other things. The air pressure equalization between the middle ear and external environmental air may not be performed efficiently, a most necessary condition for normal hearing. Of course, the middle ear is also an attractive location for infections that in turn lead to hearing impairment.

THE INNER EAR

The inner ear is a closed system of fluid-filled canals. The inward movements by the footplate of the

Table 7.1. Muscles of the Middle Ear

Muscle	Origin	Insertion	Action	Nerve
Stapedius	Pyramidal eminence	Posterior surface of neck of stapes	Moves stapes laterally, immobilizes oval footplate	Cranial VII
Tensor tympani	Edge of auditory tube opening, greater wing of sphenoid, petrous portion of temporal bone	Manubrium of malleus	Tenses tympanic membrane, moves manubrium of malleus medially	Cranial V

stapes bone, developed from the mechanical vibratory patterns of the ossicles, set up waves of pressure within the fluids of the inner ear. Certain of these ultimately stimulate sensory nerve endings. The acoustic stimuli then are transformed into auditory nerve impulses that reach the brain, and the individual hears.

Usually, the inner ear is said to consist of those canals within the petrous portion of the temporal bone that house the vestibular (equilibrium) mechanisms and the organ of hearing. There is a demonstrable anatomic connection between these structures and the chambers they occupy. However, there is little connection between their normal functions.

The *oval,* or *vestibular, window,* into which the oval footplate of the stapes bone is attached, opens into the fluid-filled space known as the *vestibule.* The fluid is *perilymph.* The vestibule is an entry-room leading into other chambers. One of these chambers is the group known as the *vestibular mechanism,* a complex arrangement of chambers whose primary function is to house the sensory end organs responsive to positional changes of the head. Thus, it is the end organ for equilibrium.

A large part of this equilibrium mechanism is housed in two membranous capsules within the vestibule, the *saccule* and the *utricle.* These capsules are filled with a fluid called *endolymph.* From the saccule, the utricle, and the vestibule extend three other membranous canals (the *semicircular canals*) housed within somewhat larger bony canals. The three canals are nearly circular, reentering the vestibule through enlarged areas

called *ampullae.* Each of the semicircular canals is oriented at right angles to the other two. Each membranous portion, as well as the membranous saccule and utricle, contains sensory end organs of equilibrium. The canals are so placed that movement of the head in any direction will move the contents of one or more of the semicircular canals and stimulate the sensory fibers therein.

Clinical Note

The vestibular system is a sensory system sending nerve impulses to the brain whenever the head position is changed. The brain then makes appropriate interpretation of these signals, often by causing postural changes of the body to accommodate the head position changes. Ocular (eye) changes may take place as well, some eye movements becoming important for adaptation of the individual for head, and body, position changes. Pathologically, the vestibular system may send messages that are interpreted as dizziness or vertigo (including nausea). Special tests, often done by audiologists, may determine the functional status of the vestibular system. Some tests are rotatory (body spinning) or caloric (hot or cold liquids inserted into the external auditory canal), while a more objective instrumental procedure is electronystagmography. As might be exptected, some pathologic conditions of the vestibular system may concurrently disturb the auditory system; a common example is Meniere's disease.

The auditory function of the inner ear is initiated first via an anterior fluid-filled opening from the vestibule. This opening is into the *cochlea,* the spiral chamber that houses the sensory end organ for audition. The entrance from the vestibule continues as a canal of the cochlea, which is appropriately called the *vestibular canal (scala)* and it too is filled with perilymph. Paralleling the vestibular canal as it spirals through the hard petrous portion is the membrane-walled canal of the cochlea, the *scala media* (or *cochlear duct*). This duct is filled with *endolymph,* the same type of fluid that fills the vestibular membranous system.

In the cochlea the vestibular canal spirals about two and a half times before it reaches the cochlear apex. There the canal reverses its direction, like a garden hose bent back on itself (Figs. 7.1 and 7.5). The canal returns to the general area of the base of the cochlea, again spiraling two and a half times. The region of reversal of the canal is called the *helicotrema.* From that point downward, the canal is called the *tympanic canal (scala)* because it terminates in the round window of the tympanum. This little window, which is closed by the *secondary tympanic membrane,* can be found just below the promontory of the medial wall of the middle ear.

In summary, the cochlea is composed, first, of a perilymph-filled canal system within the petrous portion of the temporal bone. This system starts at the vestibule of the inner ear, travels in a spiral fashion through two and a half turns, reverses its direction to return to the base of the cochlea, and terminates in a closed round window. The two canals, vestibular and tympanic, share the cochlea with a third canal that is partially sandwiched between them, the scala media, which is a membrane-walled canal filled with endolymph. The size of these canals varies from base to apex, with the diameter being widest at the base.

The middle canal, the scala media, is of great importance in hearing. Within it is the *organ of Corti,* a spiraling prominence extending along its length from base to apex. This long, complex structure is the specific receptor of hearing, the sensory end organ for audition. It rests upon the *basilar membrane* of the scala media, which is the boundary wall between the cochlear duct and the tympanic canal. This membrane has some 20,000 fibers in parallel, organized in such a way as to serve as a critical sound analyzer. The roof over the scala media, separating it from its neighbor (the vestibular canal), is the *vestibular membrane,* also known as *Reissner's membrane.*

The two boundary membranes, the basilar and the vestibular, form two of the walls of the endolymph-filled, triangular scala media. The third and outermost wall is the bony housing for the cochlea itself. This wall is covered by the *spiral ligament,* which holds the basilar membrane firmly to that outer wall, and by the *spiral stria (stripe),* which is vascular and supplies nutrients to the cochlea. The inner end of the basilar membrane is attached to the *osseus spiral lamina,* a bony shelf extending from the inner wall of the cochlea. This lamina varies in its extent, decreasing from base to apex.

A cross-section of the cochlea (Fig. 7.6) reveals that most of the cochlea is perilymphatic. The smaller membranous portion is the scala media, located on the outer portion of the cochlear canal system, spiraling around two and a half times; it begins and ends as a closed canal. Its lower wall, the basilar membrane, supports the sensory end organ, the organ of Corti.

Clinical Note

Because the two fluids of the inner ear, the perilymph and the endolymph, conduct the sound wave from the oval window to the sensory end organ (the organ of Corti), it serves as an important functioning avenue for the transmission of sound as well as possible locus of disorder. The fluids of the cochlea are continuous with those of the semicircular canals and in some instances, as in some of the Meniere's diseases, increase in fluid pressures may well result in disturbed functioning

1

2

3

4

5

12

11

10

9

8

7

6

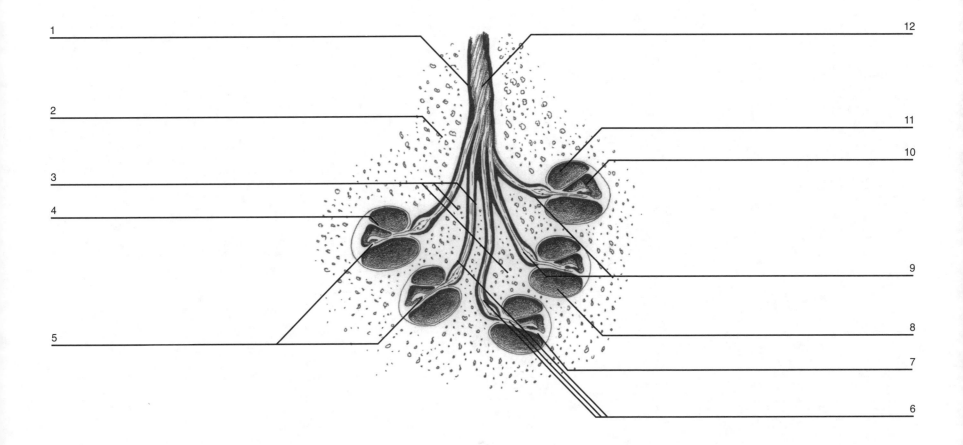

Figure 7.5 Cochlear Turns

1

2

3

4

5

6

7

8

9

10

20

19

18

17

16

15

14

13

12

11

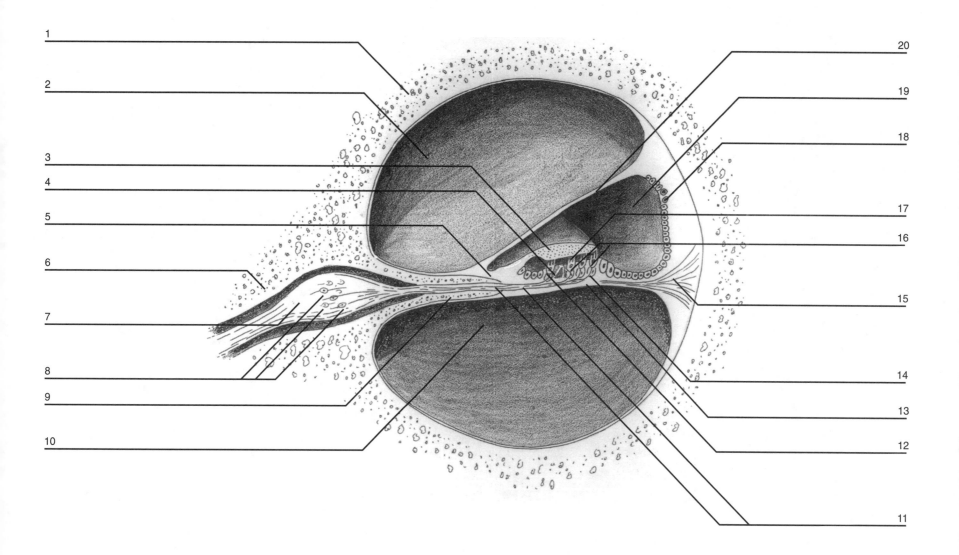

Figure 7.6   Cochlea (Cross-Section)

of either or both systems. Thus, sensory disorders such as dizziness or vertigo may be accompanied by hearing disorder, transitory or permanent. Also, the sometimes overly vigorous energies of the sound waves (as in very intense noises such as jet engines) may be carried through the fluids into the delicate sound reception system, the hair cells, and cause permanent damage and thus hearing impairment.

The *organ of Corti* is composed of a number of different kinds of extremely specialized cells. Two structures give rigidity to the organ of Corti, the *pillars of Corti*. These calcium salt structures lean together to form the *inner tunnel of Corti*. At their tops, they are continuous with the *reticular membrane,* a network of tissue with patterns of holes. Through these holes from below pass the rows of hairs that arise from the *hair cells.* Medially from the *inner pillar of Corti* are found the *inner supporting cells,* and their capping *inner hair cells,* with their multitudinous tiny hairs (cilia) extending through the reticular membrane above into the endolymph. Outward from the *outer pillar of Corti* are found several rows of *outer supporting cells,* cupped at their tops to hold the *outer hair cells,* with their hairs extending superiorly also. There are three to five rows of outer hair cells (base to apex), nearly 25,000 in all, with some 7,000 occurring in the group of inner hair cells.

More medially in the cochlear duct, on the superior surface of the osseus spiral lamina, will be found the *spiral limbus.* This thickened structure extends into the endolymph. From its superior margin projects the gelatinous tectorial membrane, an extremely flexible and mobile structure that extends over the reticular membrane. The tiny hairs from the hair cells below reach up toward this *tectorial membrane.* On the upper surface of each hair cell the hairs are arranged so the outermost ones reach and penetrate the tectorial membrane, while the more medial hairs do not quite reach it in the resting position.

The hairs and their hair cells, the supporting cells, the basilar membrane, and the other membranes, as well as the fluids of the cochlea, make up a structure that can be set into vibration. The kinds and the degrees of vibration are different from base to apex because of differences in structure along the way. Different sounds stimulate different regions along the organ of Corti. For example, at the base of the cochlea, the beginning of the spiraling chambers, the end organ is particularly sensitive to rapid vibrations (i.e., high frequency or high-pitched sounds), while the apex of the cochlea responds more to low frequency sounds.

It is the hair cells that respond to vibration as they are moved by the basilar membrane on which they sit. Inner and outer hair cells differ to some extent, with audition itself strongly centered on the inner cells. As the tiny hairs and the tectorial membrane are disturbed by the sound wave in the fluids, the cell body holding those hairs is also disturbed. The electrical and chemical characteristics of the cell's wall (membrane) change. The electrochemical difference triggers *terminal buttons,* and nerve fibers fire. An electrical potential resulting from chemical changes becomes the nerve impulse representing the sound.

In summary, the sound wave enters the inner ear through a rocking movement of the oval footplate of the stapes bone into the perilymph of the vestibule. This creates a wave of disturbance (sound) that passes to and through the perilymph of the vestibular canal and is transmitted to the vestibular membrane along its length. In turn, the wave then affects the endolymph of the cochlear duct, the tectorial membrane within that fluid, and the basilar membrane. This causes distortions of the hairs of certain hair cells, depending upon the nature of the sound and the structure of the organ of Corti. Distorting the hairs causes a distortion of the membranes of the hair cells. The nerve endings attached to the cell membranes are electrochemically stimulated by the distortion, and a nerve impulse is triggered.

Clinical Note

The condition of the cochlea, the supporting cells, the hair cells, and the nature of the fluids all play roles in the act of hearing. Problems can arise with respect to each of these factors, and auditory deficits can result. Intense or loud sounds may injure the hair cells or affect their ties with the tectorial membrane, infections of the cochlea or its parts may develop, pharmaceuticals of certain types can cause tissue changes, endolymph content might increase, and the aging process can involve the loss of hair cells and nerve fibers. In such cases, some much more common than others, hearing losses can occur.

THE NEURAL EAR

The sound passing through the neural ear (Figs. 7.1 and 7.7) does so as nerve impulses, electrochemical changes traveling along nerve fibers en route to the brain. From the beginnings of this system at the hair cells of the organ of Corti, the nerve fibers pass toward the core of the cochlea, the *modiolus,* which is physically oriented toward the brain. As the nerve fibers enter this core, their cell bodies are gathered together to form the *spiral ganglion.* From here, the nerve fibers continue through the modiolus to enter into the *internal acoustic meatus (canal)* as a single large nerve along with the *vestibular nerve.* Both are parts of the vestibulocochlear nerve (Cranial VIII). The major group of fibers from the cochlea serving audition is known as the *cochlear nerve* or the *auditory nerve.* Also within the internal acoustic meatus is the facial nerve (Cranial VII), serving facial and oral regions.

Cranial VIII is composed of the cochlear and the vestibular divisions, together having about 50,000 individual nerve fibers. The cochlear nerve consists of about 30,000 fibers, and the vestibular nerve has about 20,000 fibers. In comparison with other cranial nerves, these are small (the optic nerve, for example, contains over a million nerve fibers). The fibers in the auditory nerve are true bipolar neurons; that is, there is a peripheral process (fiber), the dendrite, extending toward the sensory end organ from the cell body and a central process (fiber), the axon, directed toward the brain from the cell body.

The cochlear nerve leaves the internal acoustic meatus and enters the brainstem laterally at the level of the juncture of the medulla and the pons. It separates from the vestibular division just before entering. The cochlear nerve divides once it enters the brain. One division is directed toward the posterior aspect and the other toward the anterior aspect of the brainstem. The fibers from the organ of Corti terminate in the brain within the *ventral* or the *dorsal cochlear nuclei (centers).* These fibers, from hair cell to cochlear nucleus, are the *first order neurons* of the auditory nervous system. At the two nuclei, the first order neurons pass on their nerve impulses to other neurons through synapses, the electrochemical (but not physical) connection between neurons. Then *second order neurons* carry the auditory impulse more centrally, en route to the cerebral cortex, where it will be perceived.

The second order neurons from the dorsal cochlear nucleus generally cross to the opposite side of the brainstem through the *trapezoid body,* with some fibers synapsing at the nucleus of the trapezoid body of the opposite side. Fibers of the second order from the ventral cochlear nucleus cross in the trapezoid body also, and some of their number, too, may synapse within the nucleus of the trapezoid body of the opposite side. From both the ventral and dorsal cochlear nuclei, fibers may start their pathway homolaterally (same side) to the cortex.

This path to the cortex rostrally is called the *lateral lemniscus* and is a grouping of second order auditory fibers. Along this pathway, a group of auditory nerve fibers pass directly to the nucleus of the facial nerve (Cranial VII). This connection provides a simple explanation of one of the acoustic reflexes, the palpe-

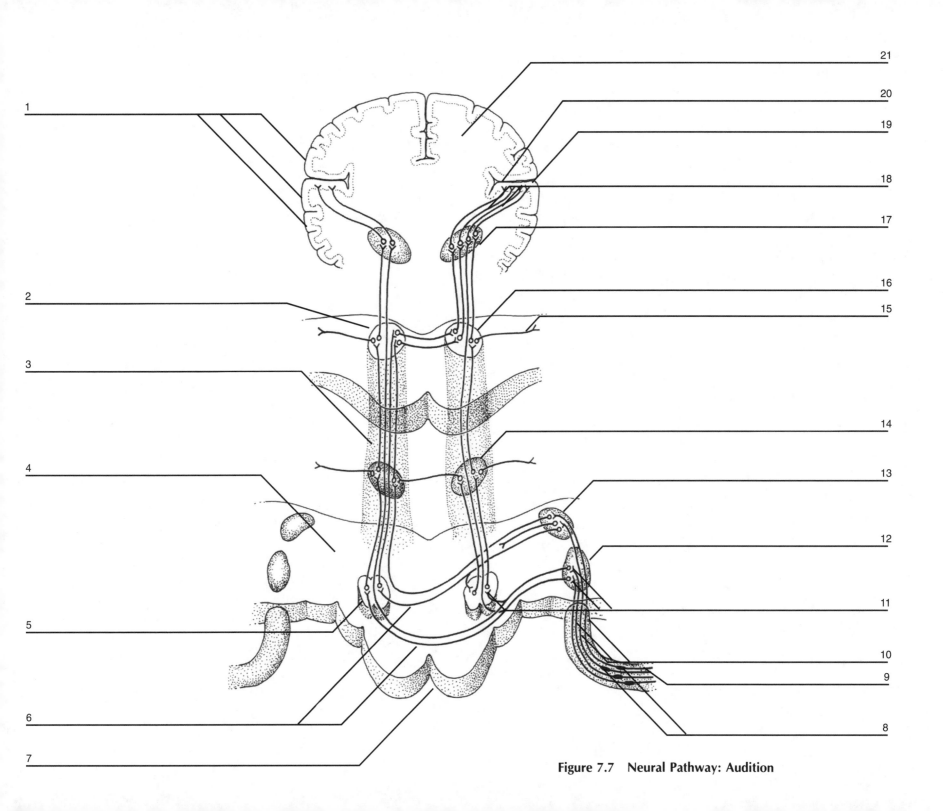

Figure 7.7   Neural Pathway: Audition

broacoustic, or blinking, reflex (startle response) to acoustic stimuli of unexpected onset and considerable intensity. The lateral lemniscus also provides a center for synapses for some fibers along the way. From this nucleus some of the nerve fibers cross to the opposite side before continuing to the cerebral cortex.

The next major way station on the auditory pathway in the brain is the *inferior colliculus,* at the level of the mesencephalon (midbrain). Here, too, some auditory fibers synapse with others; such groups may continue toward the same side of the cortex, or they may decussate (cross). The inferior colliculus serves as another center for reflexes in response to sound.

From the inferior colliculus all of the auditory fibers pass to synapse in the *medial geniculate body,* an important auditory center located in the *thalamus.* From here, all of the nerve fibers of the next (and last) order extend through the region known as the *auditory radiations,* where there is some fanning of the fibers. They terminate in the *temporal lobe* of the cerebral cortex, in the two *transverse temporal gyri.* Each ear is bilaterally represented in this region of the cortex as a result of the several crossings from one side to the other as the impulses travel toward the cortex.

The various parts of the cerebral cortex are interconnected by association fibers, so that the entire cortex can act as a unit. However, some specific areas of auditory function have been identified. The *auditory reception area* is in the anterior portion of the temporal lobes on either side of the brain. The auditory area as a whole, however, goes well beyond this. Blending with the reception area are more posterior and superior auditory areas of the cortex. These carry on the functions of recognition, association, and recall.

Clinical Note

An injury to the cortical auditory area does not necessarily result simply in an auditory dysfunction, because of the great number of interconnections with surrounding areas. The term *aphasia* refers to difficulties on the part of the injured individual in recalling, associating, or sometimes even recognizing auditory stimuli that have passed through an otherwise normal auditory system. *Wernicke's aphasia* is an auditory receptive disorder; *receptive aphasia* is more or less the same thing; and sometimes *paraphasia* is considered to be essentially an auditory disorder in that the person is unable to monitor his/her own language behavior satisfactorily. Injuries to the auditory area are found rather commonly among the population having aphasia. The proximity of the auditory area in the cerebral cortex to the various motor areas is such that an injury to one region might well produce damage in the adjacent one. The result is an extremely complex pattern of disorders of oral communication.

The auditory neural system also contains an *efferent* component. The *olivocochlear (Rassmussen's) bundle* commences, apparently, in the *olivary complex,* a center having numerous connections with other brain areas, such as the cerebellum, the thalamus, and the cortex. The olivary complex provides efferent fibers to the auditory system that relate to the inhibition of the system (it sends fibers via a complicated route to the cochlea and its hair cells, especially the outer hair cells).

AUDITORY ABILITIES

The animal ear must be a receptor system with broad capabilities. Often, the very life of the animal depends upon how well it hears. It must differentiate between the everyday rustle of leaves in a breeze and the rustle of leaves rubbing the skin of a passing predator. It must pick up the distant tinkle of falling water in a creek and be aware of the noise of a great waterfall. It must identify the scream of a high-flying eagle and the clucking of a nearby sage hen. It should differentiate between the call of a potential mate and that of a hunting killer.

The human ear must be sensitive not only to the sound of the approaching train but to that of the distant airplane, to the chirping cricket and the barking dog, to the dripping faucet and the rushing flood, to the shout for help and the whisper of endearment, to the rumbling tympani and the shrill flute.

Human hearing can be described quantitatively, which allows for important studies and provides a means of comparison between the hearing skills of normal people and those of people with a hearing loss. The two major auditory measurements are pitch and loudness.

Pitch is the brain's perception of the rate of vibration of sound. The unit of measure is *mel*. Pitch is the psychologic counterpart of *frequency,* which can be measured by instruments that count the number of vibratory events per unit of time. The unit of measure of frequency is *cycles per second,* or *Hertz (Hz)*.

Loudness is the brain's perception of the intensity of sound, the amount of energy it is producing. The unit of measure is *sone*. The physical counterpart of loudness is *sound pressure level* (SPL), the amount of pressure exerted by the vibrating air molecules as they strike the measuring device. Relative sound pressure levels are measured in *bels* or *decibels (dB),* a logarithmic representation of pressure relationships.

The frequency range to which the human ear is sensitive varies from 16 to 20 Hz to 20,000 Hz, with individual variation. The vocal tract produces sounds in a much narrower range; 500 to 2000 Hz is the range of *speech frequencies*.

The sound pressure level to which the human ear responds varies from that of a just detectable sound to that of a sound creating pain in the ears. In terms of decibels, if the normal just detectable level is arbitrarily set at 0 dB, the pain level can be as much as 130 dB. Discomfort occurs at about 120 dB. Two people speaking to each other in a quiet room may be speaking at sound pressure levels of between 45 and 60 dB.

Many other important auditory skills demonstrate the remarkable abilities of the ear. Skills of detectability are joined by those of intelligibility (assigning meaning to sound), discrimination (recognizing differences between sounds), masking (distinguishing sounds that interfere with one another), localization (identifying the direction of the source of a sound), and so on. These skills and other auditory behaviors are evaluated by means of *audiometry*.

Audiology is the study of normal and abnormal audition; it has become an important field of study. Many clinical audiologists expend much effort in the assessment, habilitation, and rehabilitation of persons disturbed by auditory deficits.

VESTIBULAR SYSTEM

Within the inner ear are the sensory end organs for body equilibrium. Because a large part of these bilateral structure are found within the vestibule of the inner ear, the system is termed the *vestibular system*. It gives its name to the cranial nerve carrying its message to the brain, the *vestibulocochlear nerve* (Cranial VIII).

This system serves both static equilibrium (how the body via the head relates to gravity) and dynamic equilibrium (how the body adjusts to changes in head position). Normally, there is little functional relationship between the vestibular end organ and the cochlear end organ functions; there may be, however, important aspects of the two requiring investigation when there is suspicion of inner ear pathology.

The end organs themselves are located in membranous sacs in the three *ampullae* of the *semicircular canals* as well as the *saccule* and *utricle* of the vestibule. These contain endolymph, while in the bony canals is perilymph. Two types of end organs may be found, the *macula* and the *crista*. Movement of the surrounding head causes the endolymph to flow to bend the end organ or to change the relationship between the hair cells there and the gelatinous material and the calcium carbonate *otoliths;* whichever occurs, the end result is a stimulation of the hair cells to initiate a nerve impulse.

Nerve fibers join to form the *vestibular division* of the vestibulocochlear nerve within the internal acoustic canal, where it passes with the cochlear division as well as the facial nerve. Most of the fibers from the end organ synapse in the several *vestibular nuclei;* from here are numerous neural connections to the spinal cord. More important to audiologists, however, are the connections to the nuclei of the cranial nerves that control movements of the eyes.

Clinical Note

As part of their clinical responsibilities, some audiologists evaluate not only the auditory abilities of their patients, but the functioning of the vestibular systems. Here, it is of importance to explore possible pathologies affecting the two inner ear systems, the vestibular and the cochlear. One test utilizes highly specialized instrumentation involved in elecronystagmography (ENG). It seeks to identify the presence of and the nature of any of several kinds of nystagmus, unusual eye movements following stimulation of the vestibular end organs.

Another group of connections from the vestibular nuclei have important connections with the *cerebellum.* This structure maintains control over static equilibrium by its constant sensory imput and coordinating that input to relay orders to the cerebrum for body muscle adjustment. Dynamic equilibrum is maintained via a similar pathway so that changes in body status, which usually are associated with changes in head position, are monitored by the vestibular system and the cerebellum.

SUMMARY

The auditory system, which transmits sound from the environment to the brain, consists of four parts: the external ear, the middle ear, the inner ear, and the neural ear.

The external ear channels air carrying sound into the side of the skull. The external acoustic meatus is a canal entering the side of the head from the pinna to the tympanic membrane.

The middle ear houses ossicles that pick up vibrations from the tympanic membrane and transmit them to the inner ear.

The inner ear is a closed system of fluid-filled canals. The vibrations from the middle ear set up waves in these fluids that are ultimately transformed into neural stimuli. The inner ear also contains the equilibrium mechanism.

The neural ear transmits neural impulses generated at the hair cells of the inner ear. These impulses travel by way of the auditory nerve to various parts of the brain, where they are processed and perceived as sound.

Auditory abilities are measured in terms of pitch and loudness, which are the psychologic counterparts of frequency and intensity. The study of and testing and patient management in hearing impairment is a large part of the field of audiology; a remarkable effort is made in the study of normal hearing by psychoacousticians as they study auditory perception.

Clinical Implications

An entire professional and academic field, audiology, is devoted to the study of audition and its disorders. Clinically, the evaluation of and the management of auditory problems is more than testing or of, say, fitting hearing aids. Educational management in the cases of children with hearing impairments may become personal counseling in adults with later-appearing hearing disorders.

Infants and children learn their spoken language by hearing it in their everyday environments. Thus, a first communication disorder in a child with a hearing impairment may be diminished language skills. In a similar way, the vowels and consonants and other aspects of speech production (e.g., prosody) are modeled after what the child hears. Thus, in a youngster with a hearing loss the problem may be demonstrated in speech problems or differences.

In both cases, language and/or speech problems, the rehabilitation specialist (the audiologist) may focus upon the child's learning, and utilizing those aspects of oral communication that may be limited.

In older persons, the loss of already acquired auditory skills can become an important problem to that individual. If s/he is in the earning phases of life, hearing impairments can become a more or less severe hindrance to remaining employed. One can imagine the multitude of problems ensuing should a commercial airline pilot develop a hearing impairment, for example. Such persons not only may lose gainful employment, but also may be expected to become more or less emotionally concerned, so that personal counseling as well as rehabilitation management techniques may be required.

The loss of hearing that occurs with many persons as they age is called *presbycusis*. It is common and of course may be related to a number of personal as well as vocational (and avocational) hindrances. Many other hearing problems occur, some associated with body health and some related to trauma and other causes. Diseases associated with the nervous system (such as meningitis, tumors, or measles) may be causally related to hearing disorders. Inner ear problems, such as the earlier mentioned presbycusis as well as infections or structural changes, also may develop at times and may or may not be associated with aging. Middle ear problems are common among children, of course, and lead to hearing impairments of several kinds. Ear aches, ruptured tympanic membranes, and other problems are well known to pediatricians. Older persons may have middle ear problems, outstanding among which is otosclerosis, which is a growth of new bone over the oval footplate of the stapes bone anchoring it in place to impede sound transmission into the inner ear.

Clinical audiology is replete with numbers of pathologies and with different hearing disorders, many of which are now manageable. Hearing aids, manual signing, assistive listening devices, special education, speech reading, and telephone devices for the deaf are among the many instruments and procedures used to help persons with hearing impairments.

Study Questions

1. Explain how the brain hears a single sound with each of two ears picking up a sound stimulus.

2. Consider the usefulness of turning the pinna without turning the head to listen. Which animals would find this most helpful?

3. If a child learning to talk cannot hear above 4000 Hz and if the [s] sound is produced with a frequency above 6000 Hz, will the child have trouble learning to say [s]?

4. Note how changes in air pressure in the middle ear can cause you to sense a sound, especially during a semiyawn.

5. In a location with sounds around you, close off one ear with a finger and see what effect this has upon your ability to locate the source of different sounds.

6. Open and close your ears during a conversation with a friend. What effect does loss of hearing have upon your ability to follow the conversation?

7. Some bats can hear sounds of four to six times the frequency of sounds that humans can hear. Why?

8. How would a middle ear that was filled with fluid interfere with hearing?

9. Consider the effect on hearing of the great difference in size between the large tympanic membrane and the small oval footplate.

10. Would cementing the joints of the ossicular chain affect hearing?

Chapter 8

The Nervous System

GENERAL INTRODUCTION

Living organisms are equipped to protect their existence with mechanisms that maintain homeostasis of the individual. Homeostasis is the biologic tendency of the organism (an animal, plant, or the human body) to maintain a state of physiologic stability or equilibrium in its internal environment (that is, in such conditions as body temperature, blood pressure, chemical balances, etc.) under changes of both external and internal environmental influences. An essential mechanism dedicated to the maintenance of homeostasis is the nervous system. The human nervous system also provides for the somewhat unique capabilities such as short and long-term storage and memory/recall.

The developed nervous system can be studied as having two functionally and structurally related divisions, the *central nervous system* and the *peripheral nervous system* (Table 8.1). The central nervous system (CNS) is composed of the *brain,* found within the protective shell of the cranial bones, and the *spinal cord,* located within the vertebral canals of adjacent vertebrae. The brain and the spinal cord are not structurally separate but together form the continuous CNS through the foramen magnum of the occipital bone.

Clinical Note

The speech-language pathologist who meets with a patient who has paralyzed speech muscles because of a fractured skull would probably guess that the broken cranial bones further damaged the brain within. That portion of the brain that was damaged, then, might well have housed brain centers controlling muscle actions. The study that occurs involves examining the damaged functions, the remaining intact functions, estimating return of function by training, and entering a plan of rehabilitation with the patient.

The peripheral nervous system (PNS) interconnects structurally and functionally with the CNS and it has two divisions largely identified by their functional statuses. The *sensory* (or *afferent*) division reacts to internal (within the body) and to external (outside the body) conditions or events. Internal conditions include hunger, need for increased oxygen, pain within body organs, and the like. External events include sound, light, outside heat or cold, among others. The sensory division delivers a signal *(nerve impulse)* into the central nervous system to initiate neurologic activities to maintain homeostasis.

The *motor* (or *efferent*) division of the PNS signals, via nerve impulses, reactive mechanisms (e.g., muscles) in their homeostatic purposes. The motor division has two subdivisions, the *somatic* and the *autonomic* efferent systems. The somatic (body functions under generally voluntary control) causes skeletal muscles to contract to perform their work. The autonomic division signals involuntary mechanisms (such as smooth muscle of the

Table 8.1. Divisions of the Nervous System

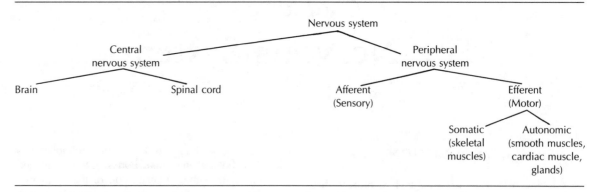

digestive tract or digestive glands or cardiac muscle) to react so as to maintain homeostasis.

In general, then, we might identify at least three important functions of the nervous system as a whole: (1) sensory, that reacts to both internal and external events; (2) interpretive, that analyzes (e.g., by learning, memory, or cognitive abilities) the incoming sensations; and (3) responsive, by voluntarily or involuntarily initiated motor action to muscles and glands. The organization of behavior becomes increasingly complex and amazing the "higher" the development of the organism, assuming that the human animal is at the apex of organizational development.

The two larger structural divisions of the nervous system are, as noted above, the brain and the spinal cord. The brain is the first important focus of attention for reasons that will become clear; the spinal cord will be examined later.

THE DEVELOPMENT OF THE BRAIN

This large structure is housed within and protected by the cranial bones. One can identify four regions (Table 8.2) of the adult brain to which many special functions are assigned. The largest portion is the *cerebrum,* expanded and spreading over the other divisions much like the upper portion of a mushroom. Internally to the two hemispheres (connected through the *corpus callosum*) of the cerebrum is the second, the *diencephalon,* an older term designating the *thalamus* and the *hypothalamus,* to which we will return later. The third region of the brain is the *brainstem,* a bilaterally fused, inferiorly oriented portion that includes the *medulla oblongata,* the *pons,* and the *midbrain.* The fourth region is the *cerebellum,* located posteriorly in the cranium and protected largely by the occipital bone.

The diencephalon was noted in the preceding paragraph as "an older term." The word "older" here refers to older developmentally, for it is one of several terms referring to the embryologic divisions of the nervous system (Table 8.3). The Greek origins of these terms are descriptive; they identify critical areas during the early development of the organisms and have become established in reference to adult brain areas by some authorities.

In about the 4th week of embryonic development, there appear three rudimentary regions (*vesicles*): the *prosencephalon* (or the forebrain), the *mesencephalon* (or the midbrain), and the *rhombencephalon* (or the hindbrain). In placing terms suggesting locations here, one might be reminded that similar regions develop in lower animals whose brains may well be organized in a more

Table 8.2. Divisions of the Brain

Larger Divisions	Subdivisions
Cerebrum	Hemispheres and lobes
Diencephalon	Thalamus and hypothalamus
Brainstem	Medulla, pons, midbrain
Cerebellum	

horizontal plan than is the human with its above-and-below organization.

The embryologic development continues rapidly from this three-vesicle arrangement. At about the 5th week of gestation, the prosencephalon now can be seen to have a telencephalon (or endbrain) from which will derive the *cerebrum,* the *corpus callosum,* and the *basal ganglia* in the adult. The other subdivision of the prosencephalon is the *diencephalon* (or between-brain) from which develop several adult areas including the *thalamus* and the *hypothalamus.*

The second brain vesicle is the mesencephalon. This does not undergo further regional division. Even the adult brain maintains that area and that term, although one commonly hears it called *midbrain.*

The third vesicle of the embryonic brain (the rhombencephalon) at about the 5th week of development also forms two regions or secondary vesicles. One is the *metencephalon* (or afterbrain). From this are formed the adult *pons* and the *cerebellum.* Also developing during the 5th week as part of the primary vesicle is the *myelencephalon* (or the rarely used term "marrow brain"). Among the regions of the adult brain associated with this area is the *medulla oblongata.* This lowermost portion of the brainstem is continuous with the spinal cord through the foramen magnum.

Embryologically, the spinal cord (*medulla spinalis*) does not show the vesicles or regions that are in the brain, but it does demonstrate minimal evidence of segmentation. This portion of the CNS is housed in the protective vertebral canal, and in the embryo is contained therein from foramen magnum to the lowermost vertebral region. It never completely fills the canal for there are protective coverings, as meninges, fatty tissues, blood vessels, among other structures, within the bony canal.

In the adult human, the spinal cord reaches only to the first or second lumbar vertebrae. It is then held to the bottommost vertebrae, the coccyx, by the *filum terminale.* By adult age, enlargements have developed along the length of the cord. As one might expect, when there is an increase in body tissues to be innervated (as in the arms and legs) there needs to be a greater quantity of nerve fibers entering and leaving the CNS to serve those limbs. Thus, we find the cervical and lumbar enlargements of the spinal cord. These represent connections to the PNS.

THE PERIPHERAL NERVOUS SYSTEM

There are arbitrary "divisions" of the entire nervous system. For the study of human communication, one can look primarily at two divisions. The two divisions of the nervous system are the peripheral and the central. Starting with the peripheral nervous system (PNS), it is evident that it is in intimate and functional contact with the other (central nervous system). The term "peripheral" suggests that the nerves serve portions of the body outside the spaces within the bones that house the CNS: the trunk, the extremities, and the head and neck. The PNS has two groups: the spinal nerves and the cranial nerves (leaving until later any consideration of the autonomic nervous system).

Clinical Note

Speaking and hearing disorders can result from damage to the peripheral nervous system. Cutting or otherwise damaging an incoming sensory nerve can cause that nerve to fail to carry nerve impulses, which would be noted as a loss of sensation of whatever type the nerve was serv-

Table 8.3. Embryologic Derivations of Major Brain Regions

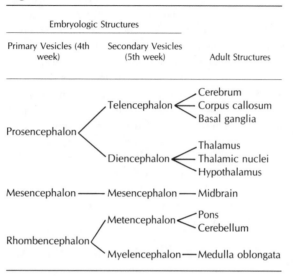

Embryologic Structures		
Primary Vesicles (4th week)	Secondary Vesicles (5th week)	Adult Structures

Prosencephalon
- Telencephalon
  - Cerebrum
  - Corpus callosum
  - Basal ganglia
- Diencephalon
  - Thalamus
  - Thalamic nuclei
  - Hypothalamus

Mesencephalon —— Mesencephalon —— Midbrain

Rhombencephalon
- Metencephalon
  - Pons
  - Cerebellum
- Myelencephalon —— Medulla oblongata

ing. For example, cutting nerve fibers carrying sensation into the central nervous system would cause the region served to become anesthetic, or numb. If an outgoing nerve fiber is damaged, a muscle could not contract because of loss of stimulation. The sensory and motor components of the peripheral nervous system carry on local or regional tasks, under the direction of the central nervous system.

Spinal Nerves

The spinal cord is a direct continuation of the brain and thus is in functional communication with higher centers (up to the cerebral cortex) and with lower centers within the cord. Understanding the voluntary muscular system and reflexes depends upon understanding the structure of the spinal cord and its nerves. The joining of the spinal nerves to the spinal cord is the joining of the peripheral with the central nervous systems (Figs. 8.1 and 8.2; see Fig. 8.4).

The segmentation noted earlier is found in the 31 pairs of *spinal nerves* along the length of the spinal cord. As the vertebral column grows vertically, with no concomitant vertical growth of the spinal cord, the spinal nerves show an increasing degree of slanting orientation outward. The cervical spinal nerves show little slanting but are oriented nearly perpendicular to the plane of the cord. In the lumbar region, however, the inclination has increased so much that the lumbar, sacral, and coccygeal nerves are vertical in the vertebral canal. Below the end of the spinal cord (at about L-2 level) there is a considerable accumulation of spinal nerves, given the name *cauda equina* (horse's tail) because of the appearance of the bundle.

As is so much of the anatomic organism, spinal nerves are paired. There are 31 pairs from the uppermost to the lowermost. Spinal nerves are named from the vertebral groups with which they are associated. There are eight pairs of cervical nerves, the first one (i.e., C-1) passing above the atlas and below the occipital bone. Below this group are the 12 pairs of thoracic nerves. Next are the five pairs of lumbar nerves, another five pairs of sacral nerves, and a single pair of coccygeal nerves.

One could conclude that each of the paired spinal nerves is identified by the adjacent vertebra. Thus, as we note cervical vertebra number three or thoracic number seven, we also name the associated spinal nerve. So, we have cervical nerve 3, or thoracic 7, etc. We can abbreviate to C-3 or T-7, of course.

The ladder-like (segmented) arrangement of the paired spinal nerves are combinations of the incoming sensory and the outgoing motor nerve portions. The sensory nerve fibers approaching the vertebral canal join with the motor nerve fibers leaving the canal at just one point, where they pass between adjacent vertebrae. At that point, they appear to be a single nerve so are named accordingly. Thus, we find lumbar four (L-4) or thoracic 11 (T-11) spinal nerves, with no separate identification of sensory or motor divisions at that point.

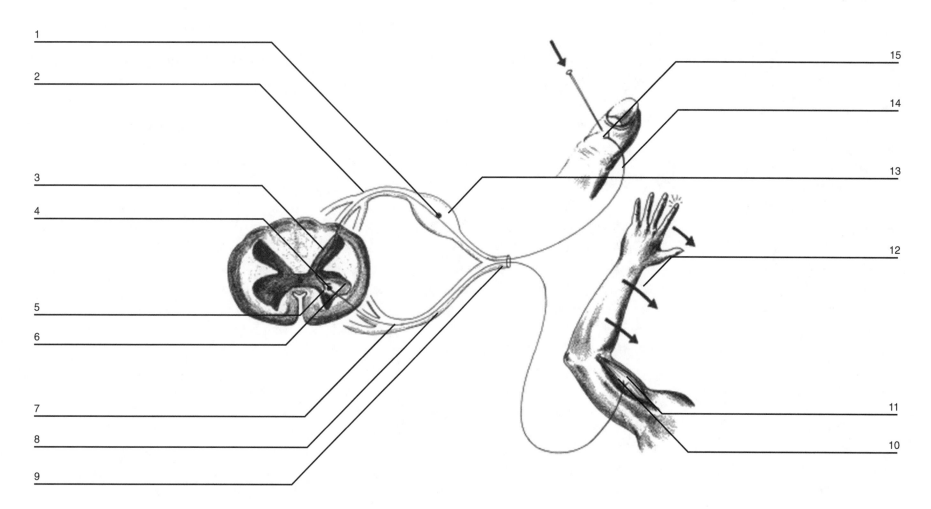

Figure 8.1   Reflex Arc

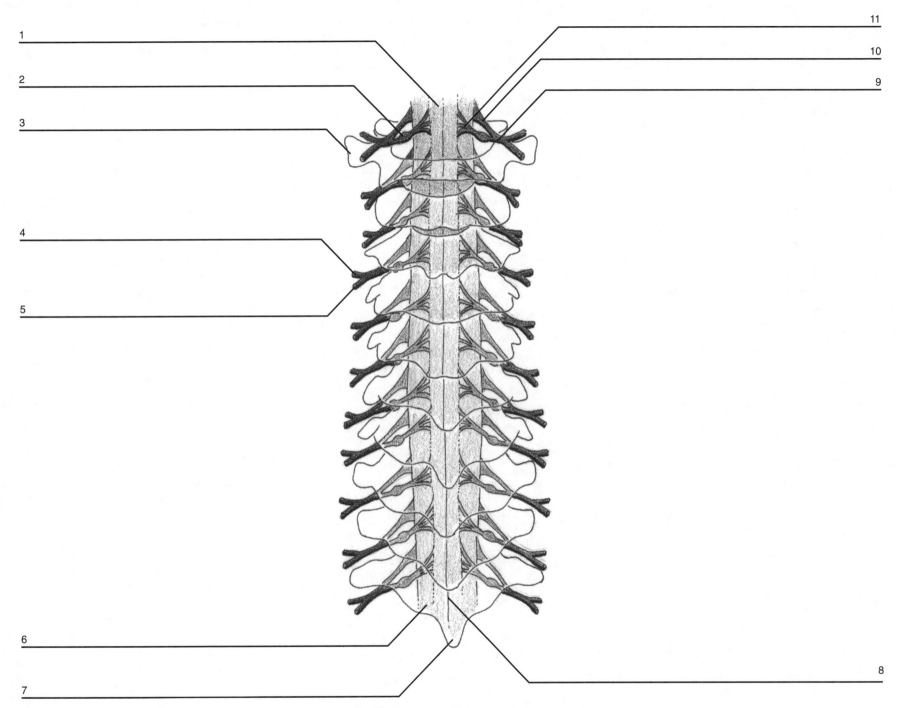

Figure 8.2   Spinal Nerves

The spinal nerves pass through the juncture of the vertebrae in the spinal column, at the intervertebral foramen and into the vertebral canal. Each spinal nerve has two portions: the dorsal portion is the *sensory root,* which enters the spinal cord; the ventral portion is the *motor root,* which leaves the spinal cord. Branching fibers also leave and form the autonomic nervous system, prior to the formation of the final spinal nerve. Entirely within the spinal cord lie millions of association neurons traveling to and from centers within the central nervous system.

On each side the sensory root presents a somewhat enlarged portion after having separated from the spinal nerve at the foramen. This enlargement is the *ganglion.* It is composed of the cell bodies of all the incoming sensory nerve fibers. From this point, centrally, the root subdivides into numerous rootlets, which ultimately form a continuous and evenly spaced line along the dorsal-lateral surface of the spinal cord. The rootlets enter the cord into an area known as the *dorsal horn,* the *dorsal column,* or because it is a part of the gray matter of the central nervous system, the *dorsal gray column.* Gray matter lacks myelin sheathing and is predominantly collections of nerve cell bodies with multitudinous synapses. This column is found through most of the spinal cord, receiving sensory impulses from all levels, starting as far caudally as its lowermost point at the level of the first lumbar vertebra. This sensory information ultimately reaches the cerebral cortex in the parietal lobe.

Clinical Note

Spinal nerves may be damaged, even incapacitated, by injury to the vertebrae. The so-called "broken backs" or "broken necks" may be such that the spinal nerves in the vicinity of the trauma are also interrupted. Should they be serving musculature of importance to speech production, such as muscles of respiration, one might expect to have that function disturbed. Recovery of function is dependent upon the recovery of the patient in terms of muscle, innervation, whether by natural healing or by surgical intervention, or some other technique.

Nerve fibers serving sensory functions form the greater portion of the nervous system, ultimately communicating with subcortical and cortical centers, where sensations are perceived and acted upon. Connections with other major pathways permit gross adjustment in the body to be accomplished without volitional involvement. Rapid *reflex activity* takes place at or about the level of the spinal nerve (Fig. 8.1).

Lower motor neurons originate in the central gray column of the spinal cord, in centers that are in contact with interconnecting fibers from the dorsal and the intermediate gray columns and with fibers (*upper motor neurons*) descending from higher centers. A *lower motor* fiber exits from the spinal cord as the ventral root, gives off collaterals that connect with the autonomic ganglia in the vicinity, and then joins with the dorsal root to form the spinal nerve of that segment of the cord.

Both the sensory and motor nerve fibers may be short, as those that leave the vertebral canal to innervate the intercostal muscles, or they may be of considerable length, as are those that travel from the vertebral canal to the toes.

There is a constant, low-level stimulation of muscle fibers by the motor nerve fibers. Thus, in every large muscle, there are always some few muscle fibers in states of contraction because of the firing of some few nerve fibers. This low-level state of contraction is termed *muscle tonicity,* or *tonus.* When large numbers of nerve fibers stimulate a muscle, the muscle as a whole contracts.

Clinical Note

In certain pathologic states neural innervation to skeletal muscles is disturbed. Speech therapists frequently are called upon to treat communicative problems stemming from such conditions. In the case of spinal nerves, the result is usually a muscular weakness; skill and understanding are needed to help a patient with paralyzed muscles and to develop adequate compensatory muscular activity. Injury to the hypoglossal nerve (Cranial XII), for example, could cause tongue muscles to be weak, which could result in a speech disorder if the tongue fails in its articulatory function.

Cranial Nerves

The peripheral nervous system is composed of cranial nerves as well as spinal nerves. There is a similarity in the functions of the two for the cranial nerves enter and exit the CNS carrying sensation or motor commands as do the spinal nerves. However, they are not as "regular" in their structures as are the spinal nerves.

The 12 pairs of cranial nerves are numbered in Roman numerals generally (as compared to the Arabic numerals used for spinal nerves). The order of numbering commences with number I at the most anterior part of the cranium, with number XII being at the most posterior-inferior portion. Some of the cranial nerves are purely sensory, carrying no motor commands; others are purely motor, carrying no entering sensory information; while a third group are mixed, carrying both sensory and motor nerve impulses. Some of the motor nerves of the cranial group are voluntary, while some are involuntary (somatic or autonomic). Some travel very short distances (e.g., nerve I is olfactory carrying the sense of smell a short distance from nose to brain). On the other hand, nerve X is vagus and travels throughout a large part of the entire body.

As you may have noted, cranial nerves are not only known by their numbers but also by names. These names may be related to their functions, to the anatomic regions they serve, or how they travel. Note in Table 8.4 the numbers and names as well as the functions for each of the cranial nerves.

The brain is the region of origin of cranial nerves (Fig. 8.3). Those serving speech and hearing rather directly include Cranials V, VII, VIII, IX, X, XI, and XII.

Cranial V is named the *trigeminal nerve* because soon after leaving the brainstem at the two sides of the pons, it divides into three parts: the ophthalmic, the maxillary, and the mandibular. Both the ophthalmic and the maxillary divisions are mainly sensory in function, running to the brain from the eye orbit and its environs—the forehead, nose, cheek, jaw, teeth, mouth, and other regions where sensation to the skin and mucosa is served. The mandibular division leaves the pons, exits from the skull through the foramen ovale, and becomes the masticator nerve, serving the muscles of mastication and other oral structures.

Cranial VII (the *facial nerve*) serves the structures of the facial region in both motor and sensory functions. The motor division leaves the central nervous system from the lower portion of the pons; it enters the internal auditory meatus, along with the cochlear and vestibular divisions of Cranial VIII, and leaves the skull at the stylomastoid foramen. It runs through the walls of the middle ear, the parotid gland, and then divides into numerous branches that serve the facial region. Most of the muscles of facial expression, the scalp, the auricle, the stapedius muscle, the stylohyoid muscle, and the posterior belly of the digastric muscle receive innervation from this major nerve. The sensory functions served by Cranial VII are mainly those of taste in the anterior two-thirds of the tongue (through the chorda tympani nerve) and the soft palate. This cranial nerve serves the salivary glands also.

Cranial VIII (the *vestibulocochlear nerve*) is primarily sensory in function; its two divisions serve the two sensations of audition and equilibrium. The cochlear division, serving the auditory function, has sensory fibers that originate at the spiral organ of Corti, pass through the spiral ganglion and the internal auditory meatus, and enter the brain between the pons and the

Table 8.4. Cranial Nerves

Cranial Nerve Number	Cranial Nerve Name	Modality Served	Functions
I	Olfactory	Sensory	Smell
II	Optic	Sensory	Vision
III	Oculomotor	Motor	Eye muscle
IV	Trochlear	Motor	Eye muscle
V[a]	Trigeminal	Mixed	Sensory to face and mouth; motor to muscles mastication
VI	Abducens	Motor	Eye muscle
VII[a]	Facial	Mixed	Sensory to taste on tongue; motor to facial muscles and salivary glands
VIII[a]	Vestibulocochlear	Mostly sensory	Audition and equilibrium
IX[a]	Glossopharyngeal	Mixed	Sensory to taste, fauces, palate, and pharynx; motor to pharynx and salivary glands
X[a]	Vagus	Mixed	Sensory to skin of ear, pharynx, larynx; motor to pharynx, larynx, viscera
XI[a]	Accessory	Motor	Pharynx and neck and shoulder muscles
XII[a]	Hypoglossal	Mostly motor	Tongue muscles, neck strap muscles

[a]Important to speech and hearing functions.

medulla. The vestibular division, serving orientation of the head in space, originates in the utricle, the saccule, the superior and lateral semicircular canals, and the ampulla of the posterior semicircular canal. Its fibers pass from the vestibular ganglion into the internal auditory meatus, along with those of the cochlear division, and enter the medulla en route to the cerebellum. The motor division of this nerve is incompletely understood.

Cranial IX (the *glossopharyngeal nerve*) is both motor and sensory in function, serving the posterior portion of the tongue and mouth and the pharynges. It has its major central nervous system origins in the medulla, leaving that region through the petrous portion of the temporal bone. Its motor fibers run to the pharyngeal musculature; its sensory fibers run to the same general area, serving taste in the posterior third of the tongue and other sensations in the fauces, tonsils, pharynx, and soft palate.

Cranial X (the *vagus nerve*), containing afferent and efferent fibers, originates at the level of the medulla and exits from the skull through the jugular foramen. At this point it is joined by the cranial portion of Cranial XI, which accompanies it throughout its passage. The vagus, whose name means *wanderer*, serves both motor and sensory functions in widely dispersed regions, from the auricle to the abdominal viscera. Its sensory fibers originate at the skin of the auricle, part of the external auditory canal, the pharynx, the larynx, and the viscera of the thorax and the abdomen. Its motor fibers serve the pharynx, the base of the tongue, and the larynx, as well as the viscera of the thorax and abdomen through autonomic nervous system ganglia. An important division of this cranial nerve, the recurrent laryngeal nerve, and its terminus, the inferior laryngeal nerve, is of considerable interest when the operations of the larynx are studied. The superior laryngeal nerve, supplying the cricothyroid muscle, is of vagus origin; the sensory division of this last branch serves the interior of the larynx to alert the organism to the presence of foreign material and to initiate a protective cough.

Cranial XI (the *accessory nerve*) is mainly a motor nerve, originating in the medulla and leaving the skull through the jugular foramen. Here it is joined with a portion derived from the first five or six spinal nerves. That portion originating in the medulla joins with the vagus and innervates muscles in the pharynx, larynx, uvula, and soft palate, perhaps also contributing to the recurrent laryngeal nerve. That portion of the accessory nerve that derives from the upper portion of the spinal cord (thus the *spinal* accessory nerve) is the efferent nerve to the large sternocleidomastoid muscle and the trapezius muscle.

Cranial XII (the *hypoglossal nerve*) is also primarily a motor nerve. Its origin is medullary, and its leaves the skull as a single nerve on each side after joining with a small group of nerve rootlets emerging from the medulla. It is motor to the intrinsic muscles of the tongue, the extrinsic muscles of the tongue (excepting the palatoglossus, which is innervated by the vagus), and the strap muscles of the neck through a loop known as the *ansa hypoglossi* and *ansa cervicalis*. This last-named structure is complex in origin, deriving from the hypoglossal nerve and the cervical nerves of the spinal cord. It innervates such muscles as the sternohyoid, sternothyroid, thyrohyoid, and omohyoid. A sensory component is thought to be present.

Clinical Note

Lesions to cranial nerves produce many and varied symptoms and signs—for example, facial paralysis when Cranial VII is involved; hearing disorders when Cranial VIII is involved; resonance and articulation disorders when Cranial IX is involved; respiration, breath support, and phonation problems when Cranial X is involved; posture problems and general tonicity of the neck regions when Cranial XI is involved; and articulation and resonance disorders when Cranial XII is involved.

THE NEURON AND NEURON CHAIN

The structural and functional unit of the nervous system is a cell, the neuron. At birth, according to estimates, there are up to 100 billion of these cells. These cells combine with the glial cells, which are supportive and protective tissues actually forming a larger portion of the CNS than do the accumulated neurons. As important as the glial cells may be, however, the functional focus is upon the neuron, for it receives the stimulus and passes that stimulus along to perform its task by electrochemical changes. To understand the activities of the nervous system, we need an exposure to its structural makeup.

A *neuron* is a cell that is stimulable and conducts nerve impulses; neurons differ from the supporting cells of nervous tissue, the *glial cells*. The neuron is composed of a cell body and its fibrous extensions. Although neurons are anatomically separate (i.e., there is no contiguity of substance between neurons), there is a functional connection between neurons, *synapses*. The message a neuron carries travels as a nerve impulse that crosses synapses and is taken up by adjoining neurons.

The extensions from the cell body are the *axons* and *dendrites*. There is generally only one axon fiber from each cell body; it can be of considerable length, up to 3 feet in some instances. The dendrites of a cell body are plural, each having numerous branchings. The axon usually carries impulses away from the cell body, whereas the dendrite carries them toward the cell body.

For the organism to receive stimuli and then react to them, there must be a series of at least two neurons in a chain: a *sensory neuron*, which is irritated by the stimulus, and a *motor neuron*, which causes a muscle (or gland) to be stimulated. The axon of one cell is in synaptic contact with the dendrite or the cell body of another cell. The direction of flow of the nerve impulse is from axon to dendrite or cell body, not the reverse. The nerve impulse traveling along the neuronal processes and through the synapse is both electrical and

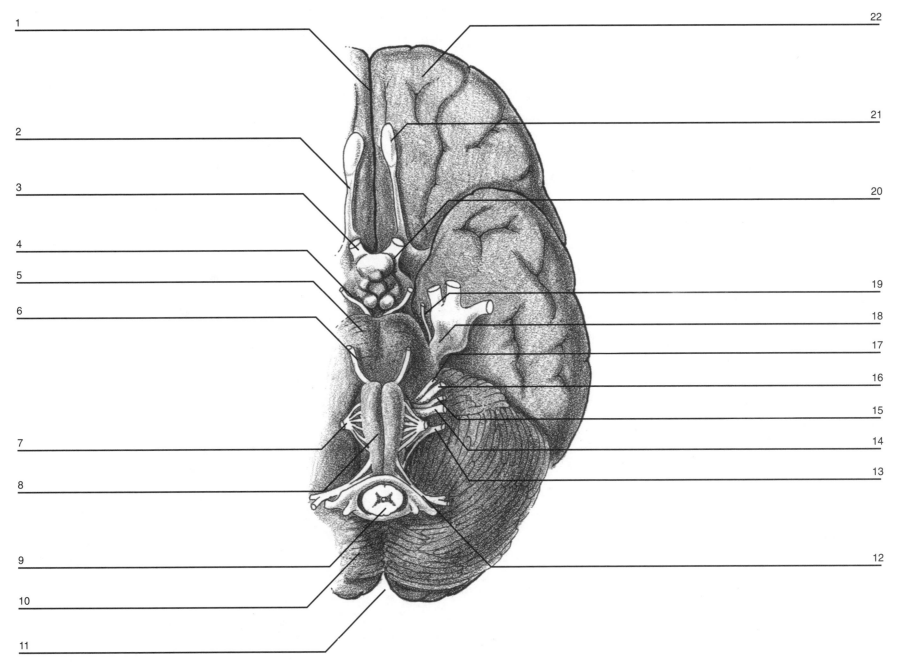

Figure 8.3   Cranial Nerves

chemical. This electrochemical transmission travels along the length of the nerve fibers and across the synapse in a rapid change of electrical polarity due to exchanges of sodium and potassium ions, the sodium-potassium pump.

The movement of sodium and potassium ions internal and external to the neuron make possible both the irritability and the conductivity of the nervous system. Because of the electrical charge that these ions carry as they move into the neural cell and return out of it, an activity that commences when the cell is stimulated, the change in the electrical potential travels along the nerve cell. This polarization is the basis for the nerve impulse and thus the irritability aspect. The conductivity aspect refers to the transmission of the nerve impulse from one nerve fiber across the synapse (the fluid-filled gap between nerve fibers) to another nerve fiber or to a muscle or gland.

The simplest type of the neuron chain is the classic *reflex arc* (Fig. 8.1). Reflexes exist and operate at various levels of the nervous system. Let us consider the kind found in the spinal system; here only two neurons are necessary. The first, in order of activity, is the sensory (afferent) neuron, with its receptor in the skin or wherever the end organ for sensation might be. This first order neuron is stimulated by an irritant (identified ultimately as pain, cold, pressure, stretch, etc.), and the resulting neural impulse is carried toward the cell body.

The route taken by the nerve impulse depends upon the type, location, and central connections of the nerve fiber. In general, the nerve fiber carrying the impulse joins with other fibers in the vicinity. A large number of such joined fibers is termed a *nerve*. The nerve passes toward the vertebral column and the spinal cord within, entering the spinal cord via the *dorsal root.*

Within the dorsal root are found the cell bodies for the entering sensory neurons. Grouped, they form the spinal ganglion. From here, the nerve fiber enters the spinal cord and penetrates to the *dorsal gray horn,* where we find the termination of the incoming sensory fibers. Most fibers divide into branches, some ascending, some descending, some traveling elsewhere as collateral branches.

In the simplest two-neuron reflex chain, or arc, the collaterals then pass to the *ventral gray horn* in the spinal cord, where the synaptic connection with the cell body of the motor (efferent) neuron is made. The wave of excitation from the sensory fiber is transferred to, and sets up another wave of excitation in, the second order neuron. The impulse, now initiated in the motor fiber, travels out of the spinal cord through the *ventral root* of the spinal nerve. It travels through body tissues and terminates in the motor end-plate (neuromuscular junction), causing the muscle to contract via a synaptic relationship with the muscle cell fiber.

Some reflex chains consist of three neurons, with the third being termed an *association neuron,* or *internuncial neuron.* In such a case the sensory fiber, having entered the spinal cord and its gray horn, synapses with the association neuron, whose cell body is in the dorsal gray horn or nearby. It sends connecting collaterals to the appropriate effector neuron, as well as to other centers and pathways of the central nervous system. It is this complex routing of the association neuron that produces the many nerve pathways of higher animals. A great number of connections among the central neurons leads to a great number of possible responses to stimuli. Thus, stereotyped behavior is much less common among animals with highly developed central nervous systems.

Reflexes are responsible for segmental patterns of movement. Thus we have flexion, or withdrawal, reflexes from irritative stimuli; there are extensor reflexes, in which posture is maintained in a gravitational field. There are other types of reflexes, too. Through association fibers, reflexes become integrated into general body behavior.

THE MOTOR SYSTEM

Control of the activities of the body, especially of the skeletal musculature, is provided through the central nervous system via an arrangement that originates in the cerebral cortex. The major center (the motor cortex) is along the bilateral *precentral gyrus,* a convolution just anterior to the *central sulcus* on either hemisphere. The balance between the motor impulses from the primary motor center and those coming from the centers for inhibition determines the efficiency of muscular activity. Imbalance produces varying degrees of inefficiency, from simple clumsiness and incoordination to complete failure of the system. It is necessary to examine the pyramidal pathway in some detail, here, and to consider the extrapyramidal system as an important associated system.

The Pyramidal Pathway

The primary motor system starts with very large cells in the precentral gyrus of the cerebral cortex (Figs. 8.4 and 8.5); these cells serve as the initiators of impulses to the musculature. Their activities develop from their many interconnections with other regions of the brain. Their axons travel from the cortex in well-defined pathways (the corticobulbar and corticospinal), most crossing to the opposite side to centers (nuclei) of origin for the cranial nerves and spinal nerves. The *pyramidal pathway* is the major route of volitional motor impulses.

Passing down through the subcortical regions of the brain (through the internal capsule, through the pons, and through the medulla), the greater portion of the motor pathway from each motor cortex crosses to the other side of the brain. This crossing (the *decussation* of the pyramids) occurs in the medulla, the lowermost region of the brain. In the medulla, the nerve fibers enter the nuclei and there synapse with peripheral nerves (cranial nerves) that innervate much of the musculature

of the vocal tract. Of course, the pyramidal pathway also serves other body muscle systems.

Because the decussation, or crossing, of the fibers from both sides produces a bulge in the brainstem at that area, the region is known as the *bulb,* or the *pyramid.* Nearly all motor fibers from the cerebral cortex decussate, although about one-fifth remain ipsilateral until they cross lower in the spinal cord. There the termination of the motor pathway is within the *ventral gray column,* the gray column that is the center of origin for the efferent spinal nerve fibers that stimulate voluntary muscles.

Clinical Note

Lesions in the nervous system are often classified as upper or lower motor neuron lesions, depending upon the site of the lesion and the nervous tissue affected. It sometimes happens that a lower motor neuron lesion produces total paralysis of the musculature served simply because it is the final and only line of innervation. Upper motor neuron lesions may produce a muscular weakness for a similar reason, but also may produce some other type of defect, such as hypertonicity or incoordination, because other neural routes to the musculature involved may be intact and continue to stimulate that region, but without the coordinated control necessary. Thus, a lesion to the recurrent laryngeal nerve on one side may well produce a paralysis of the vocal fold on that side, because that nerve is an extension of a lower motor neuron. A lesion in the brainstem or elsewhere in the central nervous system could disrupt nerve fibers going to the same laryngeal structures, but the defect could be other than simple muscle weakness.

Many of the fibers originating in the cortex travel down to the spinal cord, but a large number terminate at levels above the cord. For example, the muscles that are served by the cranial nerves receive some of their

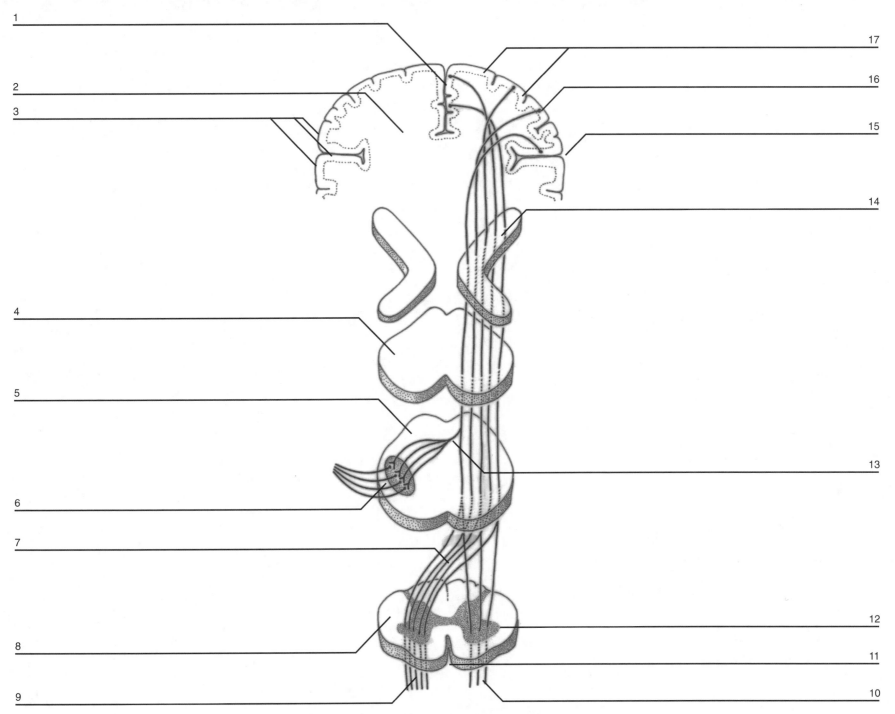

Figure 8.4 Pyramidal Pathway

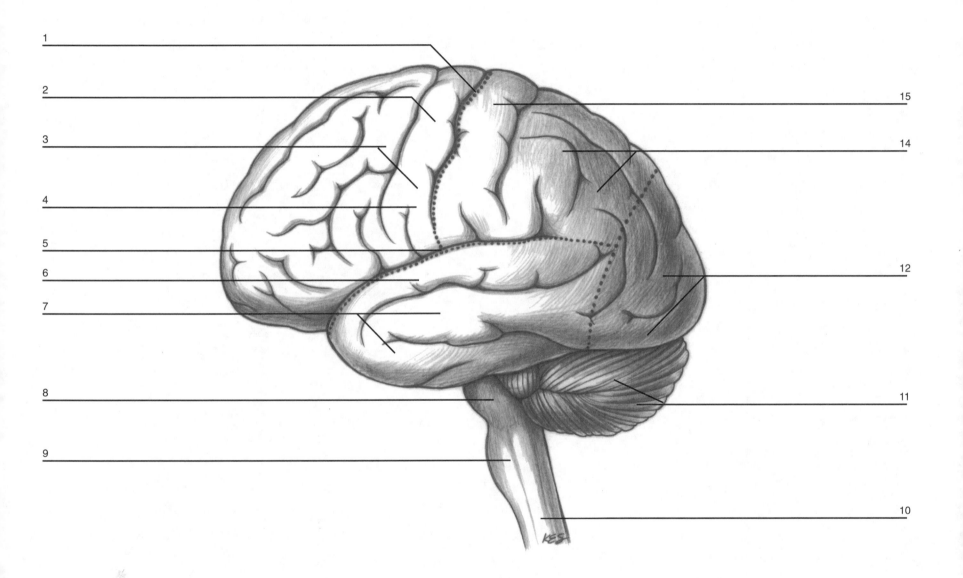

Figure 8.5 The Brain

innervation from the pyramidal pathway. Pyramidal path neurons that serve the cranial nerves terminate in contralateral centers in the pons and medulla, and are called *corticobulbar fibers;* those that continue on caudad through the decussation or otherwise are *corticospinal* fibers. Those that cross are found in the *lateral corticospinal tract* of the spinal cord, and those that remain ipsilateral are found in the *anterior,* or *ventral, cerebrospinal tract.* The latter generally serve the muscles of the trunk and decussate at the spinal level rather than at the medullary level.

The Extrapyramidal Pathway

The pyramidal pathway is the most direct system of muscle innervation from the cerebral cortex. The *extrapyramidal pathway* is an associated cooperative and coordinated system participating in body functions; it is self-directed and controls impulses from cortex to muscles. It comprises all centers other than those of the pyramidal system that send motor impulses from the brain to the spinal cord. Each of these centers relates to the cerebral cortex, as well as to other regions and centers of the brain. Together, they form a functional network. The extrapyramidal pathway is composed of special portions of the cerebral cortex, the basal ganglia (or basal nuclei), and midbrain centers (reticular areas), and is mainly a pathway for integration of motor activity. It is importantly related to complex behavior patterns usually modified by experience. Habitual and automatic activities of the body, such as those dealing with posture and reactive behavior in general, are mediated by the extrapyramidal system.

Clinical Note

Among the neuropathologies underlying speech disorders derived from lesions of the extrapyramidal system are parkinsonism, athetosis, chorea, and some forms of spasticity. Basically, the lesions occurring in various nuclei, centers, or pathways effect a release from stabilizing inhibitory mechanisms; from such lesions the various types of dysarthria, including cerebral palsy, result. Because of the many interconnections of the extrapyramidal system, elucidation of the possible pathologies is very difficult. Not only does the precentral motor area serve the efferent system in general, but there are other centers of initiation and inhibition located in the frontal lobe. Thus, some lesions may be paralytic while others may be excitatory, and the two groups may be difficult to differentiate.

THE SENSORY SYSTEM

Motor systems function in response to the influence of the sensory system, which provides means for the animal to react to its environment. Specialized neural cells respond to specific environmental changes, both external and internal. Human beings have an extremely large variety of receptors for such sensations as touch, cold, smell, hearing, and taste. The sensory system starts at the body periphery, where sensations are initiated by specialized receptors.

The receptors differ structurally, depending upon the type of stimulus to which they are responsive. Generally, there are two types. *Exteroceptors* include the sensory end organs that are cutaneous (for touch, heat, cold), those for chemical stimuli (taste and smell), and the distance receptors (vision and hearing). *Interoceptors* are represented by the proprioceptors (which respond to changes in muscle status and position) and the special receptors associated with the viscera and blood vessels (serving such sensations as hunger and thirst).

Nerve endings provide for the specificity of sensitivity. For example, the skin has corpuscles that are responsive to heat and cold, and it has free nerve endings (the most widely distributed receptors in the body) that serve pain. These are the "near" receptors. The so-called "distant" senses of vision and audition are associated with complex housings. For example, the divisions of the ear provide for certain changes in the original sound stimulus through mechanical means before the auditory receptors, the nerve endings on the hair cells of the organ of Corti, are stimulated.

Some interoceptors are associated with muscles, tendons, and joints. Others are in the viscera, blood vessels, and smooth muscle tissue. The proprioceptors are muscle spindles and tendon organs (specialized sensory end organs). When a muscle changes its tension by stretching or contracting, nerve impulses are generated that give the central nervous system information concerning that condition. This information does not usually reach consciousness, but is acted upon by subconscious processes.

Once reaching the central nervous system, sensory nerve fibers from the body enter the spinal cord via the dorsal root. Or, alternatively, they enter the brainstem through the cranial nerve serving that sensation. Ultimately, the path largely decussates (crosses to the opposite side of the spinal cord or brain) and rises rostrally in pathways. The pathways carry different modalities; for example, pain, touch, and proprioception travel in their own paths. These pathways make up some of the *white matter* in the central nervous system and include such routes as the two *spinothalamic tracts* and the *medial lemniscus.* Cranial nerves are similar to spinal nerves in how they are organized to carry sensation to the brain, and ultimately to sensory receiving areas in the cerebral cortex.

The sensory fibers generally arrive at or near the *thalamus.* Within the thalamus are several centers (nuclei) serving the different systems. Important central connections throughout the central nervous system are at the thalamus, and it is often considered the primary sensory mediating center (that is, as the place where sensations are perceived). The thalamus is responsible for relaying sensory information to the cerebral cortex and elsewhere.

The sensations reaching the cerebral cortex from the general body (*somatic sensory*) reach the parietal lobe.

Other sensory receptor areas include those for vision in the occipital lobe and audition in the temporal lobe. There are numerous association fibers interconnecting the various cortical areas, so that the import of two or more associated sensations can be fully appreciated. The great complexity with which nerve fibers from the cerebral cortex travel throughout the body provides for appropriate responses to the recognition of the incoming sensory stimuli.

SUBCORTICAL AREAS

Below the cortex and below the sensory radiations is the previously noted *thalamus,* which has numerous connections with other brain regions, including the cerebellum and the pons. There are several neural trunk lines interconnecting these regions, such as the *superior cerebellar peduncle* (also known as the *brachium conjunctivum*), between the thalamus and the cerebellum. Lower in the brainstem is the relatively large *pons,* or *bridge,* an enlarged portion of the hindbrain. The pons serves as a region from which major trunk lines depart to other important centers. It houses centers from which radiate various nerves serving the head and neck muscles, and it has interconnections to and from the cerebrum, cerebellum, and spinal cord.

A somewhat smaller region of the brainstem (sometimes considered the lowermost portion of that division and sometimes as the uppermost end of the spinal cord) is the *medulla oblongata.* The medulla is of particular importance to students of speech and hearing, for in this region are located nerve fibers and nerve centers for many of the basic functions serving communication. For example, within the medulla are located the motor nuclei of the glossopharyngeal, vagus, cranial portion of the accessory, and hypoglossal nerves. Also found in this region are the sensory nuclei of the glossopharyngeal and vagus nerves, as well as some of the vestibular centers. The cochlear (auditory) nuclei are located at the junction between the medulla and the pons. Thus, the medulla is importantly related to the functions of articulation of speech and of deglutition (swallowing); further, it is involved in coughing, sneezing, salivation, sucking, and vomiting, as well as being the motor innervator to bodily activities such as respiration, cardiovascular behavior, and digestive activities.

Clinical Note

Injuries of the subcortical regions sometimes result in problems with which the speech and hearing clinician will deal. For example, poliomyelitis may destroy nerve centers in the medulla region causing paralysis of musculature important in speech. In such cases, respiration, phonation, and articulation, among other functions, often are disturbed. In other instances, injuries or tumors to this region can result in auditory disorders. Cerebellopontine angle tumors, for example, can cause auditory disabilities.

THE CEREBRUM

The *cerebrum,* or *forebrain,* is the major portion of the brain (Fig. 8.5). It fills the upper part of the cranium and consists of two portions, called *hemispheres,* which although united at the bottom through the *corpus callosum,* are grossly separated at the midline by the longitudinal fissure.

The cerebrum consists largely of the *cerebral cortex,* plus portions of the *diencephalon.* This latter division of the brain consists of the thalamus, the epithalamus, and the hypothalamus. These serve as final mediating centers. The interior of the cerebral hemispheres housing these gray matter centers also contains white matter, consisting of supporting (glial) cells and neural pathways. These pathways for nerve impulses interconnect other CNS regions and the cerebral cortex. The cortex of the cerebrum is the outer layer of gray matter covering the entire brain. Less than one-third of the cerebral cortex is actually exposed because of the many folds, or *convolutions,* of the gray matter of this region. This important tissue is protected and separated from the bones of the skull by the three investing membranes, or *meninges;* the *pia mater,* the *arachnoid,* and the *dura mater.*

The cerebral cortex subdivides into lobes, which receive their names from the bones about them. Thus, the most anterior portion of the cortex on either side is the *frontal lobe.* Posterior to this lobe is the *parietal lobe.* At the farthest dorsal portion of the cerebrum is the *occipital lobe.* Below the frontal lobe on either hemisphere is the *temporal lobe.* The *fissure of Sylvius* separates this lobe from the frontal lobe. When this fissure is spread open, it reveals the *island (insula) of Reil* beneath.

The upper border of the fissure of Sylvius is the lower margin of the frontal lobe. The greater part of this border is called the *operculum.* Rising from the operculum, near its posterior portion, is another fissure, the *central sulcus (fissure of Rolando).* Posterior to this fissure is the parietal lobe, and anterior to it is the frontal lobe. Running up and down on either border of the central sulcus are two convolutions, or *gyri,* called the *posterior central gyrus* and the *anterior central gyrus.* These particular convolutions are of considerable importance to the speech and hearing therapist in that the anterior gyrus seems to have located in it all of the initiating nerve cells for most voluntary motor actions (i.e., the beginnings of the pyramidal tract). The posterior gyrus localizes the sensory, or somesthetic, aspects of the central nervous system. At the base of the central sulcus, encompassing a good deal of the operculum, is *Broca's area,* which is specifically related to the programming of speech production.

Clinical Note

Injuries to the regions just described often result in symptoms and syndromes amenable to speech therapeutics. Among the pathologic types are aphasia (a language disorder due to injury to the cerebral cortex) and dysarthria (a motor speech dysfunction sometimes due to injury to the anterior central gyrus or communicating subcortical regions). Cortical lesions may be expected to produce other problems accompanying communication disorders. There are important differences between the effects of lesions of the right and of the left hemispheres in terms of speech and language functions.

A large part of the frontal lobe is thought to serve functions such as memory and personality. The parietal lobe is essentially a general-body sensory lobe. The occipital lobe seems to be related primarily to vision. The temporal lobe serves audition.

The cerebrum is the highest structure of the central nervous system, and the human cerebrum is the most complex among animals. It is the region for voluntary control over functions that are often under involuntary control in other animals, the area for the reception and perception of complex stimuli, and the locale for remembering both sensory and motor experiences. It houses the areas for the linguistic or symbolic codification of experiences.

FUNCTIONAL REGIONS OF THE CEREBRAL CORTEX

Charting of the cortex involves the delineation of regions according to function. Brodmann's chart of the principal cortical areas is often used today to demonstrate generalities of function. Areas associated with oral communication can be identified by this method. These become the subject of the following.

Brodmann organized the cortex into its lobes and further subdivided the functional areas into numbered locales. Immediately anterior to the central sulcus in the frontal lobe is Area 4, the *primary motor area.* Between it and the next major region anteriorly is a strip region, sometimes called Area 4S, which borders or blends with the precentral motor area, Area 6.

Toward the front is Area 8, the frontal eye field, a special motor area. The prefrontal area of the cortex includes Areas 9, 10, 11, and 12, commonly known as the frontal association areas.

In the parietal lobe, the region between the central sulcus, the Sylvian fissure, the parietooccipital sulcus, and the midline, are several regions concerned with bodily sensation. Areas 1, 2, and 3 are in the postcentral area. These receive great numbers of projection fibers from the thalamus. Immediately posterior to these areas is the preparietal area, Area 5a, a typical sensory cortical area. Next to this is Area 5b, the superior parietal area, which is also sensory. Area 7 encompasses most of the inferior parietal region. In these three last-mentioned areas, it is thought that auditory and visual association take place, especially around the region known as the *supramarginal gyrus,* which is at the posterior-inferior part of the parietal lobe and on the left side is known as *Wernicke's area,* when it includes a part of the temporal lobe (thus it is also called the *parietotemporal area*). This is one of the most important regions for oral communication, the so-called language center.

The temporal lobe, found below the Sylvian fissure and bounded posteriorly by the parietal and occipital lobes, makes up a large portion of the cerebral cortex. Its primary function appears to be in audition. The *transverse convolutions (of Heschl)* receive acoustic radiations from the medial geniculate body of the thalamus. According to Brodmann's numbering system, this region includes Areas 41 and 42, the *primary acoustic areas.*

The occipital lobe of the cerebral cortex is the visual center of the brain. It is composed of at least three areas, 17, 18, and 19, which begin at the posterior pole of the lobe. Area 17 receives the optic radiations from the lateral geniculate bodies and is called the *primary visual cortex.* Area 18, a ring-like organization of cells immediately anterior to Area 17, is known as the *visuopsychic area.* It provides for understanding of the information received by the purely sensory receiving area, an understanding based upon past experience. Area 19 is the *preoccipital area;* it lies partly within the parietal lobe. Its function is to further the understanding of the visuopsychic region by association of visual stimuli with other sensory experiences. It operates much like the supramarginal gyrus of Area 7 in its association function.

Of special interest to the student of speech pathology is the area referred to as the *operculum,* in the third frontal convolution (Broca's area). Brodmann numbers this area in two parts, 44 and 45. The whole region may be both motor and association in function, but is definitely related to the body structures that are importantly related to the production of speech.

Clinical Note

Injuries to the cerebral cortex result from blows to the head, penetrating wounds, tumors and other neoplasms, strokes, infections, and other traumatic events. In cortical areas where function is specialized, a focal loss of function can result. For example, a local lesion in Area 17 could result in a narrow visual problem; a localized injury in Area 4 could result in a loss of muscle function in a specific part of the body. Cortical lesions in areas that bring together different functions (i.e., association areas) can result in rather complex patterns of disability (for example, the language disorder that can result from a lesion to Areas 44 or 45 or the lack of understanding of speech resulting from injury to the auditory association area).

THE AUTONOMIC NERVOUS SYSTEM

The autonomic nervous system contributes importantly to the total functioning of the body. This system of nerves is efferent and directed toward the visceral organs of the body, serving the glands, the cardiovascular system, the peripheral involuntary muscles, the intrinsic muscles of the eyes, and muscles associated with hair follicles. Most of the activities carried on in these regions are reflex mechanisms based upon sensory apparatus affiliated with the spinal nerves of the central nervous system and the central communicating regions of the spinal cord and the brainstem.

Clinical Note

Not many of the disorders associated with oral communication stem from autonomic nervous system pathologies. Clinical specialists dealing with communication disorders in medical settings (e.g., acute care hospitals) may serve patients with swallowing problems because of brainstem strokes. This neural region controls several vital functions (heart activity, respiration, and swallowing). If the muscle sphincter (cricopharyngeal) loses its neural control system, it can fail to relax and allow a food bolus to enter the esophagus. This can lead to rather dangerous consequences. Speech pathologists may serve such patients, in assessing their disorders as well as in teaching compensatory behaviors.

SUMMARY

The nervous system regulates and coordinates the activities of the organism by means of nerve impulses of the central and peripheral divisions as well as the involuntary controls imparted by the autonomic nervous system.

The structural and functional unit of the nervous system is the neuron with its cell body and its fibrous processes. The characteristic of irritability is seen in the electrochemical nerve impulse traveling along the length of the neuron. The conductivity of the nervous system is seen in the synapse, another place where the impulse is transmitted but this time across the synaptic gap in another electrochemical event.

The central nervous system is composed of the contiguous brain and its subdivisions, within the cranium, and the spinal cord within the vertebral canals. Connecting the brain to the body in general are 12 pairs of cranial nerves, some sensory only, some primarily motor, and several performing both sensory and motor function as mixed nerves. Much of the act of oral communication results from activities of the brain and the cranial nerves.

Connecting the spinal cord with much of the body are the spinal nerves. These paired divisions of the peripheral nervous system are mixed in that they carry into the spinal cord sensory impulses to reach other parts of the central nervous system as well as carrying motor impulses to muscles and glands.

Most of the muscles of the vocal tract are under voluntary control of the brain through the pyramidal tract as programmed by the speech area (Broca's). The linguistic drive comes from the language area of the cerebral cortex (Wernicke's) with input from other cortical areas (such as memory). These other areas also include sensory regions of the cortex with the auditory as a primary source, but with the other sensory areas importantly involved.

Subcortical areas serve sensory reception and perception functions, motor coordination, vital cardiac, respiratory and swallowing behaviors, among other critical activities. Within the midbrain, the pons and the medulla are the paired centers or nuclei that direct life-supporting functions. These are often associated with oral communication activities as well.

Oral communication results from a complex, well-organized vocal tract closely allied to a sophisticated auditory system under the coordinated controls of the nervous systems. It is a uniquely human activity and may well be the most important activity performed by the human body.

Clinical Implications

Demographic data suggest that the number of persons in the world over age 65 is increasing. Another group of data indicates that there appears to be an increasing number of infants born as "high risk," pointing to physical problems identified at or before birth. Many individuals with disorders of their nervous systems will be found within these two extremes of the age range in the population. These disorders may be causally related to aberrant oral communication skills; such deviations may be found in speech production, language use, or in auditory abilities.

There has long been a major effort to serve one large group of neurologically disordered persons, those with forms of cerebral palsy. Most of these persons were born with their neurogenic problems. A common anatomic site of damage is the subcortical coordinating region creating neuromotor disorders, and thus lessened skill in the use of the structures of the vocal tract, among other anatophysiologic behaviors.

In the aging population, strokes or cerebrovascular accidents rank high in the incidence of etiologic events causing brain damage and thus speech and/or language disorders. Similar brain damage may also result from degenerative conditions, from tumors invading and damaging brain tissues, as well as from accidents. Speech-language pathologists and audiologists are finding increasing numbers of patients to serve in this older age group.

Not only do such specialists provide assistance in oral communication functions, but often in other behaviors utilizing the same anatophysiologic systems. Thus, some communication specialists evaluate and manage persons with dysphagia, swallowing disorders as noted above; others operate programs in memory retraining. In many cases, oral communication problems stemming from neurologic injury are only one important aspect of a patient's total problems.

Study Questions

1. *Consider how the nervous system relaxes some muscle groups and contracts others as you take a step while maintaining balance. Note that movement does not involve only the foot moving forward, but that the body weight and posture change, as do foot and leg relationships of both extremities.*

2. *Observe how children's nervous systems mature in controlling such activities as walking or feeding. Observe how extraneous movements are extinguished and efficiency improved.*

3. *Observe an infant and its reactions to startling or other stimuli. For example, an abrupt noise can cause a whole-body reaction; a slight stroke on the sole of the foot causes an expansion of the toes. These are both reflexes.*

4. *Observe adult reflexes following a surprising loud sound. Look at changes in posture, breathing, alertness, and so on. Can you locate, in general, where in the nervous system these reflexes take place?*

5. *Experience the effects of neuromuscular breakdown by engaging in a familiar activity, but withholding involvement of some muscle groups (for example, speak a vowel sound without velopharyngeal closure, or attempt to produce consonant sounds with an immobile tongue).*

Appendix I
Drawing Keys

NOTE TO THE STUDENT

Following you will find two sets of lists of anatomic landmarks for each illustration. The first set is the Drawing Keys to the numbered leaders found on each drawing; it is the answer sheet. The second set is the alphabetized lists set. I believe this is the better learning list. The student could utilize other references, the instructor, or other assistance to locate the proper leader for each landmark identified in the alphabetized list. The student might then check his/her choices against the Drawing Keys. Instructors might prefer collecting all Drawing Keys prior to assigning landmark labeling activities and returning the Keys with the student's assignments.

DRAWING KEYS

Figure 1.2 Vocal Tract
1. Nasal Meatuses
2. Nasal Passage
3. Anterior Nares
4. Hard (Bony) Palate
5. Upper Lip
6. Teeth
7. Esophagus
8. Trachea
9. Larynx
10. Vertebrae
11. Tongue
12. Oral Cavity
13. Pharynx
14. Soft Palate
15. Sphenoid Sinus

Figure 2.1 Skull: Frontal View
1. Frontal Bone
2. Nasal Bone
3. Sphenoid Bone, Great Wing
4. Maxilla Bone, Frontal Process
5. Ethmoid Bone, Perpendicular Plate
6. Vomer Bone
7. Canine Fossa
8. Maxilla Bone, Anterior Nasal Spine
9. Maxillary Lateral Incisor Tooth
10. Mandible Bone, Oblique Line
11. Mandible Bone, Body
12. Maxillary Central Incisor Tooth
13. Mandible Bone, Mental Protuberance
14. Mandible Bone, Alveolar Process
15. Canine Tooth
16. Mandible Bone, Angle
17. Premolar Teeth
18. Molar Teeth
19. Mandible Bone, Ramus
20. Inferior Concha Bone
21. Ethmoid Bone, Middle Concha

22. Maxilla Bone, Zygomatic Process
23. Zygomatic bone (Cheekbone)
24. Ethmoid Bone
25. Lacrimal Bone
26. Temporal Bone, Squamous Portion
27. Sphenoid Bone, Great Wing
28. Parietal Bone

Figure 2.2 Skull: Lateral View
1. Parietal Bone
2. Sphenoid Bone, Great Wing
3. Temporal Bone, Squamous Portion
4. Temporal Bone, Zygomatic Process
5. Mandible Bone, Condyloid Process
6. Occipital Bone
7. External Acoustic Meatus
8. Temporal Bone, Tympanic Portion
9. Temporal Bone, Mastoid Process
10. Temporal Bone, Styloid Process
11. Sphenoid Bone, Lateral Pterygoid Plate
12. Mandible Bone, Coronoid Process
13. Mandible Bone, Ramus
14. Mandible Bone, Angle
15. Hyoid Bone
16. Mandible Bone, Mental Protuberance
17. Mandible Bone, Alveolar Process
18. Maxilla Bone, Alveolar Process
19. Maxilla Bone, Anterior Nasal Spine

20. Zygomatic (Cheek) Bone
21. Nasal Bone
22. Lacrimal Groove (Nasolacrimal Duct)
23. Lacrimal Bone
24. Maxilla Bone, Frontal Process
25. Ethmoid Bone, Orbital Lamina
26. Frontal Bone

Figure 2.3 Ethmoid Bone: Coronal View
1. Cranial Vault (Brain)
2. Horizontal (Cribriform) Plate
3. Eye Orbit
4. Air Cells
5. Superior Concha
6. Middle Concha
7. Inferior Meatus
8. Vomer Bone
9. Maxilla Bone, Palatine Process
10. Oral Cavity
11. Nasal Crest
12. Inferior Concha Bone
13. Perpendicular Plate
14. Maxillary Sinus
15. Middle Meatus
16. Superior Meatus
17. Lamina Orbitalis
18. Lateral Labyrinth
19. Olfactory Nerve Fiber Canal
20. Crista Galli

Figure 2.4A Sphenoid Bone: Superior Surfaces
1. Great Wing
2. Body
3. Sella Turcica
4. Lesser (Small) Wing

Figure 2.4B Sphenoid Bone: Anterior Surfaces
1. Lesser (Small) Wing
2. Crest

3. Vaginal Process
4. Lateral Pterygoid Plate
5. Nasal Passage
6. Hamular Process
7. Medial Pterygoid Plate
8. Rostrum
9. Sinus
10. Orbital Surface
11. Great Wing

Figure 2.5A Temporal Bone: Superior View
1. Squamous Portion
2. Petrous Portion
3. Zygomatic Process
4. Styloid Process
5. Internal Acoustic Meatus
6. Mastoid Portion

Figure 2.5B Temporal Bone: Lateral View
1. Mastoid Portion
2. Mastoid Process
3. Styloid Process
4. Tympanic Portion
5. External Acoustic Meatus
6. Zygomatic Process
7. Squamous Portion

Figure 2.6 Palatine Bone
1. Pyramidal Process
2. Horizontal Part
3. Posterior Nasal Spine
4. Vertical Part
5. Nasal Passage
6. Orbital Process
7. Sphenoidal Process

Figure 2.7A Maxilla Bone: Frontal View
1. Frontal Process
2. Anterior Nasal Spine

3. Zygomatic Process
4. Alveolar Process
5. Canine Fossa
6. Nasal Passage

Figure 2.7B Maxilla Bone: Lateral View
1. Frontal Process
2. Nasal Passage
3. Anterior Nasal Spine
4. Alveolar Process
5. Body
6. Tuberosity
7. Zygomatic Process

Figure 2.7C Maxilla Bone: Medial Surface
1. Maxillary Sinus (Antrum of Highmore)
2. Body
3. Tuberosity
4. Second Molar Tooth
5. Palatine Process
6. First Molar Tooth
7. Second Premolar Tooth
8. First Premolar Tooth
9. Canine Tooth
10. Lateral Incisor Tooth
11. Central Incisor Tooth
12. Alveolar Process
13. Anterior Nasal Spine
14. Nasal Passage
15. Frontal Process

Figure 2.8 Bony Palate and Maxillary Teeth
1. Central Incisor Tooth
2. Premaxilla (Incisive) Bone
3. Canine Tooth
4. Maxillary-Premaxillary Suture
5. Incisive Foramen
6. First Molar Tooth
7. Third Molar Tooth

8. Maxilla Bone, Tuberosity
9. Palatine Bone, Horizontal Portion
10. Palatine Bone, Posterior Nasal Spine
11. Transverse Suture
12. Second Molar Tooth
13. Maxillar Bone, Palatine Process
14. Palatine (Longitudinal) Suture
15. Second Premolar Tooth
16. First Premolar Tooth
17. Lateral Incisor Tooth
18. Maxilla Bone, Alveolar Process

Figure 2.9A Mandible Bone (Adult): Internal Aspect

1. Mandibular Notch
2. Condyloid Process
3. Ramus
4. Angle
5. Protuberance
6. Body
7. Alveolar Process
8. Mylohyoid Process
9. Tuberosity
10. Coronoid Process

Figure 2.9B Mandible Bone (Child): Lateral Aspect

1. Condyloid Process
2. Mandibular Notch
3. Coronoid Process
4. Ramus
5. Angle
6. Oblique Line
7. Body
8. Second Molar Tooth
9. Protuberance
10. Alveolar Process
11. First Molar Tooth
12. Canine Tooth

13. Lateral Incisor Tooth
14. Central Incisor Tooth

Figure 2.10 Nasal Septum

1. Frontal Sinus
2. Frontal Bone
3. Ethmoid Bone, Perpendicular Plate
4. Nasal Bone
5. Nasal Septal Cartilage
6. Greater Alar Cartilage
7. Anterior Nasal Spine
8. Maxilla Bone, Palatine Process
9. Palatine Bone, Horizontal Process
10. Vomer Bone
11. Posterior Nasal Spine
12. Vomer Bone, Ala
13. Sphenoid Bone, Body
14. Sella Turcica
15. Sphenoid Sinus
16. Sphenoid Bone, Crest
17. Ethmoid Bone, Horizontal (Cribriform) Plate
18. Ethmoid Bone, Crista Galli

Figure 3.1 Muscles of Facial Expression

1. Orbicularis Oculi Muscle
2. Zygomatic Bone (Cheekbone)
3. Levator Anguli Oris Muscle (Canine Muscle)
4. Orbicularis Oris Muscle
5. Mandible Bone
6. Risorius Muscle
7. Mental Muscle
8. Symphysis Menti
9. Platysma Muscle
10. Depressor (Quadratus) Labii Inferior Muscle
11. Depressor Anguli Oris (Triangular) Muscle
12. Buccinator Muscle
13. Zygomatic (Major) Muscle
14. Levator (Quadratus) Labii Superior Muscle

Figure 3.2A Muscles of Mastication: Masseter and Temporal Muscles

1. Parietal Bone
2. Temporal Muscle
3. Temporal Bone, Zygomatic Process
4. External Acoustic Meatus
5. Occipital Bone
6. Temporal Bone
7. Masseter Muscle
8. Mandible Bone, Angle
9. Mandible Bone, Body
10. Maxilla Bone, Body
11. Zygomatic (Cheek) Bone
12. Frontal Bone

Figure 3.2B Muscles of Mastication: Internal and External Pterygoid Muscles

1. Temporal Bone, Zygomatic Process
2. External Acoustic Meatus
3. Temporomandibular Joint, Articular Disc
4. Mandible Bone, Condyloid Process
5. External (Lateral) Pterygoid Muscle
6. Mandible Bone, Ramus
7. Mandible Bone, Angle
8. Mandible Bone, Body
9. Internal (Medial) Pterygoid Muscle
10. Maxilla Bone, Tuberosity
11. Zygomatic (Cheek) Bone
12. Sphenoid Bone, Great Wing

Figure 3.3 Muscles of the Soft Palate

1. Tensor (Veli) Palatine Muscle
2. Auditory Tube (Eustachian Tube)
3. Soft Palate
4. Velopharyngeal Sphincter Muscle
5. Levator (Veli) Palatine Muscle
6. Superior Pharyngeal Constrictor Muscle
7. Uvula
8. Pharyngopalatine (Palatopharyngeal) Muscle

9. Tonsil
10. Epiglottis
11. Pharynx
12. Glossopalatine (Palatoglossus) Muscle
13. Tongue
14. Vestibule
15. Pterygoid Hamulus
16. Uvula Muscle
17. Maxilla Bone, Alveolar Process
18. Oral Cavity Proper
19. Bony Palate
20. Posterior Nasal Spine

Figure 3.4 Auditory Tube-Related Muscles and Structures

1. Tensor (Veli) Palatine Muscle
2. Auditory Tube (Cartilage)
3. Medial Pterygoid Plate
4. Anterior Crus, Auditory Tube
5. Bony Palate
6. Hamular Process
7. Soft Palate
8. Uvula
9. Palatopharyngeal Muscle
10. Salpingopharyngeal Muscle
11. Dilator Tubae Muscle
12. Posterior Crus, Auditory Tube
13. Levator (Veli) Palatine Muscle

Figure 3.5A Tongue Muscles: Intrinsic (Lateral View)

1. Dorsum
2. Longitudinal Lingual Superior Muscle
3. Genioglossus Muscle
4. Transverse Lingual Muscle
5. Lingual Apex
6. Longitudinal Lingual Inferior Muscle
7. Superior Mental Spine

8. Geniohyoid Muscle
9. Thyroid Cartilage
10. Hyoid Bone
11. Epiglottis
12. Vallecula
13. Tongue, Pharyngeal Portion
14. Vertical Lingual Muscle

Figure 3.5B Tongue Muscles: Intrinsic (Coronal View)

1. Lingual Sulcus
2. Dorsum
3. Longitudinal Lingual Superior Muscle
4. Transverse Lingual Muscle
5. Longitudinal Lingual Inferior Muscle
6. Mylohyoid Muscle
7. Mandible Bone, Alveolar Process
8. Genioglossus Muscle
9. Lingual Septum
10. Lateral Borders

Figure 3.5C Tongue Muscles, Extrinsic (Sagittal View)

1. Soft Palate (Velum)
2. Uvula
3. Temporal Bone, Styloid Process
4. Styloglossus Muscle
5. Glossopalatine (Palatoglossus) Muscle
6. Pharynx
7. Hyoglossus Muscle
8. Hyoid Bone, Greater Cornu
9. Genioglossus Muscle
10. Mandible Bone, Superior Spine
11. Mandible Bone, Alveolar Process
12. Oral Vestibule
13. Lingual Frenulum
14. Lingual Apex
15. Oral Cavity Proper

Figure 3.6 Oral Cavity (Anterior View)

1. Soft Palate (Velum)
2. Uvula
3. Posterior Pillar of the Fauces
4. Anterior Pillar of the Fauces
5. Vallecula
6. Middle Glossoepiglottic Membrane
7. Tongue, Pharyngeal Portion
8. Vallate Papillae
9. Tongue, Dorsum
10. Tongue, Apex
11. Tongue, Sulcus
12. Foramen Cecum
13. Palatine Tonsil
14. Lingual Tonsil
15. Epiglottis
16. Oropharynx

Figure 4.1 Vocal Tract: Pharynges (Sagittal View)

1. Posterior Naris (Choana)
2. Nasal Passage
3. Oral Cavity
4. Tongue
5. Faucial Isthmus
6. Oropharynx
7. Larynx
8. Trachea
9. Esophagus
10. Laryngopharynx
11. Aditus ad Laryngis
12. Epiglottis
13. Tongue, Pharyngeal Portion
14. Soft Palate (Velum)
15. Cervical Vertebra
16. Uvula
17. Nasopharynx

18. Adenoids
19. Auditory Tube (Eustachian Tube)
20. Sphenoid Bone, Body
21. Sphenoid Sinus

Figure 4.2 Pharyngeal Constrictor Muscles (Sagittal View)

1. Oral Cavity
2. Soft Palate (Velum)
3. Superior Pharyngeal Constrictor Muscle
4. Velopharyngeal Sphincter Muscle
5. Pterygomandibular Raphe
6. Cervical Vertebrae
7. Middle Pharyngeal Constrictor Muscle
8. Inferior Pharyngeal Constrictor Muscle
9. Hyoid Bone
10. Cricopharyngeal Muscle
11. Esophagus
12. Cricoid Cartilage
13. Thyroid Cartilage
14. Epiglottis
15. Uvula
16. Tongue
17. Hard (Bony) Palate

Figure 4.3 Pharyngeal Levator Muscles

1. Auditory Tube (Eustachian Tube)
2. Temporal Bone, Styloid Process
3. Dilator Tubae Muscle
4. Stylopharyngeal Muscle
5. Palatopharyngeal Muscle
6. Faucial Isthmus
7. Tongue, Pharyngeal Portion
8. Epiglottis
9. Uvula
10. Palatal Raphe
11. Salpingopharyngeal Muscle

12. Pterygoid Hamulus
13. Vomer Bone
14. Posterior Nares

Figure 5.1 Vocal Tract: Larynx (Sagittal View)

1. Vestibular Fold (False Vocal Fold)
2. True Vocal Fold
3. Thyroid Cartilage
4. Cricoid Cartilage, Arch
5. Trachea
6. Esophagus
7. Atrium (Infraglottal Cavity)
8. Cricoid Cartilage, Lamina
9. Vestibule
10. Laryngopharynx
11. Cervical Vertebrae
12. Aditus ad Laryngis
13. Epiglottis

Figure 5.2 Skeletal Larynx

1. Triticeal Cartilage
2. Posterior Hyothyroid Ligament
3. Hyoid Bone, Greater Horn
4. Thyroid Cartilage, Superior Horn
5. Hyoid Bone, Lesser Horn
6. Hyoid Bone, Body
7. Hyothyroid Membrane
8. Middle Hyothyroid Ligament
9. Arytenoid Cartilage
10. Thyroid Cartilage, Prominence
11. Thyroid Notch
12. Thyroid Cartilage, Lamina
13. Thyroid Cartilage, Oblique Line
14. Thyroid Cartilage, Posterior Border
15. Thyroid Cartilage, Inferior Horn
16. Middle Cricothyroid Ligament
17. Cricoid Cartilage, Arch

18. Cricoid Cartilage, Lamina
19. Trachea, Cartilaginous Rings
20. Posterior Cricothyroid Ligament

Figure 5.3A Larynx (Coronal Views)

1. Epiglottic Cartilage
2. Vallecula
3. Pyriform Sinus (Recess)
4. Thyroid Cartilage
5. Laryngeal Vestibule
6. Vestibular (Ventricular) Folds
7. Laryngeal Ventricle (of Morgagni)
8. Glottis
9. Vocal Fold
10. Elastic Cone
11. Atrium
12. Cricoid Cartilage
13. Trachea

Figure 5.3B Vocal Fold Movements (Superior Views)

1. Thyroid Cartilage, Angle
2. Anterior Commissure
3. Intermembranous Glottis
4. Vocal Fold, Membranous
5. Intercartilaginous Glottis
6. Arytenoid Cartilage, Vocal Process
7. Thyroid Cartilage, Superior Horn
8. Cricoid Cartilage, Lamina
9. Thyroid Cartilage, Lamina
10. Arytenoid Cartilage, Muscular Process

Figure 5.4 Larynx (Posterior and Sagittal Views)

1. Posterior Hyothyroid Ligament
2. Triticeal Cartilage
3. Hyothyroid Membrane
4. Thyroid Cartilage, Superior Cornu
5. Corniculate Cartilage

6. Thyroarytenoid (Vocal) Ligament
7. Thyroid Cartilage, Angle
8. Arytenoid Cartilage, Apex
9. Arytenoid Cartilage, Vocal Process
10. Arytenoid Cartilage, Muscular Process
11. Cricoid Cartilage, Lamina
12. Posterior Cricoarytenoid Muscle
13. Thyroid Cartilage, Inferior Cornu
14. Trachea
15. Cricoid Cartilage, Lamina
16. Tracheal Cartilage Ring
17. Interarytenoid Muscle
18. Cricoid Cartilage, Arch
19. Atrium, Conus Elasticus
20. Ventricle (Morgagni)
21. Vocal Fold
22. Vestibular Fold (False Vocal Fold)
23. Thyroid Cartilage, Angle
24. Vestibule, Quadrangular Membrane
25. Cuneiform Cartilage
26. Aryepiglottic Fold
27. Hyoid Bone, Body
28. Hyoid Bone, Greater Cornu
29. Tongue
30. Epiglottis

Figure 5.5 Extrinsic Laryngeal Muscles
1. External Acoustic Canal
2. Temporal Bone, Mastoid Process
3. Mandible Bone, Condyloid Process
4. Temporal Bone, Styloid Process
5. Sternocleidomastoid Muscle
6. Digastric Muscle, Posterior Belly
7. Stylohyoid Muscle
8. Mandible Bone, Angle
9. Omohyoid Muscle, Inferior Belly
10. Sternohyoid Muscle

11. Thyroid Cartilage, Angle
12. Omohyoid Muscle, Superior Belly
13. Thyrohyoid Muscle
14. Hyoid Bone
15. Fascial Loop, Digastric Muscle
16. Digastric Muscle, Anterior Belly
17. Mandible Bone, Protuberance
18. Geniohyoid Muscle
19. Mylohyoid Muscle

Figure 5.6A Intrinsic Laryngeal Muscles: Superficial (Lateral View)
1. Thyroid Cartilage, Lamina
2. Thyroid Cartilage, Angle
3. Cricothyroid Muscle, Oblique Portion
4. Cricothyroid Muscle, Vertical Portion
5. Cricoid Cartilage, Arch
6. Thyroid Cartilage, Inferior Cornu
7. Cricoid Cartilage, Lamina
8. Arytenoid Cartilage
9. Corniculate Cartilage
10. Thyroid Cartilage, Superior Cornu

Figure 5.6B Intrinsic Laryngeal Muscles: Lateral Cricoarytenoid
1. Corniculate Cartilage
2. Arytenoid Cartilage, Apex
3. Arytenoid Cartilage, Vocal Process
4. Lateral Cricoarytenoid Muscle
5. Arytenoid Cartilage, Muscular Process
6. Cricoid Cartilage, Arch
7. Cricoid Cartilage, Lamina

Figure 5.6C Intrinsic Laryngeal Muscles: Posterior Cricoarytenoid
1. Cricoid Cartilage, Lamina
2. Cricoid Facet, Cricothyroid Joint
3. Posterior Cricoarytenoid Muscle

4. Arytenoid Cartilage, Muscular Process
5. Arytenoid Cartilage, Apex
6. Corniculate Cartilage

Figure 5.6D Intrinsic Laryngeal Muscles: Interarytenoid
1. Arytenoid Cartilage, Apex
2. Interarytenoid Muscle, Oblique Portion
3. Arytenoid Cartilage, Muscular Process
4. Cricoid Cartilage, Lamina
5. Interarytenoid Muscle, Transverse Portion
6. Notch
7. Corniculate Cartilage

Figure 5.6E Intrinsic Laryngeal Muscles: Thyroarytenoid
1. Thyroid Cartilage, Angle
2. Thyroid Cartilage, Lamina
3. Cricoid Cartilage, Arch
4. Arytenoid Cartilage, Vocal Process
5. Arytenoid Cartilage, Anterolateral Surface
6. Arytenoid Cartilage, Muscular Process
7. Thyroid Cartilage, Superior Cornu
8. Cricoid Cartilage, Lamina
9. Cricoarytenoid Ligament (Joint)
10. Corniculate Cartilage
11. Glottis
12. Thyroarytenoid Muscle
13. Thyroarytenoid (Vocal) Ligament
14. Vocalis Muscle
15. Anterior Commissure

Figure 5.7 Larynx Nerve Supply
1. Cerebral Cortex
2. Brain, Cerebrum
3. Nucleus Ambiguus
4. Spinal Cord
5. Hyoid Bone

6. Thyroid Cartilage
7. Cricoid Cartilage
8. Subclavicular Artery
9. Tracheal Cartilage Rings
10. Aorta, Arch
11. Recurrent (Inferior) Laryngeal Nerve
12. Superior Laryngeal Nerve, External Branch
13. Superior Laryngeal Nerve, Internal Branch
14. Superior Laryngeal Nerve
15. Vagus Nerve (Cranial X)
16. Medulla Oblongata
17. Decussation of Efferent Fibers
18. Cells of Origin

Figure 6.1 Lower Respiratory Tract
1. Trachea
2. Bronchus, Extrapulmonary
3. Bifurcation
4. Bronchus, Intrapulmonary
5. Bronchus, Lobular
6. Alveolar Sacs
7. Alveolar Duct
8. Alveoli
9. Respiratory Bronchiole
10. Terminal Bronchiole
11. Lung Base
12. Cardiac Notch
13. Inferior Lobe, Left
14. Superior Lobe, Left
15. Lung Apex

Figure 6.2 Vertebral Column
1. Atlas (First Cervical Vertebra)
2. Axis (Second Cervical Vertebra)
3. Cervical Group
4. Transverse Process
5. Thoracic Group

6. Lumbar Group
7. Sacral Group (Sacrum)
8. Coccygeal Group (Coccyx)
9. Body
10. Spinous Process

Figure 6.3 Thoracic Vertebra: Superior and Lateral Views
1. Rib Articulating Process (Transverse Process)
2. Spinous Process
3. Transverse Process
4. Lamina
5. Pedicle
6. Vertebral Canal
7. Superior Articulating Process
8. Body
9. Body, Articulating Facet
10. Spinous Process
11. Body, Articulating Facet
12. Articulating Facet, Transverse Process
13. Transverse Process
14. Superior Articulate Process
15. Body

Figure 6.4 Vertebrosternal Rib
1. Spinous Process
2. Transverse Process
3. Vertebral Articulating Process
4. Vertebral Canal
5. Body
6. Sternum Bone
7. Costal Cartilage
8. Head
9. Shaft
10. Neck
11. Angle
12. Tubercle

Figure 6.5 Rib Cage
1. Rib 1
2. Sternum Bone, Manubrium
3. Rib 4
4. Sternum Bone, Body
5. Rib 6
6. Rib 8
7. Rib 9
8. Rib 10
9. Rib 12
10. Rib 11
11. Rib 7
12. Sternum Bone, Xiphoid Process
13. Rib 5
14. Costal Cartilages
15. Rib 3
16. Sternum Bone, Angle
17. Rib 2
18. Rib, Head
19. Thoracic Vertebra 1, Transverse Process
20. Thoracic Vertebra

Figure 6.6 Pelvic Girdle
1. Ilium Bone
2. Sacrum Bone
3. Acetabulum
4. Pubis Bone
5. Ischium Bone
6. Symphysis Pubis
7. Coccyx
8. Inguinal Ligament
9. Ilium Bone, Crest

Figure 6.7 Diaphragm Muscle
1. Thoracic Vertebra 1
2. Sternum Bone, Manubrium
3. Diaphragm Muscle, Central Tendon

4. Sternum Bone, Xiphoid Process
5. Diaphragm Muscle
6. Rib 11
7. Rib 12
8. Lumbar Vertebrae
9. Rib 10
10. Rib 8
11. Rib 7
12. Costal Cartilages
13. Sternum Bone, Body
14. Costal Cartilages
15. Rib 2, Head
16. Thoracic Vertebra 2, Transverse Process

Figure 6.8 Thoracic Respiratory Muscles
1. Sternocleidomastoid Muscle
2. Pectoralis Major Muscle
3. Sternum Bone, Body
4. Serratus Anterior Muscle
5. Sternum Bone, Xiphoid Process
6. Internal Intercostal Muscles
7. External Intercostal Muscles
8. Humerus Bone
9. Pectoralis Minor Muscle
10. Ribs 1 and 2
11. Scapula Bone
12. Clavicle Bone
13. Sternum Bone, Manubrium
14. Scalene Muscles
15. Cervical Vertebrae

Figure 6.9 Abdominal Muscles
1. Sternum Bone, Xiphoid Process
2. Linea Alba
3. Costal Cartilages
4. Tendinous Aponeurosis
5. External Abdominal Oblique Muscle

6. Transverse Abdominis Muscle
7. Internal Abdominal Oblique Muscle
8. Rectus Abdominis Muscle, Tendinous Inscriptions
9. Ilium Bone, Crest
10. Rectus Abdominis Muscle
11. Inguinal Ligament
12. Pubis Bone

Figure 7.1 The Ear
1. Temporal Bone, Squamous Portion
2. Tegmen Tympani
3. Epitympanic Recess
4. Mastoid Antrum
5. Mastoid Air Cells
6. Auricle
7. Cave
8. External Acoustic Meatus, Cartilaginous Portion
9. External Acoustic Meatus, Bony Portion
10. Ceruminous (Wax) Glands
11. Tympanic Membrane
12. Middle Ear (Tympanum)
13. Nasopharynx
14. Auditory Tube (Eustachian Tube)
15. Ossicular Chain
16. Round Window
17. Cochlea
18. Internal Acoustic Meatus
19. Auditory Nerve (Cranial VIII)
20. Facial Nerve (Cranial VII)
21. Semicircular Canals
22. Temporal Bone, Petrous Portion

Figure 7.2 Pinna (Auricle)
1. Scaphoid Fossa
2. Darwin's Tubercle

3. Helix
4. Concha
5. Antihelix (Anthelix)
6. Lobule
7. Antitragus
8. Concha, Cave
9. External Acoustic Meatus
10. Tragus (Buck)
11. Helix, Crus
12. Concha, Skiff

Figure 7.3 Tympanic Membrane
1. Flaccid Portion (Shrapnell's Membrane)
2. Malleolar Fold
3. Malleus Bone, Manubrium
4. Circular Fibers
5. Radial Fibers
6. Umbo
7. Tense Portion

Figure 7.4 Middle Ear (Tympanum)
1. Mastoid Air Cells
2. Malleus Bone, Head
3. External Acoustic Meatus
4. Tensor Tympani Muscle, Tendon
5. Malleus Bone, Manubrium
6. Tympanic Membrane, Umbo
7. Stapedius Muscle, Tendon
8. Tympanic Membrane, Tense Portion
9. Middle Ear Cavity
10. Tympanic Sulcus
11. Temporal Bone, Tympanic Portion
12. Auditory Tube (Eustachian Tube), Cartilaginous Portion
13. Auditory Tube (Eustachian Tube)
14. Tensor Tympani Muscle
15. Pyramidal Eminence

16. Round (Cochlear) Window
17. Cochlea, Basal Turn
18. Oval (Vestibular) Window
19. Stapes Bone, Crura
20. Stapes Bone, Oval Footplate
21. Vestibule of Inner Ear
22. Stapes Bone, Neck
23. Incus Bone, Lenticular Process
24. Incus Bone, Long Process
25. Temporal Bone, Petrous Portion
26. Incus Bone, Body
27. Tegmen Tympani
28. Epitympanic Recess (Attic)
29. Aditus ad Antrum
30. Antrum

Figure 7.5 Cochlear Turns

1. Internal Acoustic Meatus
2. Temporal Bone, Petrous Portion
3. Modiolus
4. Vestibular Membrane (Reissner's Membrane)
5. Organ of Corti
6. Nerve Fibers
7. Basilar Membrane
8. Tympanic Canal
9. Spiral Ganglion
10. Cochlear Duct
11. Vestibular Canal (Scala)
12. Auditory Nerve (Cranial VIII), Cochlear Division

Figure 7.6 Cochlea (Cross Section)

1. Temporal Bone, Petrous Portion
2. Vestibular Canal (Scala)
3. Tectorial Membrane
4. Pillar of Corti
5. Spiral Limbus

6. Modiolus
7. Spiral Ganglion
8. Cell Bodies
9. Osseous Spiral Lamina
10. Tympanic Canal (Scala)
11. Nerve Fibers
12. Inner Hair Cell
13. Basilar Membrane
14. Supporting Cell
15. Spiral Ligament
16. Outer Hair Cells
17. Hairs
18. Spiral Stria (Stripe)
19. Cochlear Duct
20. Vestibular Membrane (Reissner's Membrane)

Figure 7.7 Neural Pathway: Audition

1. Cerebral Cortex
2. Inferior Colliculus
3. Lateral Lemniscus
4. Medulla
5. Superior Olive
6. Decussating Fibers
7. Midline
8. Cell Bodies
9. Auditory Nerve (Cranial VIII) Cochlear Division
10. Auditory Nerve Fibers
11. Synapses
12. Ventral Cochlear Nucleus
13. Dorsal Cochlear Nucleus
14. Nucleus of the Lateral Lemniscus
15. Auditory Reflex Fibers
16. Nucleus of the Inferior Colliculus
17. Medial Geniculate Body of the Thalamus
18. Auditory Radiations
19. Superior Temporal Convolution (Gyrus)

20. Lateral Sulcus
21. Cerebrum

Figure 8.1 Reflex Arc

1. Cell Body, Sensory Nerve
2. Dorsal Root, Spinal Nerve
3. Dorsal Gray Horn
4. Cell Body, Motor Nerve
5. Synapse
6. Ventral Gray Horn
7. Motor Nerve Fiber
8. Ventral Root, Spinal Nerve
9. Spinal Nerve
10. Myoneural Juncture
11. Muscle
12. Reflex Action to Stimulus
13. Dorsal Root Ganglion
14. Sensory Nerve Fiber
15. Sensory End Organ

Figure 8.2 Spinal Nerves

1. Spinal Cord
2. Dorsal Root Ganglion
3. Vertebra, Transverse Process
4. Motor Nerve Fibers
5. Sensory Nerve Fibers
6. Vertebra, Lamina
7. Vertebra, Spinous Process
8. Midline
9. Spinal Nerve
10. Ventral Root
11. Dorsal Root

Figure 8.3 Cranial Nerves

1. Longitudinal Fissure
2. Olfactory Tract (Cranial I)
3. Optic Nerve (Cranial II)

4. Oculomotor Nerve (Cranial III)
5. Pons
6. Abducens Nerve (Cranial VI)
7. Hypoglossal Nerve (Cranial XII)
8. Medulla
9. Spinal Cord
10. Cerebellum
11. Midline
12. Spinal Nerve
13. Accessory Nerve (Cranial XI)
14. Vagus Nerve (Cranial X)
15. Glossopharyngeal Nerve (Cranial IX)
16. Auditory Nerve (Cranial VIII)
17. Facial Nerve (Cranial VII)
18. Trigeminal Nerve (Cranial V)
19. Trochlear Nerve (Cranial IV)
20. Optic Chiasm
21. Olfactory Bulb (Cranial I)
22. Frontal Lobe

Figure 8.4 Pyramidal Pathway

1. Longitudinal Fissure
2. Cerebrum
3. Cerebral Cortex
4. Midbrain Level
5. Pons and Medulla Level
6. Cranial Nerves Nuclei
7. Decussations
8. Spinal Cord Level
9. Lateral Corticospinal Tract
10. Anterior (Ventral) Corticospinal Tract
11. Midline
12. Ventral Gray Column
13. Decussating Fibers
14. Internal Capsule
15. Lateral Sulcus

16. Pyramidal Cells of Origin
17. Precentral Gyrus (Area 4)

Figure 8.5 The Brain

1. Central Sulcus
2. Precentral Convolution
3. Frontal Lobe
4. Operculum
5. Lateral Sulcus
6. Superior Temporal Convolution
7. Temporal Lobe
8. Pons
9. Medulla
10. Spinal Cord
11. Cerebellum
12. Occipital Lobe
13. Parietal Lobe
14. Postcentral Convolution

ALPHABETIZED LISTS

Figure 1.2 Vocal Tract

Anterior Nares
Esophagus
Hard (Bony) Palate
Larynx
Nasal Meatuses
Nasal Passage
Nasal Passage
Oral Cavity
Pharynx
Soft Palate
Sphenoid Sinus
Teeth
Tongue
Trachea

Upper Lip
Vertebrae

Figure 2.1 Skull: Frontal View

Canine Fossa
Canine Tooth
Ethmoid Bone
Ethmoid Bone, Middle Concha
Ethmoid Bone, Perpendicular Plate
Frontal Bone
Inferior Concha Bone
Lacrimal Bone
Mandible Bone, Alveolar Process
Mandible Bone, Angle
Mandible Bone, Body
Mandible Bone, Mental Protuberance
Mandible Bone, Oblique Line
Mandible Bone, Ramus
Maxillar Bone, Anterior Nasal Spine
Maxilla Bone, Frontal Process
Maxilla Bone, Zygomatic Process
Maxillary Central Incisor Tooth
Maxillary Lateral Incisor Tooth
Molor Teeth
Nasal Bone
Parietal Bone
Premolar Teeth
Sphenoid Bone, Great Wing
Temporal Bone, Squamous Portion
Vomer Bone
Zygomatic Bone

Figure 2.2 Skull: Lateral View

Ethmoid Bone, Orbital Lamina
External Acoustic Meatus (Canal)
Frontal Bone

Hyoid Bone
Lacrimal Bone
Lacrimal Groove (Nasolacrimal Duct)
Mandible Bone, Alveolar Process
Mandible Bone, Angle
Mandible Bone, Condyloid Process
Mandible Bone, Coronoid Process
Mandible Bone, Mental Protuberance
Mandible Bone, Ramus
Maxilla Bone, Alveolar Process
Maxilla Bone, Anterior Nasal Spine
Maxilla Bone, Frontal Process
Nasal Bone
Occipital Bone
Parietal Bone
Sphenoid Bone, Great Wing
Sphenoid Bone, Lateral Pterygoid Plate
Temporal Bone, Mastoid Process
Temporal Bone, Squamous Portion
Temporal Bone, Styloid Process
Temporal Bone, Tympanic Portion
Temporal Bone, Zygomatic Process
Zygomatic (Cheek) Bone

Figure 2.3 Ethmoid Bone: Coronal View
Air Cells
Cranial Vault (Brain)
Crista Galli
Eye Orbit
Horizontal (Cribriform) Plate
Inferior Concha Bone
Inferior Meatus
Lamina Orbitalis
Lateral Labyrinth
Maxilla Bone, Palatine Process
Maxillary Sinus

Middle Concha
Middle Meatus
Olfactory Nerve Fiber Canal
Oral Cavity
Perpendicular Plate
Superior Concha
Superior Crest
Superior Meatus
Vomer Bone

Figure 2.4A Sphenoid Bone: Superior Surfaces
Body
Great Wing
Lesser (Small) Wing
Sella Turcica

Figure 2.4B Sphenoid Bone: Anterior Surfaces
Crest
Great Wing
Hamular Process
Lateral Pterygoid Plate
Lesser (Small) Wing
Medial Pterygoid Plate
Nasal Passage
Orbital Surface
Rostrum
Sinus
Vaginal Process

Figure 2.5A Temporal Bone: Superior View
Internal Acoustic Meatus
Mastoid Portion
Petrous Portion
Squamous Portion
Styloid Process
Zygomatic Process

Figure 2.5B Temporal Bone: Lateral View
External Acoustic Meatus
Mastoid Portion
Mastoid Process
Squamous Portion
Styloid Process
Tympanic Portion
Zygomatic Process

Figure 2.6 Palatine Bone
Horizontal Part
Nasal Passage
Orbital Process
Posterior Nasal Spine
Pyramidal Process
Sphenoidal Process
Vertical Part

Figure 2.7A Maxilla Bone: Frontal View
Alveolar Process
Anterior Nasal Spine
Canine Fossa
Frontal Process
Nasal Passage
Zygomatic Process

Figure 2.7B Maxilla Bone: Lateral View
Alveolar Process
Anterior Nasal Spine
Body
Frontal Process
Nasal Passage
Tuberosity
Zygomatic Process

Figure 2.7C Maxilla Bone: Medial Surface
Alveolar Process
Anterior Nasal Spine

Body
Canine Tooth
First Molar Tooth
First Premolar Tooth
Frontal Process
Lateral Incisor Tooth
Maxillary Sinus (Antrum of Highmore)
Nasal Passage
Palatine Process
Second Molar Tooth
Second Premolar Tooth
Tuberosity

Figure 2.8 Bony Palate and Maxillary Teeth
Canine Tooth
Central Incisor Tooth
First Molar Tooth
First Premolar Tooth
Incisive Foramen
Lateral Incisor Tooth
Maxilla Bone, Alveolar Process
Maxilla Bone, Palatine Process
Maxilla Bone, Tuberosity
Maxillary-Premaxillary Suture
Palatine Bone, Horizontal Portion
Palatine Bone, Posterior Nasal Spine
Palatine (Longitudinal) Suture
Premaxilla (Incisive) Bone
Second Molar Tooth
Second Premolar Tooth
Third Molar Tooth
Transverse Suture

Figure 2.9A Mandible Bone (Adult): Internal Aspect
Alveolar Process
Angle

Body
Condyloid Process
Coronoid Process
Mandibular Notch
Mylohyoid Ridge
Protuberance
Ramus
Tuberosity

Figure 2.9B Mandible Bone (Child): Lateral Aspect
Alveolar Process
Angle
Body
Canine Tooth
Central Incisor Tooth
Condyloid Process
Coronoid Process
First Molar Tooth
Lateral Incisor Tooth
Mandibular Notch
Oblique Line
Protuberance
Ramus
Second Molar Tooth

Figure 2.10 Nasal Septum
Anterior Nasal Spine
Ethmoid Bone, Crista Galli
Ethmoid Bone, Horizontal (Cribriform) Plate
Ethmoid Bone, Perpendicular Plate
Frontal Bone
Frontal Sinus
Greater Alar Cartilage
Maxilla Bone, Palatine Process
Nasal Bone
Nasal Septal Cartilage

Palatine Bone, Horizontal Process
Posterior Nasal Spine
Sella Turcica
Sphenoid Bone, Body
Sphenoid Bone, Crest
Sphenoid Sinus
Vomer Bone
Vomer Bone, Ala

Figure 3.1 Muscles of Facial Expression
Buccinator Muscle
Depressor Anguli Oris (Triangular) Muscle
Depressor (Quadratus) Labii Inferior Muscle
Levator Anguli Oris Muscle (Canine Muscle)
Levator (Quadratus) Labii Superior Muscle
Mandible Bone
Mental Muscle
Orbicularis Oris Muscle
Platysma Muscle
Risorius Muscle
Symphysis Menti
Zygomatic Bone (Cheekbone)
Zygomatic (Major) Muscle

Figure 3.2A Muscles of Mastication: Masseter and Temporal Muscles
External Acoustic Meatus
Frontal Bone
Mandible Bone, Angle
Mandible Bone, Body
Masseter Muscle
Maxilla Bone, Body
Occipital Bone
Parietal Bone
Temporal Bone
Temporal Muscle
Temporal Bone, Zygomatic Process
Zygomatic (Cheek) Bone

Figure 3.2B Muscles of Mastication: Internal and External Pterygoid Muscles

External Acoustic Meatus
External (Lateral) Pterygoid Muscle
Internal (Medial) Pterygoid Muscle
Mandible Bone, Angle
Mandible Bone, Body
Mandible Bone, Condyloid Process
Mandible Bone, Ramus
Maxilla Bone, Tuberosity
Sphenoid Bone, Great Wing
Temporal Bone, Zygomatic Process
Temporomandibular Joint, Articular Disc
Zygomatic (Cheek) Bone

Figure 3.3 Muscle of the Soft Palate

Auditory Tube (Eustachian Tube)
Bony Palate
Epiglottis
Glossopalatine (Palatoglossus) Muscle
Levator (Veli) Palatine Muscle
Maxilla Bone, Alveolar Process
Oral Cavity Proper
Pharyngopalatine (Palatopharyngeal) Muscle
Pharynx
Posterior Nasal Spine
Pterygoid Hamulus
Soft Palate
Superior Pharyngeal Constrictor Muscle
Tensor (Veli) Palatine Muscle
Tongue
Tonsil
Uvula
Uvula Muscle
Velopharyngeal Sphincter Muscle
Vestibule

Figure 3.4 Auditory Tube-Related Muscles and Structures

Auditory Tube (Cartilage)
Anterior Crus, Auditory Tube
Bony Palate
Dilator Tubae Muscle
Hamular Process
Levator (Veli) Palatine Muscle
Medial Pterygoid Plate
Palatopharyngeal Muscle
Posterior Crus, Auditory Tube
Salpingopharyngeal Muscle
Soft Palate
Tensor (Veli) Palatine Muscle
Uvula

Figure 3.5A Tongue Muscles, Intrinsic (Lateral View)

Dorsum
Epiglottis
Genioglossus Muscle
Hyoid Bone
Lingual Apex
Longitudinal Lingual Inferior Muscle
Longitudinal Lingual Superior Muscle
Superior Mental Spine
Thyroid Cartilage
Tongue, Pharyngeal Portion
Transverse Lingual Muscle
Vallecula
Vertical Lingual Muscle

Figure 3.5B Tongue Muscles, Intrinsic (Coronal View)

Dorsum
Genioglossus Muscle
Lateral Borders
Lingual Septum

Lingual Sulcus
Longitudinal Lingual Inferior Muscle
Longitudinal Lingual Superior Muscle
Mandible Bone, Alveolar Process
Mylohyoid Muscle
Transverse Lingual Muscle

Figure 3.5C Tongue Muscles, Extrinsic (Sagittal View)

Genioglossus Muscle
Glossopalatine (Palatoglossus) Muscle
Hyoglossus Muscle
Hyoid Bone, Greater Cornu
Lingual Apex
Lingual Frenulum
Mandible Bone, Alveolar Process
Mandible Bone, Superior Spine
Oral Cavity Proper
Oral Vestibule
Pharynx
Soft Palate (Velum)
Styloglossus Muscle
Temporal Bone, Styloid Process
Uvula

Figure 3.6 Oral Cavity (Anterior View)

Anterior Pillar of the Fauces
Epiglottis
Foramen Caecum
Lingual Tonsil
Middle Glossoepiglottic Membrane
Oropharynx
Palatine Tonsil
Posterior Pillar of the Fauces
Soft Palate (Velum)
Tongue, Apex
Tongue, Dorsum

Tongue, Pharyngeal Portion
Tongue, Sulcus
Uvula
Vallate Papillae
Vallecula

Figure 4.1 Vocal Tract: Pharynges (Sagittal View)
Adenoids
Aditus ad Laryngis
Auditory Tube (Eustachian Tube)
Cervical Vertebra
Epiglottis
Esophagus
Faucial Isthmus
Laryngopharynx
Larynx
Nasal Passage
Nasopharynx
Oral Cavity
Oropharynx
Posterior Naris (Choana)
Soft Palate (Velum)
Sphenoid Bone, Body
Sphenoid Sinus
Tongue
Tongue, Pharyngeal Portion
Trachea
Uvula

Figure 4.2 Pharyngeal Constrictor Muscles (Sagittal View)
Cervical Vertebrae
Cricoid Cartilage
Cricopharyngeal Muscle
Epiglottis
Esophagus
Hard (Bony) Palate

Hyoid Bone
Inferior Pharyngeal Constrictor Muscle
Middle Pharyngeal Constrictor Muscle
Oral Cavity
Pterygomandibular Raphe
Soft Palate (Velum)
Superior Pharyngeal Constrictor Muscle
Thyroid Cartilage
Tongue
Uvula
Velopharyngeal Sphincter Muscle

Figure 4.3 Pharyngeal Levator Muscles
Auditory Tube (Eustachian Tube)
Dilator Tubae Muscle
Epiglottis
Faucial Isthmus
Palatal Raphe
Palatopharyngeal Muscle
Posterior Nares
Pterygoid Hamulus
Salpingopharyngeal Muscle
Stylopharyngeal Muscle
Temporal Bone, Styloid Process
Tongue, Pharyngeal Portion
Uvula
Vomer Bone

Figure 5.1 Vocal Tract: Larynx (Sagittal View)
Atrium (Infraglottal Cavity)
Aditus ad Laryngis
Cricoid Cartilage, Arch
Cricoid Cartilage, Lamina
Epiglottis
Esophagus
Laryngopharynx
Thyroid Cartilage
Trachea

True Vocal Fold
Vestibular Fold (False Vocal Fold)
Vestibule

Figure 5.2 Skeletal Larynx
Arytenoid Cartilage
Cricoid Cartilage, Arch
Cricoid Cartilage, Lamina
Hyoid Bone, Body
Hyoid Bone, Greater Horn
Hyoid Bone, Lesser Horn
Hyothyroid Membrane
Middle Cricothyroid Ligament
Middle Hyothyroid Ligament
Posterior Cricothyroid Ligament
Posterior Hyothyroid Ligament
Thyroid Cartilage, Inferior Horn
Thyroid Cartilage, Lamina
Thyroid Cartilage, Posterior Border
Thyroid Cartilage, Oblique Line
Thyroid Cartilage, Prominence
Thyroid Cartilage, Superior Horn
Thyroid Notch
Trachea, Cartilaginous Rings
Triticeal Cartilage

Figure 5.3A Larynx (Coronal Views)
Atrium
Cricoid Cartilage
Elastic Cone
Epiglottic Cartilage
Glottis
Laryngeal Ventricle (of Morgagni)
Laryngeal Vestibule
Pyriform Sinus (recess)
Thyroid Cartilage
Trachea
Vallecula

Vestibular (Ventricular) Folds
Vocal Fold

Figure 5.3B Vocal Fold Movements (Superior Views)
Anterior Commissure
Arytenoid Cartilage, Muscular Process
Arytenoid Cartilage, Vocal Process
Cricoid Cartilage, Arch
Cricoid Cartilage, Lamina
Intercartilaginous Glottis
Intermembranous Glottis
Thyroid Cartilage, Angle
Thyroid Cartilage, Lamina
Vocal Fold, Membranous

Figure 5.4 Larynx (Posterior and Sagittal Views)
Aryepiglottic Fold
Arytenoid Cartilage, Apex
Arytenoid Cartilage, Muscular Process
Arytenoid Cartilage, Vocal Process
Atrium, Conus Elasticus
Corniculate Cartilage
Cuneiform Cartilage
Cricoid Cartilage, Arch
Cricoid Cartilage, Lamina (2)
Epiglottis
Hyoid Bone, Body
Hyoid Bone, Greater Cornu
Hyothyroid Membrane
Interarytenoid Muscle
Posterior Cricoarytenoid Muscle
Posterior Hyothyroid Ligament
Thyroarytenoid (Vocal) Ligament
Thyroid Cartilage, Angle
Thyroid Cartilage, Angle (Interior)
Thyroid Cartilage, Inferior Cornu
Thyroid Cartilage, Superior Cornu

Tongue
Trachea
Tracheal Cartilage Ring
Triticeal Cartilage
Ventricle (Morgagni)
Vestibular Fold (False Vocal Fold)
Vestibule, Quadrangular Membrane
Vocal Fold

Figure 5.5 Extrinsic Laryngeal Muscles
Digastric Muscle, Anterior Belly
Digastric Muscle, Posterior Belly
External Acoustic Meatus
Fascial Loop, Digastric Muscle
Geniohyoid Muscle
Hyoid Bone
Mandible Bone, Angle
Mandible Bone, Condyloid Process
Mandible Bone, Protuberance
Mylohyoid Muscle
Omohyoid Muscle, Inferior Belly
Omohyoid Muscle, Superior Belly
Sternocleidomastoid Muscle
Sternohyoid Muscle
Stylohyoid Muscle
Temporal Bone, Mastoid Process
Temporal Bone, Styloid Process
Thyrohyoid Muscle
Thyroid Cartilage, Angle

Figure 5.6A Intrinsic Laryngeal Muscles: Superficial (Lateral View)
Arytenoid Cartilage
Corniculate Cartilage
Cricoid Cartilage, Arch
Cricoid Cartilage, Lamina
Cricothyroid Muscle, Oblique Portion
Cricothyroid Muscle, Vertical Portion

Thyroid Cartilage, Angle
Thyroid Cartilage, Inferior Cornu
Thyroid Cartilage, Lamina
Thyroid Cartilage, Superior Cornu

Figure 5.6B Intrinsic Laryngeal Muscles: Lateral Cricoarytenoid
Arytenoid Cartilage, Apex
Arytenoid Cartilage, Muscular Process
Arytenoid Cartilage, Vocal Process
Corniculate Cartilage
Cricoid Cartilage, Arch
Cricoid Cartilage, Lamina
Lateral Cricoarytenoid Muscle

Figure 5.6C Intrinsic Laryngeal Muscles: Posterior Cricoarytenoid
Arytenoid Cartilage, Apex
Arytenoid Cartilage, Muscular Process
Corniculate Cartilage
Cricoid Cartilage, Lamina
Cricoid Facet, Cricoarytenoid Joint
Notch
Posterior Cricoarytenoid Muscle

Figure 5.6D Intrinsic Laryngeal Muscles: Interarytenoid
Arytenoid Cartilage, Apex
Arytenoid Cartilage, Muscular Process
Corniculate Cartilage
Cricoid Cartilage, Lamina
Interarytenoid Muscle, Oblique Portion
Interarytenoid Muscle, Transverse Portion

Figure 5.6E Intrinsic Laryngeal Muscles: Thyroarytenoid
Anterior Commissure
Arytenoid Cartilage, Anterolateral Surface
Arytenoid Cartilage, Muscular Process
Arytenoid Cartilage, Vocal Process

Corniculate Cartilage
Cricoarytenoid Ligament (Joint)
Cricoid Cartilage, Arch
Cricoid Cartilage, Lamina
Glottis
Thyroarytenoid Muscle
Thyroarytenoid (Vocal) Ligament
Thyroid Cartilage, Angle
Thyroid Cartilage, Lamina
Thyroid Cartilage, Superior Cornu
Vocalis Muscle

Figure 5.7 Larynx Nerve Supply
Aorta, Arch
Brain, Cerebrum
Cells of Origin
Cerebral Cortex
Cricoid Cartilage
Decussation of Efferent Fibers
Hyoid Bone
Medulla Oblongata
Nucleus Ambiguus
Recurrent (Inferior) Laryngeal Nerve
Spinal Cord
Subclavian Artery
Superior Laryngeal Nerve
Superior Laryngeal Nerve, External Branch
Superior Laryngeal Nerve, Internal Branch
Thyroid Cartilage
Tracheal Cartilage Rings
Vagus Nerve (Cranial X)

Figure 6.1 Lower Respiratory Tract
Alveoli
Alveolar Duct
Alveolar Sacs

Bifurcation
Bronchus, Extrapulmonary
Bronchus, Intrapulmonary
Bronchus, Lobular
Cardiac Notch
Inferior Lobe, Left
Lung Apex
Lung Base
Respiratory Bronchiole
Superior Lobe, Left
Terminal Bronchiole
Trachea

Figure 6.2 Vertebral Column
Atlas (First Cervical Vertebra)
Axis (Second Cervical Vertebra)
Body
Cervical Group
Coccygeal Group (Coccyx)
Lumbar Group
Sacral Group (Sacrum)
Spinous Process
Thoracic Group
Transverse Process

Figure 6.3 Thoracic Vertebra: Superior and Lateral Views
Articulating Facet, Transverse Process
Body
Body, Articulating Facet
Lamina
Pedicle
Rib Articulating Process (Transverse Process)
Spinous Process
Superior Articulating Process

Transverse Process
Vertebral Canal

Figure 6.4 Vertebrosternal Rib
Angle
Body
Costal Cartilage
Head
Neck
Shaft
Spinous Process
Sternum Bone
Transverse Process
Tubercle
Vertebral Articulating Process
Vertebral Canal

Figure 6.5 Rib Cage
Costal Cartilages
Rib 1
Rib 2
Rib 3
Rib 4
Rib 5
Rib 6
Rib 7
Rib 8
Rib 9
Rib 10
Rib 11
Rib 12
Rib, Head
Sternum Bone, Angle
Sternum Bone, Body
Sternum Bone, Manubrium
Sternum Bone, Xiphoid Process

Thoracic Vertebra 1
Thoracic Vertebra 1, Transverse Process

Figure 6.6 Pelvic Girdle
Acetabulum
Coccyx
Ilium Bone
Ilium Bone, Crest
Inguinal Ligament
Ischium Bone
Pubis Bone
Sacrum Bone
Symphysis Pubis

Figure 6.7 Diaphragm Muscle
Costal Cartilages
Diaphragm Muscle
Diaphragm Muscle, Central Tendon
Lumbar Vertebrae
Rib 2, Head
Rib 8
Rib 9
Rib 10
Rib 11
Rib 12
Sternum Bone, Body
Sternum Bone, Manubrium
Sternum Bone, Xiphoid Process
Thoracic Vertebra 1
Thoracic Vertebra 2, Transverse Process

Figure 6.8 Thoracic Respiratory Muscles
Cervical Vertebrae
Clavicle Bone
External Intercostal Muscles
Humerus Bone
Internal Intercostal Muscles
Pectoralis Major Muscles

Pectoralis Minor Muscle
Ribs 1 and 2
Scalene Muscles
Scapula Bone
Serratus Anterior Muscle
Sternocleidomastoid Muscle
Sternum Bone, Body
Sternum Bone, Manubrium
Sternum Bone, Xiphoid Process

Figure 6.9 Abdominal Muscles
Costal Cartilages
External Abdominal Oblique Muscle
Ilium Bone, Crest
Inguinal Ligament
Internal Abdominal Oblique Muscle
Linea Alba
Pubis Bone
Rectus Abdominis Muscle
Rectus Abdominis Muscle, Tendinous Inscriptions
Sternum Bone, Xiphoid Process
Tendinous Aponeurosis
Transverse Abdominis Muscle

Figure 7.1 The Ear
Auditory Nerve (Cranial VIII)
Auditory Tube (Eustachian Tube)
Auricle
Cave
Ceruminous (Wax) Glands
Cochlea
Epitympanic Recess
External Acoustic Meatus, Bony Portion
External Acoustic Meatus, Cartilaginous Portion
Facial Nerve (Cranial VII)
Internal Acoustic Meatus
Mastoid Air Cells
Mastoid Antrum

Middle Ear (Tympanum)
Nasopharynx
Ossicular Chain
Round Window
Semicircular Canals
Tegmen Tympani
Temporal Bone, Petrous Portion
Temporal Bone, Squamous Portion
Tympanic Membrane

Figure 7.2 Pinna (Auricle)
Antihelix (Anthelix)
Antitragus
Concha
Concha, Cave
Concha, Skiff
Darwin's Tubercle
External Acoustic Meatus
Helix
Helix, Crus
Lobule
Scaphoid Fossa
Tragus (Buck)

Figure 7.3 Tympanic Membrane
Circular Fibers
Flaccid Portion (Shrapnell's Membrane)
Malleolar Fold
Malleus Bone, Manubrium
Radial Fibers
Tense Portion
Umbo

Figure 7.4 Middle Ear (Tympanum)
Aditus ad Antrum
Antrum
Epitympanic Recess (Attic)
Auditory Tube (Eustachian Tube)

Auditory Tube (Eustachian Tube), Cartilaginous Portion
Cochlea, Basal Turn
External Acoustic Meatus
Incus Bone, Body
Incus Bone, Lenticular Process
Incus Bone, Long Process
Malleus Bone, Head
Malleus Bone, Manubrium
Mastoid Air Cells
Middle Ear Cavity
Oval (Vestibular) Window
Pyramidal Eminence
Round (Cochlear) Window
Stapes Bone, Crura
Stapes Bone, Neck
Stapes Bone, Oval Footplate
Stapedius Muscle, Tendon
Tegmen Tympani
Temporal Bone, Petrous Portion
Temporal Bone, Tympanic Portion
Tensor Tympani Muscle
Tensor Tympani Muscle, Tendon
Tympanic Membrane, Tense Portion
Tympanic Membrane, Umbo
Tympanic Sulcus
Vestibule of Inner Ear

Figure 7.5 Cochlear Turns
Auditory Nerve (Cranial VII), Cochlear Division
Basilar Membrane
Cochlear Duct
Internal Acoustic Meatus
Modiolus
Nerve Fibers
Organ of Corti
Spiral Ganglion

Temporal Bone, Petrous Portion
Tympanic Canal
Vestibular Canal (Scala)
Vestibular Membrane (Reissner's Membrane)

Figure 7.6 Cochlea (Cross-Section)
Basilar Membrane
Cell Bodies
Cochlear Duct
Hairs
Inner Hair Cell
Modiolus
Nerve Fibers
Osseous Spiral Lamina
Outer Hair Cells
Pillar of Corti
Spiral Ganglion
Spiral Ligament
Spiral Limbus
Spiral Stria (Stripe)
Supporting Cell
Tectorial Membrane
Temporal Bone, Petrous Portion
Tympanic Canal (Scala)
Vestibular Canal (Scala)
Vestibular Membrane (Reissner's Membrane)

Figure 7.7 Neural Pathway: Audition
Auditory Nerve Fibers
Auditory Nerve (Cranial VIII) Cochlear Division
Auditory Radiations
Auditory Reflex Fibers
Cell Bodies
Cerebral Cortex
Cerebrum
Decussating Fibers
Dorsal Cochlear Nucleus

Inferior Colliculus
Lateral Lemniscus
Lateral Sulcus
Medial Geniculate Body of the Thalamus
Medulla
Midline
Nucleus of the Inferior Colliculus
Nucleus of the Lateral Lemniscus
Superior Olive
Superior Temporal Convolution (Gyrus)
Synapses
Ventral Cochlear Nucleus

Figure 8.1 Reflex Arc
Cell Body, Motor Nerve
Cell Body, Sensory Nerve
Dorsal Gray Horn
Dorsal Root Ganglion
Dorsal Root, Spinal Nerve
Motor Nerve Fiber
Muscle
Myoneural Juncture
Reflex Action to Stimulus
Sensory End Organ
Sensory Nerve Fiber
Spinal Nerve
Synapse
Ventral Gray Horn
Ventral Root, Spinal Nerve

Figure 8.2 Spinal Nerves
Dorsal Root
Dorsal Root Ganglion
Midline
Motor Nerve Fibers
Sensory Nerve Fibers
Spinal Cord

Spinal Nerve
Ventral Root
Vertebra, Lamina
Vertebra, Spinous Process
Ventral Root

Figure 8.3 Cranial Nerves
Abducens Nerve (Cranial VI)
Accessory Nerve (Cranial XI)
Auditory Nerve (Cranial VIII)
Cerebellum
Facial Nerve (Cranial VII)
Frontal Lobe
Glossopharyngeal Nerve (Cranial IX)
Hypoglossal Nerve (Cranial XII)
Longitudinal Fissure
Medulla
Midline
Oculomotor Nerve (Cranial III)
Olfactory Bulb (Cranial I)
Olfactory Tract (Cranial I)
Optic Chiasm

Optic Nerve (Cranial II)
Pons
Spinal Cord
Spinal Nerve
Trigeminal Nerve (Cranial V)
Trochlear Nerve (Cranial IV)
Vagus Nerve (Cranial X)

Figure 8.4 Pyramidal Pathway
Anterior (Ventral) Corticospinal Tract
Cerebral Cortex
Cerebrum
Cranial Nerves Nuclei
Decussating Fibers
Decussations
Internal Capsule
Lateral Coricospinal Tract
Lateral Sulcus
Longitudinal Fissure
Midbrain Level
Midline

Pons and Medulla Level
Precentral Gyrus (Area 4)
Pyramidal Cells of Origin
Spinal Cord Level
Ventral Gray Column

Figure 8.5 The Brain
Central Sulcus
Cerebellum
Frontal Lobe
Lateral Sulcus
Medulla
Occipital Lobe
Operculum
Parietal Lobe
Pons
Postcentral Convolution
Precentral Convolution
Spinal Cord
Superior Temporal Convolution
Temporal Lobe

Appendix II
Glossary

NOTE

Here are presented a few of the terms in this text that may require definition or example. For a more complete terminologic reference, see Nicolosi L, Harryman E, Kreshek J: *Terminology of communication disorders. Speech-language-hearing* 3rd edition. Baltimore: Williams & Wilkins, 1989, and Dox I, Melloni BJ, Eisner GM: *Melloni's illustrated medical dictionary.* Baltimore: Williams & Wilkins, 1979.

Abduction: to draw away from the midline.

Acromion (ac-ROW-me-on): the point of the shoulder.

Adduction: to draw toward the mid-line.

Adipose (ADD-i-pos): usually related to various tissues that store fat cells.

Aditus (ADD-i-tuss): an entrance, usually related to the opening into the laryngeal area called *aditus ad laryngis,* to *aditus ad antrum,* or to *aditus* of mastoid air cells.

Afferent (AFF-erent): that which conducts toward the center; sensory.

Ala (AY-lah): a structure that has wing-like characteristics; the wings or laminae.

Alveolus (al-VEE-o-luss): a sac or socket of teeth, lungs, or glands.

Amorphous (ah-MORE-fuss): shape-less; without distinct form.

Ansa (AN-sah): any loop-like structure of bone or nerve.

Anterior: toward the front or abdomen, in man.

Antrum (AN-trum): a hollow or cavity, usually applied to those cavities or sinuses located in the various bones.

Apex: the topmost part of a structure that is conical or pyramidal in shape.

Aponeurosis (apo-new-ROW-sis): a tendon that is usually flat, broad, and sheet-like.

Appendix: any extension of a structure that acts as an appendage.

Approximation: any action that brings two or more structures into an adjoining position.

Areolar (ah-REE-o-lar): related usually to a mesh-like organization of connective tissue that occupies various spaces in the body.

Articular: pertaining to surfaces or structures that meet to form a joint.

Articulation: a joint, as seen between two bones or cartilages; a diarthrosis or synarthrosis (in bony joints).

Astrocytes (AS-tro-sites): nerve cells or bone corpuscles that are star-shaped.

Atlas: term given to the first cervical vertebra.

Atrium (AY-tree-um): chamber or space in the heart, lungs, ear, and larynx.

Auricular (aw-RICK-you-lar): the center portion of the external auditory meatus, or to the external ear in general.

Autonomic: a self-controlling structure or system; usually related to a an involuntary portion of the nervous system uncontrolled by the brain or spinal cord.

Axis: the name given to second cervical vertebra; also the pivot-point; the center.

Axon: the portion of the neuron that carries stimuli away from the cell body, usually the longest portion of the neuron.

Bicuspid: teeth that have two prominent cusps or heads.

Bifurcate (BY-fur-kate): to divide into two portions, as in the trachea.

Brachial (BRAY-key-ull): usually applied to structures and tissues of the arm.

Bronchiole: each of the smaller divisions resulting from the forking of the trachea and bronchi.

Buccinator (BUCK-sin-ay-tore): a flat muscle located in the cheek, compresses the cheeks and holds food between the teeth.

Canine: the longer, pointed teeth used for holding and tearing (cuspid).

Capillary: the smallest vessel of the vascular system that aids in conducting blood from arteries to veins, and v.v.

Capitulum (kah-PIT-you-lum): a small, round protuberance on a bone surface.

Capsule: an encapsulating membrane acting as a container.

Cardiac: pertaining to the heart.

Carotid (kah-ROT-id): the arteries that run to the brain, or to the head in general.

Cartilage: a body tissue intermediary between bone and epithelium, which furnishes strength, shape, and flexibility.

Caudal (KAW-dull): toward the tail or lower end.

Caudate (KAW-date): resembling or possessing a tail.

Centrosome (SEN-tro-sohm): a concentration of cytoplasm that houses the agent responsible for sexual division of cells.

Cephalad (SEF-ahl-ahd): toward the head or upper end.

Cerebellum (ser-eh-BELL-um): the small portion of the brain located behind and below the cerebrum. Its major responsibility is coordination of bodily actions.

Cerebrum (sir-EE-brum): the largest portion of the brain. It is incompletely divided into two major hemispheres and contains many convolutions and fissures.

Cervical (SIR-vi-kull): related to the region of the cervix or neck; usually applied to bones and nerves.

Choana (ko-AY-nah): the nostril, naris, or posterior opening of the nasal cavity.

Cilia: small hairs located on cell borders and responsible for movement of food and wastes; also applied to the sensory nerve fibers located within the cochlea of the inner ear.

Cochlea (KOE-kle-a): spiral; that part of the inner ear housing the auditory sensory mechanisms.

Collagenous (ko-LAJ-en-us): usually white tissue that has a high concentration of the protein collagen; also, usually applied to the white, fibrous connective tissue.

Concha (KON-cha): the pit, hollow, or cavity of the external ear.

Condyle (KON-di-al): a round protuberance usually located at bone ends, as on the mandible.

Corniculate (kore-NICK-you-let): cartilaginous nodules located on the arytenoid cartilages in the larynx.

Cornu (KORE-new): a structure shaped like a horn.

Coronal: the anatomic plane that divides the body into front and back sections.

Corpus: any body.

Corpuscle: a small body; usually applied to specialized bodies located in nerves, epithelium, bone, blood, etc.

Cortex: any outer layer of substance; applied to the outer layer of the brain (cerebral cortex) or of bone.

Costal (KOS-tuhl): that which pertains to the rib; applied to the cartilages that connect the ribs and the sternum.

Cranial: related to the head or upper end.

Cricoid (CRY-koid): signet-shaped; usually applied to the cricoid cartilage in the larynx that acts to support the thyroid and arytenoid cartilages.

Cuneiform (cue-KNEE-i-form): a wedge-shaped structure; cartilages located near the arytenoid cartilages of the larynx.

Cutaneous (cue-TAY-knee-us): pertaining to the first layer of the skin.

Cytology: the study of cellular structures.

Decussate (DEH-cuss-ate): a crossing action that results in an X formation; usually applied to nerve groups of the central nervous system.

Deferens (DEAF-er-ens): that which carries away from the center; usually applied to nerves or ducts.

Deglutition (deh-glue-TISH-un): the act of swallowing.

Dendrite (DEN-drite): the portion of the neuron that carries stimuli toward the cell body, usually a short portion.

Diaphragm: a large muscle of respiration that separates thoracic and abdominal cavities.

Diaphysis (die-AFF-i-sis): the portion of a growing bone called the *shaft*.

Diarthrosis (die-are-THROW-sis): a freely moving joint such as the elbow, wrist, shoulder, etc. (also, *diarthrodial*).

Digastric (die-GAS-trick): double-bellied muscle of mastication located below the tongue.

Distal (DIS-tull): away from the point of attachment, away from the midline.

Dorsal: toward the back or rear side.

Dorsum: the superior and rear surface of a portion, especially of the tongue.

Ectoplast (EK-toe-plast): the outer layer of the protoplasm that forms a cell membrane.

Efferent: that which conveys away from the center; usually applied to motor nerves.

Embryology: the study of cell growth and the development of an organism.

Endo-: prefix meaning within or inner.

Epi-: prefix meaning upon, above, or upper.

Epiphysis (ee-PIFF-i-sis): the ends of a growing bone that form the boundaries for the diaphysis or shaft.

Epithelium (epeh-THEE-lee-um): the cellular, outer

substance of skin and mucous membrane that is without blood supply.

Esophagus: part of the digestive system; the tube connecting the pharynx and the stomach.

Eustachian tube (you-STAY-kee-un): the tube that leads from the middle ear to the pharynx; named in honor of Eustachius, Italian anatomist of the sixteenth century. Now termed auditory tube.

Falciform (FALL-si-form): sickle-shaped.

Fascia (FASH-ah): a band or sheet of fibrous connective tissue that encloses muscles and some organs.

Fasciculus (fas-IK-you-lus): a bundle or cluster of nerve or muscle fibers that gather to make up whole nerves or muscles.

Fauces (FAW-seez): the space between mouth and pharynx.

Fenestra (fen-ES-tra): window or opening; usually applied to the openings found in the middle ear that lead to the inner ear.

Fissure: a groove or sulcus; usually applied to those clefts found in tissues.

Fixate: the act of making static, fixed, or relatively immovable.

Flaccid (FLAK-sid): soft, inert; usually applied to muscles that have lost their quality or tonus.

Follicle: a small sac or gland capable of excretion.

Foramen (fore-AY-men): a window or hole that is a regular part of a structure.

Fossa (FOSS-ah): a pit, cavity, or depression that is a regular part of a structure.

Frenum (FREE-num): a fold or ridge; mucous membrane ridge that connects the tongue with the floor of the mouth; frenulum.

Fusiform (FEW-zi-form): anything that has a spindle shape.

Ganglion (GANG-lee-on): a concentration of nerve-cell bodies that serve as nervous centers.

Gastric: pertaining to the stomach.

Gestalt (gesh-TALT): usually related to a philosophy or action that is total and wholistic.

Gingiva (JIN-ji-vah): the membranous covering of the alveolar ridge; the gum.

Gladiolus (glad-EYE-oh-luss): body or main portion.

Glossal (GLAH-sull): pertaining to the tongue.

Glottis (GLAH-tis): the opening between the vocal folds.

Gyrus (JIE-rus): a rise, hill, or promontory located in membranous tissue; usually applied to the convolutions located in the brain.

Hamulus (HAM-you-luss): any hook-shaped structure; usually applied to the pterygoid process of the sphenoid bone.

Hiatus (hie-A-tuss): a space, gap, groove, or opening in any structure.

Histology: the study of tissues.

Hormone: a chemical secretion of the ductless glands that is carried in the blood stream and that acts to stimulate the activity of organs.

Humerus: the upper arm bone.

Hyaline (HIE-a-lynn): type of white cartilage commonly found throughout the body.

Hyoid (HIE-oid): the U-shaped bone located below the tongue and above the thyroid cartilage.

Hyper-: prefix meaning in excess of some normal state.

Hypo-: prefix meaning less than some normal state.

Illium (ILL-ee-um): the hip bone.

Incus (ING-kuss): anvil-shaped bone of the middle ear.

Inferior: below; toward the caudal end of the body.

Infundibulum (in-fun-DIB-you-lum): a funnel, canal, or extended cavity; usually applied to a passage connecting the nasal cavity with ethmoid bone or with the area at the upper end of the cochlear canal.

Inguinal (IN-gwi-null): pertaining to the groin.

Innervate (IN-nerve-ate): to stimulate or to supply with nervous stimulation.

Insertion: point of attachment for muscles; usually applied to the most movable attachment.

Integument (in-TEG-you-ment): the outermost surface of the body, or skin.

Interstitial (in-ter-STISH-ull): located in the spaces between cells.

Intrinsic: anything wholly contained within another structure; usually applies to muscles that are exclusively attached to one organ or structure, as intrinsic muscles of the tongue.

Jugular: pertaining to the neck; usually applied to the large vein of the neck.

Karyotheca (kare-ee-OH-thee-kah): term applied to the membrane separating the nucleus from the cytosome of a cell.

Labial (LAY-bee-ull): pertaining to the lips.

Lacrimal (LACK-ri-mull): pertaining to the tears and the ducts from which they arise.

Lacuna (lah-KOO-nah): a small pit or cavity; usually applied to bone cavities.

Lamina (LAM-i-nah): a plate or flat layer of bone.

Larynx (LEH-rinks): the structure responsible for voice; composed of cartilages and muscles; colloquially the voice-box.

Laryngectomy: surgical removal of the larynx.

Lateral: away from the midline, toward the periphery.

Ligament: tough, fibrous connective bands that support or bind bones and various organs.

Linea alba (LIN-ee-ah AHL-bah): a white line; usually applied to major tendinous structure running down the front of the abdominal cavity.

Lingual (LING-gwull): pertaining to the tongue.

Lobe: a regular part of an organ usually delineated by fissures or cleavages.

Lumbar (LUM-bar): pertaining to the portion of the back located between the thorax and the pelvis, commonly referred to as the loins.

Lumen (LOO-men): a transverse or cross-sectional area in a tubular structure.

Lymph (LIMF): a clear, watery fluid secreted by the lymph glands in order to expedite the removal of waste from tissue cells.

Malleus (MALL-ee-us): mallet-shaped bone of the middle ear.

Mandible: major bone of the lower jaw.

Manubrium (mah-NEW-bree-um): a handle; usually applied to the uppermost portion of the breast bone and the inferior portion of the malleus.

Mastoid: nipple-shaped; usually applied to a process of the temporal bone.

Meatus: (mee-AY-tuss): any passage; usually applied to the passage of the ear or nose.

Media: middle.

Medial: toward the midline or median plane.

Mediastinum (meed-di-ah-STIE-num): a median partition; usually applied to the median region that divides the thorax into two lateral cavities.

Medulla oblongata (meh-DOOL-ah ahb-long-GAH-tah): the most inferior portion of the brain; the uppermost portion of the spinal cord that connects with the pons.

Membrane: a thin sheet of tissue that sheaves or divides organs and surfaces.

Meninges (meh-NIN-jeez): specialized membranes that encase the brain and spinal cord.

Mental: relating to the chin or genu of the mandible.

Metabolism: the regular chemical modifications of substances that occur in the growth and development of the body.

Modiolus (mo-DIE-o-luss): the central pillar of the cochlea.

Morphology: the study of forms and structure.

Mucus (MEW-cuss): the secretion that covers the membranes of many cavities and passages that are exposed to the external environment; mucous membrane.

Muscle: specialized fibers, tissues, and organs that can contract and furnish the body with motive power.

Myo-: prefix pertaining to muscle.

Nares (NAY-reez): the anterior openings of the nasal cavities that communicate with the external environment, i.e., the nostrils.

Nasopharynx: the part of the pharynx located above the velum or soft palate.

Neuron (NEW-ron): the basic structural unit of the nervous system; composed of a cell body, axon, and dendrites.

Nucleus (NEW-klee-us): a small round body within every cell that acts as the functional control center; refers also to a mass of cell bodies in the brain or spinal cord.

Occlusion (uk-KLOO-shun): the act of closing or the state of being closed, as in the teeth.

Orbicular (or-BICK-you-lar): circular; usually applied to the orbicularis oris muscle encircling the mouth.

Orifice (OR-i-fiss): an entrance or opening into a body cavity.

Origin: the relatively fixed muscular connection.

Oropharynx: the part of the pharynx located between the velum, or soft palate, and the hyoid bone.

Ossicle (AHS-i-kull): a small bone; usually applied to the bones of the ear.

Ossify: the act of becoming bone.

Osteoblasts (AHS-tee-o-blasts): cells that are formed into bone.

Osteology: (ahs-tee-AH-low-gee): study of bone.

Ostium (AHS-tee-um): an entrance or opening.

Otosclerosis (oh-toe-skler-ROW-sis): formation of spongy bone in the ear.

Papilla (pah-Pill-ah): a small elevation on epithelial tissue.

Paranasal: alongside the nose, as in paranasal sinuses.

Parietal (pah-RIE-eh-tull): pertaining to the walls of organs or cavities; as applied to the parietal bones of the cranium or to the lobes of the brain lying near these bones.

Pectoralis (peck-toe-RAH-liss): pertaining to the chest; usually applied to the muscles that form the chest.

Pedicle (PED-i-cull): stalk-like process or stem.

Peduncles (pee-DUNG-culls): a supporting part of another structure; usually applied to the bands running between sections of the brain.

Pelvis (PEL-viss): a basin; usually applied to the hip region.

Pericardium (per-i-CAR-dee-um): the membranous sac that ensheathes and contains the heart.

Perilymph (PER-il-imf): the fluid that fills the space in the outer canals of the inner ear.

Periosteum (per-ee-OSS-tee-um): the fibrous sheath that covers all bones.

Peristalsis (per-i-STAHL-sis): a wave of contraction passing along a tube, as in the digestive tract.

Peritoneum (per-i-toe-KNEE-um): the membrane that lines the abdominal cavity.

Pharyngeal (fah-RIN-gee-ull): pertaining to the pharynx or throat.

Phrenic (FREN-ik): pertaining to the diaphragm; usually applied to the spinal nerve that supplies the diaphragm muscle.

Pinna: the skin-covered cartilaginous sound collector of the outer ear; also auricle.

Plasma: the fluid portion of the blood during circulation.

Platysma (plah-TIZZ-mah): a plate; usually applied to the neck muscle connected to the mandible and the clavicle.

Pleura (PLOOR-ah): pertaining to the ribs; usually applied to the chest or thoracic cavity; refers also to the membranes that line the cavity.

Plexus (PLEK-suss): a collection, concentration, or network of parts of the nervous or vascular systems.

Pons: a bridge; usually applied to that portion of brainstem that is between the medulla oblongata and the midbrain.

Posterior: toward the back or rear side.

Protoplasm: the basic material of every living cell.

Proximal: toward the point of attachment.

Pterygoid (TER-i-goid): wing-shaped; usually applied to the sphenoid bone and to the muscles that are connected beneath the skull to the mandible.

Pulmonary: pertaining to the lungs.

Ramus (RAY-muss): a branch; usually applied to parts of nerves, vessels, or bone.

Raphe (ruh-FAY): a line formed by the union of two parts.

Rectus: straight; applied to the rectus abdominis muscles connected to the pubis and the lower costal cartilages.

Reticular: like a network; usually applied to the network of fibers passing between the pons and the medulla oblongata.

Rostral (RAHS-trull): toward the head end.

Sagittal (SAJ-i-tull): straight; usually applied to the plane that divides the body into right and left portions.

Sarcolemma (sar-ko-LEM-mah): a membranous sheath encasing a muscle.

Scala: chamber, as in scala media of the cochlea.

Scalenus (skay-LEE-nuss): uneven; applied to the muscles of the neck that connect to the first rib and the cervical vertebrae.

Scaphoid (SKAF-oid): a bone, fossa or process shaped like a small boat.

Segmentation: division into small parts or segments.

Sensory: nerves, organs, or structures related to the process of sensation and carrying stimuli from the exterior toward the cerebrospinal system; afferent.

Septum: a partition or dividing wall; such as the nasal septum.

Sinus: a depression, hollow, or cavity; usually applied to those located in the bones around the nose (paranasal sinuses).

Sphenoid (SFEE-noid): wedge-shaped; usually applied to the complex bone of the cranium.

Sphincter (SFING-ter): any muscle or combination of muscles that provides a closure for a natural body opening.

Stapes (STAY-peez); a small, stirrup-shaped bone of the ear.

Sternum: the breast bone.

Striated: streaked or striped; usually applied to a special type of muscular fiber that effects voluntary movement.

Styloid (STY-loid); pin-shaped; usually applied to a part of the temporal bone that furnishes attachment for muscles and ligaments.

Sulcus (SULL-kuss): a fissure or groove in bone or membranous tissue.

Superior: above; toward the head or cephalic end.

Suture (SOO-cher): a seam; usually applied to a juncture of cranial or facial bones.

Symphysis (SIM-fi-sis): usually applied to a line formed by the union of two bones; more definite than a suture.

Synapse (SIN-aps): the functional junction between the axon of one nerve cell and the dendrite of another.

Synarthrosis (sin-are-THROW-sis): restricted movement or complete lack of movement in a joint.

Synchondrosis: restricted movement of a cartilaginous joint.

Synergy (SIN-er-jee): a coordination or cooperation that results in smooth economical activity.

Synostosis (sin-os-TOE-sis): restricted or lack of movement of a joint due to a bony connection.

Synovial (sin-OH-vee-ull): pertains to a fluid secreted in joints, bursae, and around certain tendon sheaths.

Systemic: affecting the body as a whole.

Tendon: a cord-like, fibrous material connecting muscles with points of origin and insertion.

Therapy: the treatment of a pathologic condition.

Thorax: pertains to the region of the body that is located between the clavicle and the diaphragm.

Thyroid: the shield-like cartilage of the larynx that rests on the cricoid cartilage and furnishes an attachment for the vocal folds; also a gland.

Tonus: a state of partial contraction of a muscle that produces a healthy, resilient quality in the muscle.

Trachea (TRAY-kee-ah): the cartilaginous and membranous tube extending from the larynx to the bronchial tubes, commonly referred to as the windpipe.

Transverse: usually applied to a plane that extends horizontally from one side of a structure to the other.

Tricuspid (try-CUSS-pid): having three cusps or heads; usually applied to molars.

Tuberosity (too-ber-OSS-i-tee): protuberance or eminence; usually applied to bones.

Turbinate (TER-bi-nate): any structure shaped like a top and filled with pits, hollows, or swirls; usually applied to bones of the nasal chamber.

Tympanum: a drum, especially the middle ear.

Vaginal (VAJ-i-null): pertaining to any sheath or sheath-like structure.

Vein: a vessel that conveys blood toward the heart.

Velum (VEE-lum): the soft palate; the posterior muscular portion of the roof of the mouth.

Ventral: toward the front or abdomen.

Ventricle: a small cavity.

Vertex (VER-tex): the topmost part; usually applied to the top of the head.

Vestibule: an antechamber; usually applied to special chambers in the nose, ear, and larynx.

Viscera (VISS-er-ah): generic term for the organs of any large body cavity; most frequently applied to the organs in the abdomen.

Xiphoid process (ZIF-oid): the most inferior portion of the sternum; the tip of the breast bone.

Appendix III
Physiologic Phonetics

BASIC ASSUMPTIONS

The following charts attempt to present primary muscular activity in the production of speech sounds. They are the result of essentially a deduced analysis that is incompletely substantiated by research or clinical evidence. The reader must assume the following:

1. He is dealing with a normal, average speaker of general American speech, who has no known defects or deviations.
2. In all cases, the inspiration of the air to the lungs has been completed.
3. The articulators under consideration are in a dynamically neutral position, with
    a. the mouth closed,
    b. velopharyngeal aperture open,
    c. the tongue blade horizontally flat.
4. Static positions indicated are preceded and followed by dynamic synergic activities such as facial movement or exhalation of air.

In reading the charts, reference to phonation (Section I) or to resonance (Section II) must be made at the indicated analysis to complete the description of the articulatory act.

The reader should refer to the text for complete descriptions of the musculature, including origins and insertions as well as neural innervation of the muscles listed. Also, the listed bilateral structures are ordered according to an arbitrary importance of the muscles. Individual differences, among persons as well as sounds, dictate the degree of participation of each muscle in the action indicated. The listing only indicates that a muscle does participate, not the extent to which it contributes to the completed phonetic act. Fixation of antagonistic muscles or muscle groups is assumed to maintain an equilibrium in the articulatory system. Effort has been made to present the essential muscles that effect the movement; in each case, contraction of closely related muscles probably assists the activity.

I. THE PHONATORY PROCESS

Action	*Musculature*

A. Glottal closure (vocal fold adduction)	1. Intermembranous adduction
	    a. Lateral cricoarytenoid
	    b. Thyroarytenoid
	2. Intercartilaginous adduction
	    a. Interarytenoid

Action	*Musculature*
B. Vocal fold tension and lengthening	1. Cricothyroid
	2. Vocalis
C. Vocal fold mass change	1. Vocalis
	2. Cricothyroid
	3. Thyroarytenoid
D. Increase of air pressure	1. Controlled relaxation of
	a. Diaphragm
	b. Thoracic
	2. Abdominal group
	a. External oblique
	b. Internal oblique
	c. Rectus
	d. Transverse

II. THE RESONANCE PROCESS

Action	*Musculature*
A. Velopharyngeal closure	1. Velopharyngeal sphincter
	2. Levator veli palatine
	3. Superior pharyngeal constrictor
	4. Palatopharyngeus
	5. Uvula
B. Tongue movement[1]	
1. Position	1. Extrinsic
2. Shape (contour)	1. Intrinsic
C. Mouth opening	
1. Jaw depression	1. External pterygoid
	2. Digastric (anterior belly)
	3. Mylohyoid
	4. Geniohyoid
	5. Platysma
2. Lip opening	
a. Upper lip	1. Levator labii

---

[1] For detailed analysis, see specific speech sounds.

Action	*Musculature*
	2. Zygomatic
	3. Levator anguli
b. Lower lip	
	1. Depressor anguli
	2. Depressor labii
	3. Mentalis

III. VOWEL SOUND PRODUCTION[2]

Sound	*Action*	*Musculature*
[i]	A. Slight parting of lips	1. Levator labii
		2. Depressor labii
	B. Strong retraction of lips	1. Risorius
		2. Zygomatic
	C. Slight depression of mandible	1. External pterygoid
		2. Digastric (anterior belly)
		3. Mylohyoid
		4. Geniohyoid
	D. Strong depression of tongue apex	1. Longitudinal inferior
		2. Genioglossus (anterior fibers)
		3. Hyoglossus
	E. Strong elevation of posterior tongue dorsum	1. Palatoglossus
		2. Styloglossus
[I]	A. Slight parting of lips	1. Depressor labii
		2. Levator labii
	B. Slight depression of mandible	1. External pterygoid
		2. Digastric (anterior belly)
		3. Mylohyoid
		4. Geniohyoid
	C. Slight depression of tongue apex	1. Longitudinal inferior
		2. Genioglossus (anterior fibers)
		3. Hyoglossus
	D. Slight elevation of posterior tongue dorsum	1. Palatoglossus
		2. Styloglossus
[e]	A. Slight parting of lips	1. Depressor labii
		2. Levator labii

---

[2]Basic assumptions: (1) all vowels are phonated (see Section I); (2) velopharyngeal closure occurs for all vowels (see Section I A).

Sound	*Action*	*Musculature*
	B. Slight retraction of lips	1. Risorius
		2. Zygomatic
	C. Moderate depression of mandible	1. External pterygoid
		2. Digastric
		3. Mylohyoid
		4. Geniohyoid
		5. Platysma
	D. Moderate depression of tongue apex	1. Longitudinal inferior
		2. Genioglossus (anterior fibers)
		3. Hyoglossus
	E. Slight elevation of posterior tongue dorsum	1. Palatoglossus
		2. Styloglossus
[ɛ]	A. Moderate parting of lips	1. Levator labii
		2. Depressor labii
		3. Levator anguli
		4. Depressor anguli
		5. Zygomatic
		6. Mentalis
	B. Moderate depression of mandible	1. External pterygoid
		2. Digastric (anterior belly)
		3. Mylohyoid
		4. Geniohyoid
		5. Platysma
	C. Slight elevation of posterior tongue dorsum	1. Palatoglossus
		2. Styloglossus
	D. Slight retraction of lips	1. Risorius
		2. Styloglossus
[æ]	A. Considerable mandibular depression	1. External pterygoid
		2. Digastric (anterior belly)
		3. Mylohyoid
		4. Geniohyoid
		5. Platysma
	B. Retraction of angles of lips	1. Risorius
		2. Zygomatic
	C. Strong depression of anterior tongue dorsum	1. Genioglossus (anterior and middle fibers)
		2. Hyoglossus
[a]	A. Moderate mandibular depression	1. External pterygoid
		2. Digastric (anterior belly)
		3. Mylohyoid

Sound	*Action*	*Musculature*
		4. Geniohyoid
		5. Platysma
	B. Moderate depression of anterior tongue dorsum	1. Genioglossus (anterior and middle fibers)
		2. Hyoglossus
[ɔ]	A. Slight mandibular depression	1. External pterygoid
		2. Digastric (anterior belly)
		3. Mylohyoid
		4. Geniohyoid
	B. Moderate labial protrusion	1. Orbicularis oris
		2. Mentalis
		3. Levator labii
		4. Depressor labii
	C. Slight tongue apex depression	1. Genioglossus (anterior fibers)
		2. Longitudinal inferior
		3. Hyoglossus
	D. Slight depression of anterior tongue dorsum	1. Hyoglossus
		2. Genioglossus (middle and posterior fibers)
[o]	A. Slight mandibular depression	1. External pterygoid
		2. Digastric (anterior belly)
		3. Mylohyoid
		4. Geniohyoid
	B. Moderate labial protrusion	1. Orbicularis oris
		2. Mentalis
		3. Levator labii
		4. Depressor labii
	C. Tongue dorsum depression	1. Genioglossus (anterior and middle fibers)
		2. Hyoglossus
[U]	A. Slight mandibular depression	1. External pterygoid
		2. Digastric (anterior belly)
		3. Mylohyoid
		4. Geniohyoid
	B. Moderate labial protrusion	1. Orbicularis oris
	C. Depression of anterior tongue dorsum	1. Genioglossus (anterior and middle fibers)
		2. Hyoglossus
		3. Longitudinal lingual inferior
[u]	A. Slight mandibular depression	1. External pterygoid
		2. Digastric (anterior belly)
		3. Mylohyoid
		4. Geniohyoid

Sound	*Action*	*Musculature*
	B. Strong labial protrusion	1. Orbicularis oris
		2. Mentalis
		3. Levator labii
		4. Depressor labii
	C. Depression of anterior tongue dorsum	1. Genioglossus (anterior and middle fibers)
		2. Hyoglossus
		3. Longitudinal lingual inferior
[ə]	A. Slight mandibular depression	1. External pterygoid
[ʌ]		2. Digastric (anterior belly)
		3. Mylohyoid
		4. Geniohyoid
	B. Depression of anterior tongue dorsum	1. Genioglossus (anterior and middle fibers)
		2. Hyoglossus
		3. Longitudinal lingual inferior
[ɝ]	A. Slight mandibular depression	1. External pterygoid
[ʌ]		2. Digastric (anterior belly)
		3. Mylohyoid
		4. Geniohyoid
	B. Slight lip protrusion	1. Orbicularis oris
		2. Mentalis
		3. Levator labii
		4. Depressor labii
	C. Tongue border elevation	1. Palatoglossus
		2. Styloglossus
		3. Transverse lingual

IV. CONSONANT SOUND PRODUCTION

Sound	*Action*	*Musculature*
[b]	A. Strong lip compression	1. Orbicularis oris
	B. Slight mandibular depression (on release)	1. External pterygoid
		2. Digastric (anterior belly)
		3. Mylohyoid
		4. Geniohyoid
	C. Velopharyngeal closure	(See Section IIA)
	D. Phonation	(See Section I)
[p]	A. Strong lip compression	1. Orbicularis oris
	B. Slight mandibular depression (on release)	1. External pterygoid

Sound	Action	Musculature
		2. Digastric (anterior belly)
		3. Mylohyoid
		4. Geniohyoid
	C. Velopharyngeal closure	(See Section IIA)
[t]	A. Elevation of tongue tip and lateral margins	1. Superior longitudinal lingual
		2. Styloglossus
	B. Velopharyngeal closure	(See Section IIA)
	C.³	
[d]	A. Elevation of tongue tip and lateral margins	1. Superior longitudinal lingual
		2. Styloglossus
	B. Velopharyngeal closure	(See Section IIA)
	C. Phonation	(See Section I)
	D³	
[k]	A. Elevation of tongue middle, from border to border	1. Palatoglossus
		2. Styloglossus
	B. Velopharyngeal closure	(See Section IIA)
	C³	
[g]	A. Elevation of tongue middle, from border to border	1. Palatoglossus
		2. Styloglossus
	B. Velopharyngeal closure	(See Section IIA)
	C. Phonation	(See Section I)
	D³	
[s]	A. Lips slightly apart	1. Levator labii
		2. Depressor labii
	B. Dental occlusion (jaws together)	1. Internal pterygoid
		2. Temporalis
		3. Masseter
	C. Extension of tongue apex	1. Genioglossus
	D. Narrow grooving of tongue dorsum	1. Transverse lingual
	E. Velopharyngeal closure	(See Section IIA)
[z]	A. Lips slightly apart	1. Levator labii
		2. Depressor labii
	B. Dental occlusion (jaws together)	1. Internal pterygoid
		2. Temporalis
		3. Masseter
	C. Extension of tongue apex	1. Genioglossus

³ Indicates release as in [p].

Sound	Action	Musculature
	D. Narrow grooving of tongue dorsum	1. Transverse lingual
	E. Velopharyngeal closure	(See Section IIA)
	F. Phonation	(See Section I)
[f]	A. Slight mandibular retraction	1. Internal pterygoid
	B. Slight mandibular depression	1. Digastric (anterior belly)
		2. Mylohyoid
		3. Geniohyoid
		4. External pterygoid
	C. Tension of lower lip	1. Buccinator
		2. Risorius
		3. Orbicularis oris (lower portion)
	D. Slight elevation of lower lip	1. Those listed in C
		2. Mentalis
	E. Velopharyngeal closure	(See Section IIA)
[v]	A. Slight mandibular retraction	1. Internal pterygoid
	B. Slight mandibular depression	1. Digastric (anterior belly)
		2. Mylohyoid
		3. Geniohyoid
		4. External pterygoid
	C. Tension of lower lip	1. Buccinator
		2. Risorius
		3. Orbicularis oris (lower portion)
	D. Slight elevation of lower lip	1. Those listed in C.
		2. Mentalis
	E. Velopharyngeal closure	(See Section IIA)
	F. Phonation	(See Section I)
[m]	A. Strong lip compression	1. Orbicularis oris
	B. Phonation	(See Section I)
[n]	A. Slight mandibular depression	1. Digastric (anterior belly)
		2. Mylohyoid
		3. Geniohyoid
		4. External pterygoid
	B. Strong elevation of tongue apex	1. Longitudinal lingual superior
		2. Styloglossus
	C. Phonation	(See Section I)
[ŋ]	A. Slight mandibular depression	1. Digastric (anterior belly)
		2. Mylohyoid
		3. Geniohyoid
		4. External pterygoid

Sound	*Action*	*Musculature*
	B. Strong elevation of tongue middle	1. Palatoglossus 2. Styloglossus
	C. Phonation	(See Section I)
[tʃ]	A. Elevation of tongue tip, lateral margins, and central apical portion	1. Superior longitudinal lingual 2. Styloglossus
	B. Velopharyngeal closure C⁴	(See Section IIA)
[dʒ]	A. Elevation of tongue tip, lateral margins, and central apical region	1. Superior longitudinal lingual 2. Styloglossus
	B. Velopharyngeal closure	(See Section IIA)
	C. Phonation D⁵	(See Section I)
[θ]	A. Slight mandibular depression	1. Digastric (anterior belly) 2. Mylohyoid 3. Geniohyoid 4. External pterygoid
	B. Protrusion of tongue tip	1. Genioglossus (medial and posterior fibers) 2. Longitudinal superior lingual
	C. Flattening of tongue dorsum	1. Vertical lingual
	D. Velopharyngeal closure	(See Section IIA)
[ð]	A. Slight mandibular depression	1. Digastric (anterior belly) 2. Mylohyoid 3. Geniohyoid 4. External pterygoid
	B. Protrusion of tongue tip	1. Genioglossus (medial and posterior fibers) 2. Longitudinal lingual superior
	C. Flattening of tongue dorsum	2. Vertical lingual
	D. Velopharyngeal closure	(See Section IIA)
	E. Phonation	(See Section I)
[ʃ]	A. Slight mandibular depression	1. Digastric (anterior belly) 2. Mylohyoid 3. Geniohyoid 4. External pterygoid
	B. Slight labial protrusion	1. Orbicularis oris 2. Mentalis

---

⁴Indicates release as in [p].

---

⁵Indicates release as in [p].

Sound	*Action*	*Musculature*
		3. Levator labii
		4. Depressor labii
	C. Flattening of tongue dorsum	1. Vertical lingual
	D. Depression of tongue apex	1. Genioglossus (anterior fibers)
		2. Longitudinal inferior lingual
		3. Hyoglossus
	E. Velopharyngeal closure	(See Section IIA)
[ʒ]	A. Slight mandibular depression	1. Digastric (anterior belly)
		2. Mylohyoid
		3. Geniohyoid
		4. External pterygoid
	B. Slight labial protrusion	1. Orbicularis oris
		2. Mentalis
		3. Levator labii
		4. Depressor labii
	C. Flattening of tongue dorsum	1. Vertical lingual
	D. Depression of tongue apex	1. Genioglossus (anterior fibers)
		2. Longitudinal lingual inferior
		3. Hyoglossus
	E. Velopharyngeal closure	(See Section IIA)
	F. Phonation	(See Section I)
[l]	A. Slight mandibular depression	1. Digastric (anterior belly)
		2. Mylohyoid
		3. Geniohyoid
		4. External pterygoid
	B. Elevation of tongue apex	1. Longitudinal lingual superior
		2. Styloglossus
	C. Elevation of tongue borders	1. Transverse lingual
		2. Palatoglossus
	D. Velopharyngeal closure	(See Section IIA)
	E. Phonation	(See Section I)
[r]	A. Slight mandibular depression	1. Digastric (anterior belly)
		2. Mylohyoid
		3. Geniohyoid
		4. External pterygoid
	B. Slight protrusion of lips	1. Orbicularis oris
		2. Mentalis
		3. Levator labii
		4. Depressor labii

Sound	Action	Musculature
	C. Elevation of posterior tongue borders	1. Palatoglossus
		2. Transverse lingual
	D. Depression of tongue apex	1. Genioglossus (anterior fibers)
		2. Longitudinal lingual inferior
		3. Hyoglossus
	E. Velopharyngeal closure	(See Section IIA)
	F. Phonation	(See Section I)
[j]	A. Slight mandibular depression	1. Digastric (anterior belly)
		2. Mylohyoid
		3. Geniohyoid
		4. External pterygoid
	B. Protrusion of lips	1. Orbicularis oris
		2. Mentalis
		3. Levator labii
		4. Depressor labii
	C. Tongue grooved	1. Transverse lingual
		2. Palatoglossus
	D. Velopharyngeal closure	(See Section IIA)
	E. Phonation	(See Section I)
[hw]	A. Slight mandibular depression	1. Digastric (anterior belly)
		2. Mylohyoid
		3. Geniohyoid
		4. External pterygoid
	B. Strong protrusion of lips	1. Orbicularis oris
		2. Mentalis
		3. Levator labii
		4. Depressor labii
	C. Velopharyngeal closure	(See Section IIA)
[w]	A. Slight mandibular depression	1. Digastric (anterior belly)
		2. Mylohyoid
		3. Geniohyoid
		4. External pterygoid
	B. Strong protrusion of lips	1. Orbicularis oris
		2. Mentalis
		3. Levator labii
		4. Depressor labii
	C. Velopharyngeal closure	(See Section IIA)
	D. Phonation	(See Section I)

Sound	Action	Musculature
[h]	A. Slight mandibular depression	1. Digastric (anterior belly)
		2. Mylohyoid
		3. Geniohyoid
		4. External pterygoid
	B. Velopharyngeal closure	(See Section IIA)
	C. Partial vocal fold adduction	1. Lateral cricoarytenoid
		2. (Inter)arytenoid

References

The student of anatomy can find references of many varieties to clarify, expand and illustrate the concepts any text introduces. There are several anatomy books for speech and hearing science students specifically; it is with these that the annotated list commences.

Speech and Hearing Sciences

Dickson DR, Maue WM: Human vocal anatomy. Springfield, IL: Charles C Thomas, 1973.

The drawings in this text can be of considerable help to a student; however, some presentations can be confusing. The text is minimal, limited to abbreviated descriptions of areas and terms identified on drawings, much as is done in a glossary.

Dickson DR, Maue-Dickson W: Anatomical and physiological bases of speech. Boston: Little, Brown, 1982.

This is a carefully and moderately detailed presentation of the anatomic bases of both speech and hearing. Each section provides references to pertinent basic research, line drawings, plates, cadaveric dissection, and even radiologic presentations. Physiology is simply but carefully presented at the level of discussion of the anatomic entity, as well as at the summary level.

Kahane JC, Folkins JF: Atlas of speech and hearing anatomy. Columbus, OH: Merrill, 1984.

The illustrations of this atlas are largely photographic, although some few line drawings are presented. The text,

as in most atlases, is minimal. The photography of actual dissections is excellent. This book may best be used as supplementary to a more discursive text.

Kaplan HM: Anatomy and physiology of speech, 2nd ed. New York: McGraw-Hill, 1971.

This is a worthy reference, clear and straightforward, with not only basic anatomic information but uncomplicated physiologic elaboration. It utilizes pathology to provide interest and to explain the material. The appendix has an excellent tabular review of the muscles described in the text, a comprehensive glossary of terms, and a reference listing of texts and journal articles, foreign and in English.

Minifie FD, Hixon TJ, Williams F: Normal aspects of speech, hearing and language. Englewood Cliffs, NJ: Prentice-Hall, 1973.

This popular and classic text is not a typical anatomy text, although anatomy and physiology play important roles in its pages. It is efficiently integrated along with acoustics and physics. The text represents the true scientific character of the speech and hearing sciences.

Perkins WH Kent RD: Functional anatomy of speech, language, and hearing. a primer. San Diego: College-Hill, 1986.

This is a basic text for speech and hearing science students emphasizing anatomy, essential physiology, and additional materials (e.g., acoustics). Added are detailed glossaries, tables and self-study tests. It is a bit more than a simple

atlas, for there are ample explanations of complex activities and functions.

Zemlin WR: Speech and hearing science. Anatomy and physiology. 2nd ed. Englewood Cliffs, NJ: Prentice-Hall, 1981.

This may be the most popular of the focused speech and hearing anatomy and physiology texts. It is filled with line drawings, cadaveric photographs, frames from motion photography as well as extensive discussion of the physics and physiology of regions presented. Also provided are an extensive glossary, references lists, and summaries of structures and systems.

General Anatomy Texts

The student will find many different types of general, whole-body, anatomy texts. Perhaps browsing through a medical section of a library to identify references promising more immediate and direct help would be a profitable initial activity. One will find that there are several groups of such texts. One, the gross anatomy books are those that present information about the entire body generally covering those aspects that are visible to the unaided eye. These will present the bones, the muscles, the nerves, and all other major tissues in some detail; one possible drawback to their use might be the fewer and smaller and more detailed illustrations many present. There are a number of very popular and historically accepted gross anatomy texts;

each is probably in editions that may number in the 30s, as in the case of Gray's, or in fewer, as in the case of Tortora's. Further, one will probably note that a different editor for different editions will be identified on the cover as well as the title page; as the years pass, the publisher sees a need for a new edition and seeks an editor who will assume the great task of selecting chapter (or special topic) writers.

So, one might find the commonly known Gray's Anatomy, published by Lea & Febiger, edited by Goss (as in, say, the 28th edition), or another editor in subsequent ones (for students in speech and hearing sciences, sometimes the latest edition is not entirely essential and certainly is more costly). Morris's Human Anatomy published by Blakiston is another popular reference, also in the multiedition condition. A third possibility is Cunningham's Textbook of Anatomy, published by Oxford, is a British reference of considerable value and of multieditions. In the United States, probably the most popular gross anatomy text is that by Tortora, *Principles of Human Anatomy,* published by Harper & Row and reaching toward its 10th edition.

A second type of gross anatomy reference is the atlas. These consist of illustrations, sometimes photographs and sometimes artistic renditions of anatomic structure, with minimal text. An old popular one, in multieditions, is Grant's Atlas of Human Anatomy, published by Williams & Wilkins, and in multieditions as well. A recent one is McMinn and Hutching's Color Atlas of Human Anatomy in a revised and updated second edition by Year Book Medical Publishers. This reference is largely photographic with outstandingly clear photographs and identification leaders. Another atlas is represented by the series produced by Frank Netter (also in multieditions) with special texts for special systems; thus, one would find his Volume I Nervous System as part of the Ciba Collection of Medical Illustrations, also in multieditions. Dr. Netter also has a single-volume atlas of gross anatomy in his usual inimitable style that is very attractive.

A word of warning about anatomic references: there are many other types that are highly specialized. For example, one might find a radiologic atlas designed to acquaint students of x-ray examination in how to identify spaces and structures via x-rays. Or, dental anatomy references are common, providing focused attention upon dentition. There are embryonic as well as new-born references for those with interest in that age-related anatomy and there are specialized texts for special student groups, such as neuroanatomy for the nursing student.

Lastly, the student should become acquainted with dictionaries of various types, as noted earlier. These also may be in the multiedition condition. Perhaps the latest editions would provide for new terms in special areas, such as new definitions relating to the mushrooming pharmacologic fields. Some common dictionaries are Dorland's, Blakiston's and Taber's (some being in "pocket book" editions). One that is helpful for the relatively unsophisticated student is Melloni's Illustrated Medical Dictionary, published by Williams & Wilkins (1979), having extremely helpful drawings on half of each page and very simple definitions below. The special terminology reference by Nicolosi, Harryman and Kresheck (Terminology of Communication Disorders, 3rd edition, Williams & Wilkins, 1989) not only has basic anatomic and physiologic terms defined but also presents many other technical and specialized terms in all aspects of speech, language, and hearing.

Index

Page numbers in *italics* denote figures; those followed by "t" denote tables. Terms are listed under nouns; e.g., "cricoid cartilage" is found under "Cartilages."